EYE MOVEMENTS AND THE HIGHER PSYCHOLOGICAL FUNCTIONS

EYE MOVEMENTS AND THE HIGHER PSYCHOLOGICAL FUNCTIONS

edited by

JOHN W. SENDERS
University of Toronto

DENNIS F. FISHER
RICHARD A. MONTY
U. S. Army Human Engineering Laboratory

SPONSORED BY THE U. S. ARMY
HUMAN ENGINEERING LABORATORY

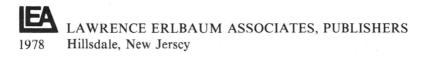

LAWRENCE ERLBAUM ASSOCIATES, PUBLISHERS
1978   Hillsdale, New Jersey

DISTRIBUTED BY THE HALSTED PRESS DIVISION OF
JOHN WILEY & SONS
New York   Toronto   London   Sydney

Lawrence Erlbaum Associates, Inc., Publishers
62 Maria Drive
Hillsdale, New Jersey 07642

Distributed solely by Halsted Press Division
John Wiley & Sons, Inc., New York

Library of Congress Cataloging in Publication Data

Main entry under title:

Eye movements and the higher psychological functions.

Bibliography: p.
Includes indexes.
1. Eye—Movements—Congresses. 2. Visual percep-
tion—Congresses. 3. Higher nervous activity—Con-
gresses. I. Senders, John W., 1920– II. Fisher,
Dennis F. III. Monty, Richard A. IV. United States.
Army Human Engineering Laboratories.
QP477.5.E93   152.1'4   78-15618
ISBN 0-470-26489-6

Printed in the United States of America

In any scientific endeavor,
You must have men who are clever
And men who are nice
As well, like John Weisz.
Without whose support and encouragement
it would have been impossible
to put this book together.

JOHN W. SENDERS

Participants and Contributors

Numbers in parentheses indicate the pages on which authors' contributions begin.

James E. Anliker, NASA Ames Research Center, Menlo Park, California

James K. Arima, Naval Postgraduate School, Monterey, California

Mary Anne Baker, Indiana University Southeast, New Albany, Indiana

Captain John Bermudez, Department of Behavioral Sciences and Leadership, USAF Academy, Colorado

Gordon W. Bronson, Department of Psychology, Mills College, Oakland, California

Virginia Brooks, Department of Psychology, Columbia University, New York (293)

Dennis P. Carmody, Radiology Research Laboratory, Temple University School of Medicine, Philadelphia, Pennsylvania (241)

Patricia A. Carpenter, Psychology Department, Carnegie-Mellon University, Pittsburgh, Pennsylvania (115, 157)

Michael R. Clark, Stanford Research Institute, Menlo Park, California (77)

Roger M. Cooper, Stanford Research Institute, Menlo Park, California

Hewitt D. Crane, Stanford Research Institute, Menlo Park, California (77)

Ann Crichton-Harris, Toronto, Ontario, Canada

Merle E. Day, North Chicago, Illinois

Peter Dixon, Department of Psychology, Carnegie-Mellon University, Pittsburgh, Pennsylvania

Dennis F. Fisher, Behavioral Research Directorate, U. S. Army Human Engineering Laboratory Aberdeen Proving Ground, Maryland

Barbara N. Flagg, Harvard University, Cambridge, Massachusetts (65, 279)

Leo Ganz, Department of Psychology, Stanford University, Stanford, California (55)

Susanne M. Gatchell, Industrial & Operations Engineering, University of Michigan, Ann Arbor, Michigan

Lester A. Gerhardt, Electrical and Systems Engineering Department, Rensselaer Polytechnic Institute, Troy, New York

Samuel Y. Gibbon, Children's Television Workshop, New York, New York

Michael E. Goldberg, Armed Forces Radiobiology Research Institute, Bethesda, Maryland (3)

J. C. Gutmann, Virginia Polytechnic Institute and State University, Blacksburg, Virginia

Roger I. C. Hansell, Department of Zoology, University of Toronto, Toronto, Ontario, Canada

Ronald M. Hansen, Psychology Department, Northeastern University, Boston, Massachusetts (15)

Edward M. Herman, Radiology Research Laboratory, Temple University School of Medicine, Philadelphia, Pennsylvania

Julian Hochberg, Department of Psychology, Columbia University, New York, New York (293)

Frank Holly, USAARL, Fort Rucker, Alabama

Margaret H. Jones, Department of Pediatrics, UCLA Medical School, Pacific Palisades, California

Marcel Just, Psychology Department, Carnegie-Mellon University, Pittsburgh, Pennsylvania (115, 157)

Patricia A. Kinney, New Mexico Department of Transportation, Santa Fe, New Mexico (259)

Eileen Kowler, Department of Psychology, University of Maryland, College Park, Maryland

Harold L. Kundel, Department of Radiology, Temple University School of Medicine, Philadelphia, Pennsylvania (241, 317)

Eugene Kwatny, Krusen Center for Research and Engineering, Philadelphia, Pennsylvania

Robert H. Lambert, Behavioral Research Directorate, U. S. Army Human Engineering Laboratory, Aberdeen Proving Ground, Maryland

Lester A. Lefton, Psychology Department, University of South Carolina, Columbia, South Carolina (225)

Gerald Leisman, Department of Health Sciences, Brooklyn College, CUNY, Brooklyn, New York (195)

Dean LeMaster Air Force Human Resources Laboratory, Williams AFB, Arizona (259)

George S. Leonard, Gulf & Western Applied Science Laboratories, Waltham, Massachusetts

Edward Llewellyn-Thomas, Institute of Biomedical Engineering, University of Toronto, Toronto, Ontario, Canada

Ethel Matin, C. W. Post Center of Long Island University, Greenvale, New York

Joseph Mazurczak, Behavioral Research Directorate, U. S. Army Human Engineering Laboratory, Aberdeen Proving Ground, Maryland

Edward D. McDowell, Industrial and General Engineering, Oregon State University, Corvallis, Oregon (329)

John B. Mocharnuk, Engineering Psychology Department, McDonnell Douglas Astronautics Co., St. Louis, Missouri

Richard A. Monty, Behavioral Research Directorate, U. S. Army Human Engineering Laboratory, Aberdeen Proving Ground, Maryland

Robert K. Moore, Hunter Lab, Brown University, Providence, Rhode Island (35)

Ronald R. Mourant, Wayne State University, Detroit, Michigan

Douglas E. Neil, Naval Postgraduate School, Monterey, California

Sandra Newsome, Psychology Department, New Mexico State University, Las Cruces, New Mexico

Calvin F. Nodine, Department of Educational Psychology, Temple University, Philadelphia, Pennsylvania (241, 317)

Kenneth Paap, Psychology Department, New Mexico State University, Las Cruces, New Mexico

Lawrence C. Perlmuter, Psychology Department, Virginia Polytechnic Institute and State University, Blacksburg, Virginia

Mary C. Potter, Massachusetts Institute of Technology, Cambridge, Massachusetts

Lorrin A. Riggs, Department of Psychology, Brown University, Providence,
  Rhode Island (35)
David Lee Robinson, Armed Forces Radiobiology Research Institute,
  Bethesda, Maryland
Gordon H. Robinson, Department of Industrial Engineering, University of
  Wisconsin, Madison, Wisconsin
Thomas H. Rockwell, Industrial and Systems Engineering, Ohio State University,
  Columbus, Ohio (329)
Larry D. Rosen, Psychology Department, California State College,
  Dominguez Hills, California
Ernst Z. Rothkopf, Bell Laboratories, Murray Hill, New Jersey (209)
J. Edward Russo, Graduate School of Business, University of Chicago,
  Chicago, Illinois (89)
Jock C. H. Schwank, DFBL, USAF Academy, Colorado
Leonard F. Scinto, Laboratory of Human Development, Harvard University,
  Cambridge, Massachusetts (175)
John W. Senders, Department of Industrial Engineering, University of Toronto,
  Toronto, Ontario, Canada
Wayne L. Shebilske, University of Virginia, Department of Psychology,
  Charlottesville, Virginia
David Sheena, Gulf & Western Applied Science Laboratories, Waltham,
  Massachusetts (65)
Marian Sigman, Department of Pediatrics, UCLA Medical School, Los Angeles,
  California
Ronald R. Simmons, USAARL, Fort Rucker, Alabama
Alexander A. Skavenski, Psychology Department, Northeastern University, Boston,
  Massachusetts (15)
Harry L. Snyder, Virginia Polytechnic Institute, Blacksburg, Virginia
Amos Spady, NASA—Langley Research Center, Hampton, Virginia
Lawrence Stark, University of California, Berkeley, California
Robert M. Steinman, Department of Psychology, University of Maryland,
  College Park, Maryland
John A. Stern Department of Psychology, Washington University, St. Louis,
  Missouri (145)
Warren H. Teichner, Department of Psychology, New Mexico State University,
  Las Cruces, New Mexico (259)
Jonathan Vaughan, Psychology Department, Hamilton College, Clinton, New York (135)
Frances C. Volkmann, Clark Science Center, Smith College, Northampton,
  Massachusetts (35)
Marvin Waller, NASA—Langley Research Center, Hampton, Virginia
Ed Wells, Radiology Research Laboratory, School of Medicine, Temple University,
  Philadelphia, Pennsylvania
Charles W. White, Graduate Faculty, New School for Social Research, New York,
  New York
Keith D. White, University of Florida, Gainesville, Florida (35)
Evelyn Williams, Department of Psychology, New Mexico State University,
  Las Cruces, New Mexico
Robert Wisher, Navy Personnel Research and Development Center, San Diego,
  California
Kenneth Ziedman, Southern California Research Institute, Los Angeles, California
Helmut T. Zwahlen, Department of Industrial and Systems Engineering,
  Ohio University, Athen, Ohio

Contents

Preface

This volume represents the edited proceedings of the second symposium on eye movements and behavior sponsored by the U. S. Army Human Engineering Laboratory. The conference was held at the Naval Postgraduate School in Monterey, California on February 6–9, 1977.

This volume is intended to serve as a complementary volume to R. A. Monty and J. W. Senders (Eds.), *Eye Movements and Psychological Processes,* published by Lawrence Erlbaum Associates (1976), rather than as a revision or update of it.

We wish to thank the U. S. Army Human Engineering Laboratory for sponsoring the symposium. In particular, we once again wish to express our deep appreciation to Dr. John D. Weisz, Director of the Human Engineering Laboratory, for his continued encouragement and support. It is to him that we have dedicated this volume.

We are also deeply indebted to Dr. Francis C. Volkmann for organizing and chairing the first session, and to the staff of the Naval Post Graduate School, especially Ms. Ruth Guthrie and Dr. J. Kenneth Arima, who made this one of the smoothest running symposia we have ever witnessed. We are grateful to Ms. Judy Weishampel for keeping the work of the first editor on an even keel and for maintaining liaison among us. Once again, special thanks go to B. Diane Eberly (now operating under the alias of Mrs. B. Diane Barnette), who since the last volume has advanced from the role of secretary to mathematics aide. She, nevertheless, was responsible for handling a myriad of details surrounding planning of the symposium and the resulting publication.

JOHN W. SENDERS
DENNIS F. FISHER
RICHARD A. MONTY

Introduction

This volume reflects the proceedings of a conference held in February 1977 at the Naval Postgraduate School at Monterey, California, and is the natural successor to an earlier volume of the proceedings of a conference in Princeton, New Jersey entitled *Eye Movements and Psychological Processes* (Monty & Senders, 1976). The earlier conference and book were organized with what we, as organizers and editors, hoped was a logical sequence, beginning with a common base of nomenclature, information, and understanding of the underlying mechanisms of oculomotor control, then progressing through a series of topics relating eye movements to processes that, at least conceptually, advanced from simple to more complex.

To quote from the preface of the earlier volume: "Our purpose was to bring together investigators representing different theoretical positions and methodological approaches to present their recent findings, to debate the theoretical points of view, and to identify and discuss the major research problems." That is, of course, an adequate statement of the purposes of the second conference as well. Parts of the first conference were devoted to search and scanning, to reading, and (Part 7) to eye movements and higher mental processes. The second conference was aimed at providing a greater opportunity for discussing these "higher mental processes." In view of the fact that there were many people at the second conference who had not attended the first or who may not have read the first proceedings, we thought it necessary to have one half day devoted to reviewing topics presented during two whole days at the first meeting.

Part I of this volume is devoted to an intensive review of the underlying processes and psychological functions of eye movements. It includes discussions of the relationships of cortical and subcortical visual areas to eye movements and visual processing associated with them; information about the position of the eye in the head and the perception of visual space; saccades and visual functioning; and masking. These four papers were essentially didactic in nature. All persons working in the area of eye movements must be aware of the status of knowledge relating to those topics in order to be able to design experiments appropriately and to interpret results accurately. Another session was devoted to methodology and models in order to update information since the earlier conference and published proceedings.

Beginning with the third session, questions of the effects of tasks on eye movements and the effects of eye movements on tasks were addressed. Here, out of necessity, higher mental processes include dealing with particular kinds of application: reading, watching television, flying aircraft, looking for objects, counting things, and the like. Although not all papers presented at the meeting are included in this volume, all were informative and made a contribution to the participants' understanding of the complex relationships between eye movements and behavior. Obviously, behavior and eye movements are the variables which could be compared and correlated. For most of the participants, of course, the behavior was then interpreted in terms of "higher mental processes." It seems appropriate once again to quote from the earlier volume:

> Now we are concerned with the question of what people do with eye movements.
>
> It is an important question. We spend our time, as Steinman has pointed out, sometimes voluntarily selecting places in the visual field to look at, and at other times allowing a process to go on that one is nearly unaware of, in which the eye successively fixates different parts of an apparently nicely stabilized visual field. From these "looks" we continually reconstruct, renew, and refresh some internal map of what is "out there."
>
> There has been continuing study over the last 25 years of how people look at dynamical things, for example, dials on an aircraft instruments panel [when one is flying], or faces if one is engaged in conversation or lecturing. They change when one is not looking at them; sometimes they change while one is looking at them. Certain rules can be established relating the content of dynamic displays to the distribution of visual attention across these displays.
>
> Another aspect of the visual world is the static aspect. We look at a landscape and things mostly stay where they are. Trees don't get up and walk around; paintings and cast-iron eagles, in particular, tend to stay exactly as they have been. Yet the eye does come back from time to time to look once again at a piece of the visual field which it has just recently visited and from which it has departed. A very interesting problem is that of the relationship between the content and structure of a [static] visual field, and the way in which one distributes visual attention over that field.

And further:

> The possibility of keeping physical records as aids to memory by the use of spatially organized materials must have occurred very early to ancient man. The

particular ways in which these materials are specially organized, however, has varied through all possible arrangements. Languages may be written from left to right or right to left and top to bottom or bottom to top, in vertical lines and in horizontal lines, and there is no particular reason to assume that any one way of organizing material is better than any other. However, some serial arrangement in one sense or another must be imposed if the written material is to be interpreted correctly. The degree, however, to which positional structure within sentences is important depends upon the degree to which the language is inflected. English is a highly positional language in which the meanings of sentences are determined both by the words within the sentence and by the positions they hold relative to the other words. This is not necessarily true of all languages.

Even more interesting, of course, is the higher mental process involved in the extraction of meaning from written language. Much of the work in this area is related to the hypothetical internal representation of the material that is read and the relationship of that material to the eye movements made during the reading as well as subsequent to it, as was the case for some of the chapters in the earlier volume. Virtually all the chapters beyond the first set in this volume imply that there is "a strong direct link between the way in which the eye moves and the fact of its moving at all, and the kind of perceptual and memory structure which is being used by the observer to store and organize information."

Where it has made a contribution to the reader's understanding of the content of a paper, we have preserved the discussion with only a few deletions. In some cases, the points raised during the discussions were as important to those present as the paper itself. Although all the papers presented at this meeting had been prepared in advance, unlike those of the first meeting, we have attempted to preserve, through the discussions, the spirit of intense involvement and serious give-and-take that pervaded the whole meeting. We hope that the chapters and comments presented here will encourage subsequent research efforts using eye movements, so that the state of the art and understanding of the processes are continually advanced.

* * * * *

WARREN H. TEICHNER, 1921–1978

Just before this book went to press, the editors learned of the death of Warren H. Teichner, who was a participant in the symposium and a contributor to this volume. We were saddened to lose a good friend and colleague who had contributed so much to Experimental and Engineering Psychology.

EYE MOVEMENTS
AND THE HIGHER
PSYCHOLOGICAL FUNCTIONS

Part I

BASIC PROCESSES

I.1

The Visual Substrate of Eye Movements

David Lee Robinson
Michael E. Goldberg
Armed Forces Radiobiology Research Institute

The visual system is continually bombarded with stimuli. Not all of these stimuli are of equal significance; some are ignored whereas others elicit a shift of attention and an eye movement. The visual processing preceding such a movement requires analysis of the visual stimulus in terms of three questions: where is it, what is it, and is it behaviorally significant? Recent work has attempted to analyze several cortical and subcortical visual areas in order to determine their contributions to the visual processing preceding eye movements. We will discuss these questions with reference to the superior colliculus, the striate cortex (area 17), the posterior parietal cortex (area 7), and the frontal visual area (area 8, "the frontal eye fields") of the rhesus monkey.

SUPERIOR COLLICULUS

The cells in the superficial grey and optic layers of the monkey superior colliculus respond to visual stimuli (Cynader & Berman, 1972; Goldberg & Wurtz, 1972a; Humphrey, 1968; Schiller & Koerner, 1971). Unlike cells in striate cortex (Hubel & Wiesel, 1968; Wurtz, 1969a), visual cells in the superior colliculus are not sensitive to the shape or orientation of stimuli. Instead, these respond to the onset of small spots of light within their receptive field, and also to stimuli moving over a wide range of directions and stimulus velocities (Goldberg & Wurtz, 1972a) as shown in Fig. 1. They have large receptive fields, and receptive field size increases with depth in the colliculus (Goldberg & Wurtz, 1972a; Humphrey, 1968). It is highly unlikely that cells in the colliculus can provide much qualitative information about visual stimuli, although ensembles of collicular neurons

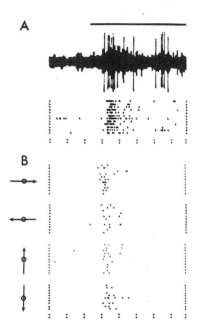

FIG. 1.   Response of a pandirectional cell to both stationary and moving stimuli. The cell was recorded from the superficial layers of the superior colliculus of an awake monkey. (A) illustrates the discharge of the cell to a stationary spot of light flashed in its receptive field. The horizontal line above the trace indicates the time of stimulus onset. The raster in (A) shows the response of the same cell to repeated presentations of the same stimulus. Each dot represents either a discharge of the cell or the beginning or end of a line. Each horizontal line of dots indicates a single fixation by the monkey and a single presentation of the stimulus. (B) depicts the response of this cell to a spot of light swept across the receptive field while the monkey fixates. The interval between pairs of dots is 50 *msec*. (From Goldberg & Wurtz, 1972a. Reproduced with permission.)

could provide some information about the spatial localization of visual stimuli (McIlwain, 1975).

Collicular neurons do have several features that may be useful in analyzing the behavioral significance of stimuli. If a visual stimulus is going to be the target for a saccadic eye movement, cells in the superficial layers of the colliculus which ordinarily respond to that stimulus will have an enhanced response. This enhancement is selective; it does not occur before eye movements to stimuli that are not in the receptive field of the cell (Goldberg & Wurtz, 1972b; Wurtz & Mohler, 1976a), as shown in Fig. 2. This pre-eye movement activity is an enhancement of the visual response. It is time-locked to the onset of the visual stimulus and does not appear if the appropriate eye movement occurs in the absence of a visual stimulus. The enhanced activity in these neurons may signal that (1) there is a stimulus in a certain part of the visual field, and (2) the eye is going to (or should) move to fixate that stimulus.

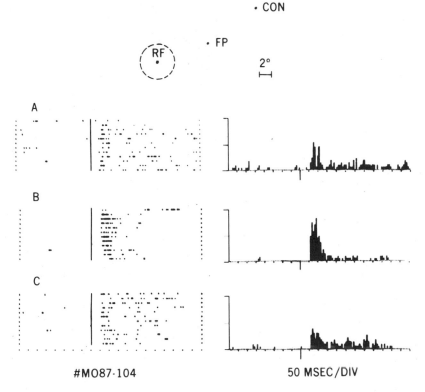

FIG. 2.   Enhancement specificity for a collicular neuron. (A) shows the response of the neuron to a spot of light flashed in the receptive field (RF) while the monkey fixates. (B) illustrates the discharge of the same cell to the same stimulus when the monkey uses that light as the target for an eye movement from the fixation point (FP) to the RF stimulus. (C) presents the response of this cell to the RF stimulus on the trials when the animal makes an eye movement to the control point (CON). Histograms sum the data in the adjacent raster; full scale of the vertical axis, 250 spikes/sec per trial. (From Wurtz & Mohler, 1976a. Reproduced with permission.)

Moving objects are powerful stimuli for collicular neurons. During an eye movement the entire visual field moves across the retina allowing stimuli that would not have been salient when the eye was stationary to become so. The brain must have a system that can differentiate between real stimulus movement in the environment and artifactually salient stimulus movement caused by movement of the eye across a stationary field. Many cells in the superficial layers of the superior colliculus that respond to real stimulus movement do not respond to self-induced stimulus movement (Robinson & Wurtz, 1976) as shown in Fig. 3. These results are in contrast to data from the striate cortex, where cells do not distinguish between these two types of stimulus movement (Wurtz, 1969b). The ability of collicular neurons to distinguish real from self-induced

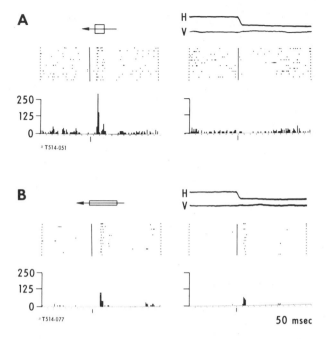

FIG. 3.   Activity of cells which do and do not distinguish real from self-induced stimulus movement. (A) left: shows the response of a collicular neuron to a stimulus swept across the receptive field at 900°/sec while the animal fixates. (A) right: shows the lack of response of the same cell to comparable stimulus movement generated by a 20° eye movement. Representative electrooculogram traces are illustrated above the raster. Raster and histograms for eye movement experiments are triggered on the beginning of the eye movement. (B) illustrates the results of similar experiments conducted on a cell which does not distinguish between these types of stimulus movement. (From Robinson & Wurtz, 1976. Reproduced with permission.)

stimulus movement is accomplished by a threshold elevation of at least one log unit that is present over a wide range of stimulus directions. It is unlikely that collicular cells fail to respond to self-induced stimulus movement because of movement of the visual background, since the differentiation is seen when peripheral visual factors are drastically reduced, as illustrated in Fig. 4. This lack of response is due to an extraretinal input. When the monkey is placed in total darkness, one can see a suppression of background activity after eye movements, noted in Fig. 5. This suppression indicates the presence of the extraretinal input. Collicular neurons which do not differentiate between real and self-induced stimulus movement do not show this background suppression in total darkness. The suppression begins at roughly the time that visual stimuli resulting from an eye movement would reach the colliculus.

The source of extraretinal suppression is not yet known. It is not proprioceptive from the extraocular muscles, since it is present when the monkey

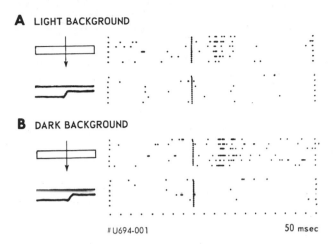

FIG. 4.   Reduction of visual factors with persistence of the differentiation between real and self-induced stimulus movement. (A) illustrates the response of a cell to rapid stimulus movement while the monkey fixates, and lack of response to stimulus movement caused by an eye movement in the light. (B) shows comparable results when these experiments are conducted after a large reduction in background illumination. (From Robinson & Wurtz, 1976. Reproduced with permission.)

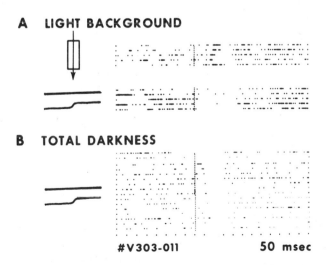

FIG. 5.   Demonstration of an extraretinal suppression for collicular neuron which distinguished between types of stimulus movement. (A) shows the response of a cell with externally generated and self-induced stimulus movement. (B) illustrates a period of suppression of background firing after eye movements made spontaneously in total darkness, indicating the presence of the extraretinal input. (From Robinson & Wurtz, 1976. Reproduced with permission.)

attempts to make an eye movement after paralysis of its extraocular muscles (Richmond & Wurtz, 1977). It must be a corollary discharge originating from some system that discharges with eye movements. One attractive candidate for such a system is the small set of cells in the frontal eye fields that discharge after eye movements (Bizzi, 1968; Bizzi & Schiller, 1970; Mohler, Goldberg, & Wurtz, 1973), since it has been shown that the frontal eye fields project to the superficial layers of the superior colliculus (Astruc, 1971; Künzle, Akert, & Wurtz, 1976). Furthermore, stimulation of the frontal eye fields of the cat produces a reduced responsiveness of collicular neurons to visual stimuli (Guitton & Mandl, 1974).

The neurons in the superior colliculus that differentiate between real stimulus movement and self-induced stimulus movement seem to be those which show enhancement of their visual response before eye movements (Robinson & Wurtz, 1976) as shown in Fig. 6. The physiology of these neurons would, therefore, lead one to postulate that they have nothing to do with qualitative analysis of the visual field, something to do with spatial localization, and a great deal to do with identifying significant stimuli as targets for eye movements. These postulates are supported by the results of ablation studies that have shown a large increase in the latency of onset of the eye movements to fixate a peripheral target (Wurtz & Goldberg, 1972), illustrated in Fig. 7, and a small decrease in the accuracy of eye movements, as indicated by an increase in the number of corrective saccades following large saccades to fixate peripheral objects (Mohler &

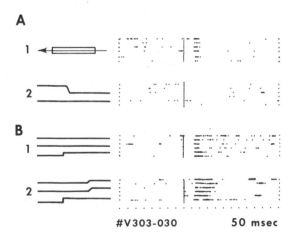

#V303-030   50 msec

FIG. 6.   Stimulus movement differentiation and response enhancement in the same collicular neuron. (A1) documents the discharge of this cell to real stimulus movement and lack of response (A2) with self-generated movement. (B1) shows the response of this cell to a stationary spot of light flashed in the receptive field while the monkey fixates. (B2) presents the enhanced response to this cell to the same stimulus when it is to be the target for a saccadic eye movement. (From Robinson & Wurtz, 1976. Reproduced with permission.)

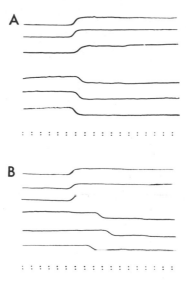

FIG. 7. Eye movements before and after a focal lesion in the superior colliculus. (A) shows a monkey's eye movements to targets 10° to the left (first three traces) and 10° to the right (second three traces). Each sweep is triggered by the saccade target onset. A microelectrode was used to find the area in the superior colliculus with neurons with visual receptive fields that included the target point, and then a focal electrolytic lesion was made through the microelectrode. (B) shows the eye movements to the same points as in (A) 24 hours after the lesion. The latency of eye movements to the target contralateral to the lesion is lengthened. (From Wurtz & Goldberg, 1972. Reproduced with permission.)

Wurtz, 1977). These data suggest that the stimulus selection process is impaired, whereas the mechanism for programming the eye movement is largely undisturbed.

STRIATE CORTEX

The work of Hubel and Wiesel (1968), among others, has shown that neurons in the striate cortex are extremely sensitive to the orientation and shape of visual stimuli. Some striate cortical neurons show presaccadic enhancement, but it is nonselective, occurring with eye movements to many points of the visual field (Wurtz & Mohler, 1976b). Although some striate neurons show a slight decrement in activity associated with eye movements in the dark when subjected to computer averaging (Duffy & Burchfiel, 1975), they do not exhibit the dramatic differentiation between real and self-induced stimulus movement that is shown by neurons in the superior colliculus (Wurtz, 1969b).

Immediately after striate cortical lesions, monkeys have a hemianopia. Within several weeks they can be trained to detect flashed stimuli in the contralateral field, and to make eye movements to them (Mohler & Wurtz, 1977). These eye movements and detections are presumably subsumed by the superior colliculus, since immediately after a subsequent collicular ablation these animals cannot perform either task and can never be trained to perform them. Neurons in the superior colliculus of animals with striate ablations still show specific presaccadic enhancement. Neurons in the striate cortex therefore contribute to eye movements by telling the brain what is in the contralateral visual field, and where it is, but they do not provide information about the behavioral significance of the target. Two other cortical areas provide information about behavioral significance of stimuli: the frontal eye fields (area 8) and the posterior parietal cortex (area 7).

FRONTAL AND PARIETAL CORTEX

Since the early stimulation experiments of Ferrier (1874), it has been assumed that the frontal eye fields functioned as a motor cortex for eye movements. Bizzi (1968) studied the relationship of frontal cortical neurons to eye movements in untrained awake monkeys and found only a few neurons which discharged after, but not before, eye movements. Bizzi and Schiller (1970) found neurons that discharged with head position, but not before eye movements. In a careful study using electrical stimulation, Robinson and Fuchs (1969) found that excitation of the frontal eye fields resulted in saccades to the contralateral visual field. These data were difficult to interpret in the absence of preoculomotor single unit activity. The relationship of the frontal eye fields to visually guided eye movements became clearer when Mohler, Goldberg, and Wurtz (1973) found that over half of the neurons they studied had visual receptive fields. Again, like the colliculus and unlike the striate cortex, neurons in the frontal eye fields have large receptive fields, as shown in Fig. 8, that are not fastidious about the qualities of the visual stimuli that excite the neurons. Many of the frontal visual neurons had presaccadic enhancement, and this enhancement is specific: like that found in the superior colliculus, it occurs only with eye movements into the receptive field (Wurtz & Mohler, 1976b). The activity responsible for the saccades induced by electrical stimulation may be the enhanced response to the target of the eye movement. No lesion studies in monkeys have tested the hypothesis that the frontal eye field's contribution to saccadic eye movements involves target selection. However, there exists a large body of clinical literature to suggest that frontal lesions in humans that seem to cause contralateral oculomotor paresis do so by inducing visual neglect (Heilman & Valenstein, 1972).

Posterior parietal cortex (area 7) has also been implicated in the control eye movements. Using untrained monkeys, Hyvärinen and Poranen (1974) found neurons that discharged before eye movements, and others that discharged in relation to the monkey's looking at his hand or at other significant visual phenomena. Mountcastle and his associates (Mountcastle, Lynch, Georgopoulos,

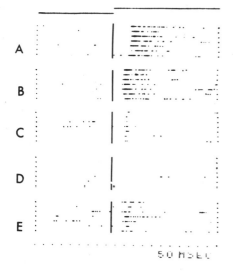

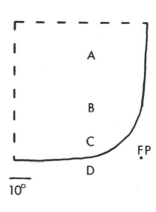

FIG. 8.   Visual response of a neuron in area 8. The drawing outlines the area of the left upper quadrant of visual field where 1° spots of light produced excitatory bursts. FP indicates the location of the fixation point. The dot patterns A–D show the responses of the neuron to stimuli at points A–D in the field. Dot pattern E shows the response of the neuron to a 20° x 20° spot centered in the receptive field. (From Mohler, Goldberg, & Wurtz, 1973. Reproduced with permission.)

Sakata, & Acuna, 1975; Mountcastle, 1976) have studied this area in more detail using trained monkeys and have found that when the animals performed a task that required them to make saccadic eye movements, neurons in area 7 discharged before the eye movements, whereas others discharged when gaze had been accomplished.

We have analyzed the visual properties of parietal neurons in some detail (Goldberg & Robinson, 1977; Robinson & Goldberg, 1977). They, like neurons in the superior colliculus and the frontal eye fields, have large visual receptive fields without significant stimulus requirements, as illustrated in Fig. 9. Few if any of these neurons have inhibitory surrounds. The response of some of these neurons is enhanced before eye movements, shown in Fig. 10. Their enhancement makes the cells appear to have a premovement discharge, an activity that is actually a stimulus-locked response similar to that in the superior colliculus. Neurons in this area which discharge during visual fixation seem to do so because the fixation involves positioning the retina in an area that stimulates the tonically responding receptive field of the neurons. A fixation response can usually be exaggerated by obliterating the animal's fixation point with a large, bright stimulus. When the animal is presented with a raisin or some other interesting stimulus, the discharge of many neurons in this area becomes quite dramatic. However, this "raisin response" can usually be duplicated by finding the proper visual stimulus.

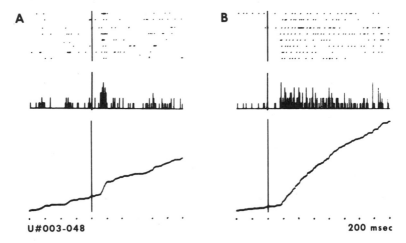

U#003-048   200 msec

FIG. 9.   Visual response of a parietal neuron to small and large stimuli. Data in (A) illustrate the response of this cell to a 0.5° x 0.5° spot of light centered on the vertical meridian 1° above the fixation point. (B) shows that a large stimulus (5° x 5°) centered at the same point still elicits a response indicating some summation within the visual receptive field and the lack of an inhibitory surround smaller than 5° x 5°. The trace at the bottom is a cumulative histogram calculated by summing the accumulated discharges in bins moving rightward. (Robinson & Goldberg, unpublished observations.)

NO SACCADE   **SACCADE**

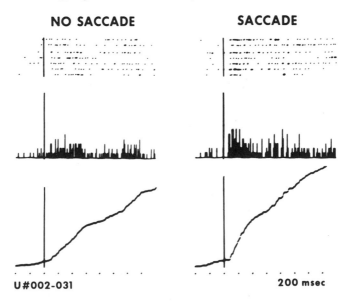

U#002-031   200 msec

FIG. 10.   Visual response enhancement for a neuron in parietal cortex. Data on the left show the response of the cell to a spot of light flashed on the screen 2° in the contralateral visual field, 2° above the horizontal meridian. The animal fixates throughout these trials. Data on the right illustrate the enhanced response to the identical stimulus when the animal is going to use it as the target for a saccadic eye movement. (Robinson & Goldberg, unpublished observations.)

CONCLUSIONS

The visual substrate of saccadic eye movements can be discussed in terms of the properties of the neurons which provide the answers to the questions *what?* and *why?* for eye movements. If one looks at a saccadic eye movement to the onset of a visual stimulus, it is clear that the striate cortex receives the information first, and then analyzes it in exceedingly fine grain, without adding any behavioral data. At the level of the superior colliculus, neurons extract less information about the qualitative aspects of the visual stimulus, but information clarifying whether the stimulus will be the target for an eye movement or whether the seemingly salient stimulus is merely the result of an eye movement is already implicit in the discharge pattern of the neuron. As the visual response appears in the frontal eye fields and in the posterior parietal cortex, this behavioral information becomes more dominant. However, at all of these levels it is apparent that the neuronal discharge is strongly locked to the visual stimulus and, at best, only modified by the behavioral input.

DISCUSSION

LEISMAN: One factor that could affect activity in the receptive field would be contrast sensitivity. First, I wonder if you made any attempt to control for the space average luminance of the stimulus array?; second, you mentioned that pupillary dilation was a possible factor. Did you make any attempt to instill a cycloplegic?; and third, you were studying the superior colliculus while the animals were involved in a search task. Do you have any data on the interaction between the animals in the type of situation they were in and reticular mechanisms as well?

GOLDBERG: We did not look particularly carefully at the fine grain receptive field properties like space luminance and contrast gradations, because once we found a stimulus that could drive a cell we were more interested in changes in response to that stimulus when the animal behaved differently towards it. We did not use cycloplegics because we doubted that a cycloplegic monkey either could do or would want to do the task. We also felt that the specific enhancement control experiment obviated the need to use a cycloplegic: if pupillary dilation were important, the cell should be enhanced when the animal fixates a spot outside of the receptive field as well as one in the receptive field. I think that reticular mechanisms would be important; reticular lesions cause visual neglect, and there are anatomical connections between the superior colliculus and the reticular formation. We didn't study the reticular system.

STARK: It seems as if the neurophysiologists' recording techniques haven't been able to find motor neurons except in the brain stem; that is, if you stimulate areas aa and so on, you do get eye movements.

GOLDBERG: If you stimulate any visual area, even striate cortex, you can get eye movements. If you think about this question evolutionarily, and therefore teleogically, the oculomotor system of animals without a particularly well developed forebrain is well developed compared to that of primates. This is in contradistinction to the hand area; the hand in primates is significantly different from that of lower animals, and we have evolved a cortex to control the hand that is new. For example, there are direct monosynaptic connections from motor neurons, but no one has ever demonstrated a cortical connection to oculomotor neurons. If the job of the cerebral cortex is to analyze the visual world in a retinotopic fashion, to identify important objects and localize them, the cortex could transmit that information to the brain stem, which would then determine the motor parameters of the eye movement. It would not be necessary for the cortex to discharge in a way predictive of the exact parameters of the movement, but it would be necessary for the cortex to discharge in a way descriptive of the stimulus.

STARK: You mean because you can't record the appropriate neurons that are firing, you feel there are no upper motor neurons?

GOLDBERG: Because neither we nor anyone else has recorded from a cortical upper motor neuron for eye movements, I made a rationalization that enables me to feel comfortable with that fact.

I.2

Role of Eye Position Information in Visual Space Perception[1]

Alexander A. Skavenski
Ronald M. Hansen
Northeastern University

In *Alice's Adventures in Wonderland* Alice asks, "Cheshire puss — Would you tell me, please, which way I ought to go from here?" To help Alice decide where to go the cat offered, "In that direction, lives a Hatter, and in that direction, lives a March Hare. Visit either you like: they're both mad." After deliberation Alice walked in the direction of the March Hare. Exactly how she could do that is a subject of some interest to us all.

Often we must feel a bit like Alice, especially when we find ourselves in new and strange environments. One of our problems is movement. The body moves, the head moves on the body, the eyes move with respect to the head. Consequently the position of a retinal image is not uniquely related to the position of an object in space but is continuously changing. Some accounting for these movements must be made and it is our task to describe what we know about the mechanism that accounts for movements of the eye.

Actually, when Carroll was writing the Alice story, Helmholtz (see Helmholtz, 1909/1962) recognized the problem and proposed a source for the eye position information used in this accounting. At that time the muscle spindle had been found but it would be nearly a half of a century before its sensory

---

[1]Much of the research in this chapter as well as the manuscript itself were supported by Research Grants EY 01049 from the National Eye Institute and BMS75-18181 from the National Science Foundation to the first author. Early work on control in the dark was supported by Grant EY 325 from the National Eye Institute to R.M. Steinman.

nature was discovered.[2] Thus, Helmholtz as early as 1862, and others before him were disposed to think that the relative positions of the eye as well as all parts of the body were known, in part, from the motor commands sent to the various muscles. Helmholtz called this the *effort of will.* Support came from his observations of the effect of oculomotor activity on *perception of direction.* Specifically, when the eye was passively displaced, images of objects in the environment appeared to move. This failure of the brain to account for externally produced eye movements has since been replicated by Irvine and Ludvigh (1936), by Brindley and Merton (1960), and by others on countless informal occasions. Helmholtz further noted that objects were perceived to move if the subject attempted to make an eye movement, but the eye itself was prevented from moving. This observation too has been replicated in several ways by Mach (1959), Kornmuller (1930), and others (see Matin, 1976, for a recent review and reinterpretation of the results of this procedure). Together, these observations led Helmholtz to conclude that, for *visual direction,* eye movements were accounted for by the effort of will put forth in moving the eye.

Three decades later histological evidence led Sherrington (1894) to deduce the sensory role of the muscle spindle. When he found these receptors in extraocular muscles (Sherrington, 1898), he speculated that they provided the eye position information used in perception of direction. Over the next three quarters of a century this speculation stimulated numerous qualitative tests of whether the eye position information arose from spindles or from the motor commands as Helmholtz (1909/1962) proposed. The bulk of evidence supported Helmholtz. None of these experiments challenged the notion that *eye position information* was needed.

The first formal proposal of a mechanism in which eye position signals were used to compensate for retinal image movement came from the work of Sperry (1950) and von Holst (1954). They attempted to account for the forced circling observed in animals whose visual systems were surgically inverted. A model of visual space perception that partially includes their suggestion is shown in Fig. 1.[3]

---

[2]According to Dickinson (1974), some controversy exists about the identity of the investigator who first discovered the muscle spindle. Various accounts credit Hassal with the discovery in 1851, Wiesman in 1861, and Kühne in 1863. However, none of these investigators were correct in their speculations about the function of these structures they found in the muscle.

[3]The model shows the oculomotor control systems using solely retinally-based signals to control eye position and thus departs from the suggestion of von Holst (1954) and Sperry (1950) who maintained that it was the perceived location and motion of objects with respect to the head ("$\Theta_{T/H}$" in Fig. 1) that served as inputs to these motor systems. This modification was made solely on the basis that it makes the models of space perception included in this manuscript more comprehensible. The reader is referred to Robinson (1975) for a discussion of the relative strengths of models of eye movement control based on perceived object location as opposed to retinal error signals.

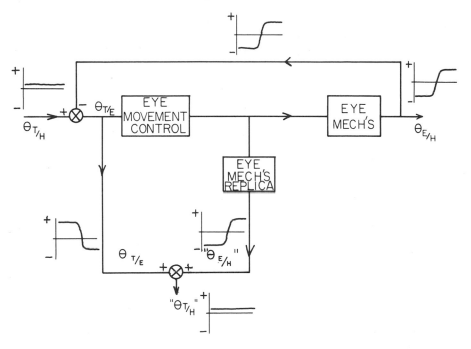

FIG. 1.   A block diagram schematizing one way the nervous system could determine the location of a seen object with respect to the head. At the top left, the position of the target with respect to the head ($\Theta_{T/H}$) is shown combining with the position of the eye in the head ($\Theta_{E/H}$) to produce retinal image position (target position with respect to eye, $\Theta_{T/E}$). This happens because the retina is mechanically attached to the eye. Retinal image position ($\Theta_{T/E}$) is used by various *Eye Movement Control* systems to produce commanded eye position: *(Command "$\Theta_{E/H}$")*, a neural pattern that will produce $\Theta_{E/H}$ when passed through mechanical characteristics of the eye muscles and supporting tissues of the globe (*Eye Mech's*). The lower paths show that neural analogues of target position on the retina ("$\Theta_{T/E}$") and position of the eye in the head ("$\Theta_{E/H}$") are added to produce a neural representation of the position of the target with respect to the head ("$\Theta_{T/H}$"). This mechanism is often described as "subtractive" for reasons one can see by examining small graphs near signal lines. The plot in the upper left shows stable target position as a function of time. When the eye executes a spontaneous saccade as shown on the right, the retinal image changes position as though the object was moved in the direction opposite to the eye movement, as shown in the bottom left plot. If this signal is added to the analogue of eye position (on the right) then stable target position is reconstructed as shown at the bottom.

The main implication of the model is that space perception depends critically on eye position signals and, primative as it appears, this model seemed consistent with perception data until only recently. To illustrate, eye position information is shown arising from the motor commands sent to the eye muscles. The most recent support for this came from quantitative replications of Helmholtz's observations done by Skavenski, Haddad, and Steinman (1972). They were led to do this experiment because Skavenski (1972) had earlier shown that subjects could use sensory information from orbital mechanoreceptors to control eye position in total darkness. Furthermore, these subjects could accurately report time and direction of passive displacement of their eyes when a forced choice psychophysical procedure was used (Skavenski, 1972). This result raised a serious question: Was it possible that proprioception made a *partial contribution* to the eye position information used in perceiving direction in Helmholtz's experiments? No one had measured the correspondence between changes in oculomotor commands and shifts in perceived direction to rule out a proprioceptive contribution. Skavenski et al. (1972) made these measurements in two experiments. First, oculomotor commands were varied while eye position was kept constant by applying known forces to a subject's right eye, while requiring him to fixate a target. The left eye was occluded. In this experiment the target remained on the same retinal locus so its perceived direction depended only on nonvisual eye position information. The diagram in Fig. 2 shows how this experiment indicates whether proprioception makes a contribution.

Figure 2 shows that a proprioceptive source of the eye position signals leads to the prediction that the target would be perceived to not change position or to move *in* the direction of the load when it was applied, while eye position information based on the effort of will predicts that the target would be perceived to move *opposite* to the direction of the load. The results shown in Fig. 3 support the "effort of will" prediction, because shifts in perceived direction were always opposite to the load.

Figure 3 shows mean shifts in the perceived direction of the fixation target for various loads applied to the left and right of the subject's right eye. In this experiment, subjects indicated shifts in the perceived direction of the fixation target by placing a second moveable target in their subjective straight ahead position. Perceived shifts were calculated from the *difference* between the mean straight position when the eye was not loaded and when it was loaded. Data points in Fig. 3 show that perceived shifts were always opposite to the direction of the load on the eye and the amplitude of the shift increased monotonically with load magnitude. In fact, the results do not depart in any systematic way from the predicted shifts in perceived direction based on the "effort of will." Essentially the same result was obtained from a second subject leading Skavenski et al. (1972) to conclude that perceived target direction was proportional to the magnitude of the command sent to the eye muscles.

In a second experiment Skavenski et al. (1972) found that systematic changes in proprioception from one eye had no effect on perceived target direction. Combined, the results of these two experiments were interpreted as indicating that the eye position signals of particular importance to perception of visual direction were based on the "effort of will."

The data shown in Fig. 3 also strongly indicate that a non-visual eye position signal is involved in visual space perception. It must be stressed that Skavenski et al. (1972) affected a change in the eye position information and measured a closely comparable change in the perceived direction of a target. Consequently,

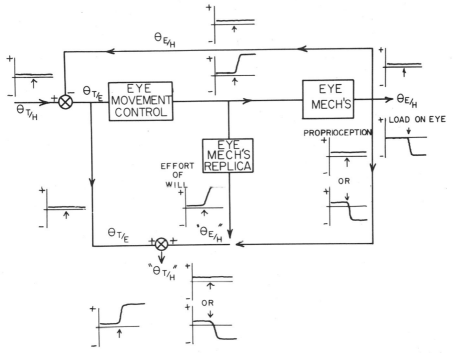

FIG. 2.   A block diagram schematizing the changes in various oculomotor signals and their consequences on the perceived direction of a fixation target when an external *load* is applied to the eye. This diagram is organized like the one in Fig. 1, except that a proprioceptive path for eye position information has been added and now small plots show the changes in signals when an external load was applied to the eye at the time indicated by arrows near the plots. When the load was applied, the subject had to change the motor commands to increase the force on the eye by an amount exactly equal to the load, but in the opposite direction, to continue fixating the target. Eye position signals based on these motor commands would indicate the eye rotated opposite to the load as shown in the *effort of will* plot. If perceived target position depended solely on the effort of will, then adding that function to retinal image position ($\Theta_{T/E}$) yields the prediction that the target should be perceived to move *opposite* to the direction of the load. Predictions for a *proprioception* source of the eye position signals are complicated, but it can be shown that proprioceptor activity would indicate that the eye did not change position if the nervous system accounted for its bias of the muscle spindle by the gamma efferent system as shown in the top *proprioception* plot (Skavenski, 1976). If the nervous system ignored its bias of the spindle, then proprioception would indicate the eye rotated in the direction of the load in the bottom proprioception plot. If the proprioceptive path were connected to perception and the effort of will is not, the predictions are that the target should be perceived to not change position or move in the direction of the load as shown in the lowest plot.

under the somewhat static conditions of fixation eye movements, eye position information has a profound influence on where seen objects are localized in visual space. It is tempting to conclude that a combination of retinal signals with eye position information, as shown in Fig. 1, completely explains how we localize objects with respect to our heads.

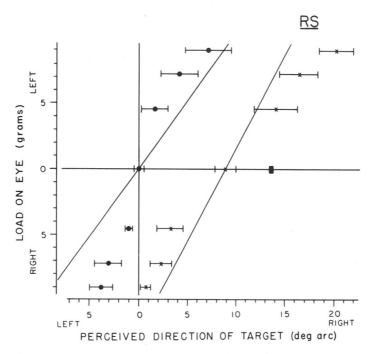

FIG. 3.   Mean perceived direction of a fixation target for various loads applied to the left and right of RS's right eye. RS's mean straight ahead position when no load was applied is shown as the intersection of the axes. Circles (●) show mean shifts in perceived direction of the fixation target when it was placed straight ahead of the subject and crosses (Xs) show mean shifts when it was placed 13.5 deg. arc to the right. Oblique lines show perceived shifts in target position predicted from the "effort of will," and the slopes of these lines are equal to the measured spring constants for this subject's eye. Predictions for a proprioceptive source of the eye position information would be no shift, (in other words, vertical lines on this plot) or that the target shifted in the direction of the load (lines roughly orthogonal to the "effort of will" lines shown). (From Skavenski, Haddad & Steinman, 1972. The extra-retinal signal for the visual perception of direction. Copyright 1972 by the Psychonomic Society. Reprinted by permission.)

The model is, however, incomplete. What happens to visual space perceptions that are forced to depend on eye position information during saccadic and smooth pursuit eye movements? In recent psychophysical studies of space perception under these *dynamic* conditions, Matin and his coworkers (see Matin, 1972 for a review of this work) found that subjects failed to accurately report the direction of test targets seen near the time of or during saccades. Matin inferred that the cause of the mislocalizations was such a serious failure of the eye position signals that these signals could not be relied on for veridical space perception.

Matin's (1972) procedure required subjects to judge the relative location of test flashes with respect to a reference target under the following conditions.

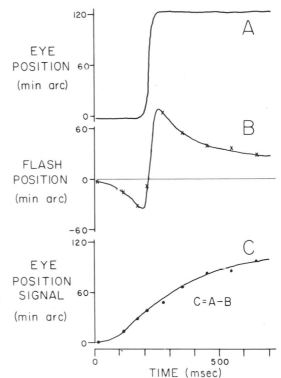

FIG. 4. A schematic drawing showing mean position of flashes (B) judged to be in the same location when seen at the time indicated relative to the saccadic eye movement shown in A. C is the position of the eye indicated by the eye position signal for the saccade in A and was calculated by subtracting B from A. See text for details and significance of this operation. (Data for this figure taken from Matin, 1972.)

Trials began with 4 sec of fixation of a visible target. This target was then switched off, and 300 msec later a second target was briefly flashed 2 deg. arc in peripheral retina. The subject made a saccade to it. At various times before, during, or after that saccade, one target out of an array of targets was flashed on and subjects judged whether it was left or right of the position of the fixation target. A schematic drawing illustrating flash positions that a representative subject could not discriminate as being left or right of the fixation position as a function of time relative to the saccade is shown in Fig. 4B.

It is immediately apparent from Fig. 4B that constancy of perceived position is not maintained during saccades; that is, subjects required quite different flash positions at various times before, during, and after the saccade for constancy of *perceived position* to occur. Matin (1972) inferred that this failure of constancy arose because the eye position information failed to keep up with eye position during rapid saccades. This can be shown by solving the model in Fig. 1 for the underlying eye position signal using the data in Fig. 4A and 4B. In these figures, perceived target position with respect to the head ("$\Theta_{T/H}$") is given by:

$$"\Theta_{T/H}" = \Theta_{T/E} + "\Theta_{E/H}" \tag{1}$$

where "$\Theta_{E/H}$" is the central representation of eye position in the head and $\Theta_{T/E}$ is the position of the target image on the retina. The position of the target image on the retina is:

$$\Theta_{T/E} = \Theta_{T/H} - \Theta_{E/H} \qquad (2)$$

where $\Theta_{T/H}$ is the position of the target with respect to the head and $\Theta_{E/H}$, eye position in the head. Substituting Eq. 2 in Eq. 1 and solving for the eye position information "$\Theta_{E/H}$" yields:

$$"\Theta_{E/H}" = \Theta_{E/H} - \Theta_{T/H} + "\Theta_{T/H}" \qquad (3)$$

In Matin's (1972) experiment "$\Theta_{T/H}$" is assumed to be a constant and can be neglected because the subject's task was to judge whether flashes were left or right of the constant initial fixation position. Thus, solving Eq. 3 by subtracting Fig. 4B from Fig. 4A yields the time course with which the eye position signal follows eye position during the saccade, and the result is shown in Fig. 4C.

It is apparent that the change in the eye position signal in Fig. 4C begins well before the saccadic eye movement in Fig. 4A (as much as 150 msec before) and slowly grows to equal eye position thereafter. For this reason Matin (1972) concluded that the eye position signal was temporally quite sluggish. In fact, Hansen and Skavenski (1977) found that exponential functions very closely describe the way the eye position signal follows eye position. These functions had exponents corresponding to time constants between 200 and 500 msec for Matin's (Matin, Matin, & Pearce, 1969; Matin, Matin, & Pola, 1970) and Pola's (1971) subjects. These are fairly long and suggest that the internal eye movement monitor is a very sluggish device. This failure of eye position signals to keep up with eye position has been replicated by Bischof and Kramer (1968) for saccades. In addition, Stoper (1973) has found that subjects also severely mislocalize targets seen during smooth pursuit eye movements. Finally, failure of the eye position signal to keep up with the smoothly moving eye has been inferred as the cause of mislocalizations or various illusions of shape or direction of movement (Festinger & Canon, 1965; Festinger & Easton, 1974; Festinger, Sedgwick, & Holtzman, 1976; Mack & Herman, 1973; Sedgwick & Festinger, 1976). Together, these data suggest that the person in our cortex who keeps track of where things are has very poor information about where the eye is when it is moving.

This conclusion led Matin (1972), MacKay (1972), and others to argue that cancellation of movements of retinal signals by an eye position signal could not explain *perceived stability*. They suggested that some other mechanism must explain why we do not ordinarily notice the visual world sweeping across the retina during saccades. This may be the case, but the implications of a sluggish change in the eye position signal go beyond understanding perceived stability. In fact it seriously challenges the idea that a nonvisual eye position signal is

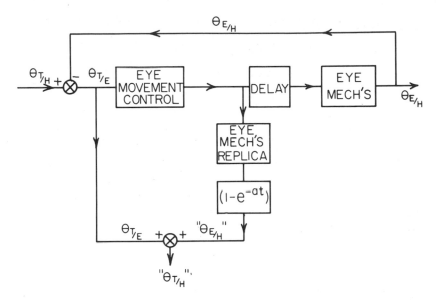

FIG. 5.   A block diagram illustrating modifications to the model shown in Fig. 1 needed to produce the psychophysical localization data observed during saccades. Features of the diagram are the same as Fig. 1 except that a pure delay has been inserted between the source of the oculomotor command, and the eye and the eye position signal ("$\Theta_{E/H}$") was made to follow $\Theta_{F/H}$ exponentially. In the exponent, a is the reciprocal of the time constant and t is time.

directly involved in space perception. The following analysis illustrates that problem. Figure 5 shows the modifications that need to be made to the perception model to produce the localization data observed during saccades.

This block diagram is similar to that shown in Fig. 1 except that a delay has been inserted between the source of the oculomotor command and the eye to account for changes in the eye position signal that preceed saccades. In addition, a function causing the eye position signal to follow eye position exponentially has been inserted between the source of the command and its influence on space perception. Figure 6 shows a computer solution of this model, illustrating where the little person in our cortex would perceive a stationary object to be located during a representative saccadic eye movement pattern if he received sluggish information about eye position.

The top trace in Fig. 6 is a representative horizontal eye movement pattern of a subject looking around the room. The middle trace shows the perceived location of a stationary object when the eye position signal begins its change 50 msec before the eye movement and slowly grows to equal eye position with a time constant of 250 msec. These parameters represent the performance of one of Matin's (1972) subjects whose eye position signal came closest to keeping up with the saccade. This trace shows that the model predicts that once the eye

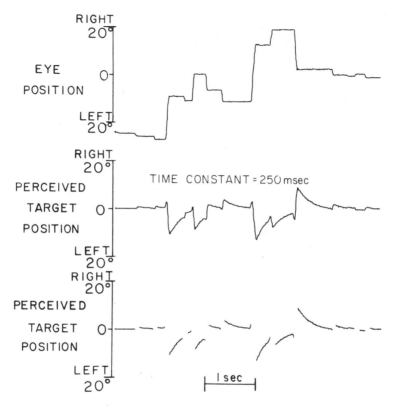

FIG. 6.   A computer solution of the model in Fig. 5 showing perceived location of a stationary object during a representative pattern of eye movements. Top trace shows horizontal eye position of a subject looking around the room and was used as input ($\Theta_{E/H}$) to the model. The middle trace shows perceived target position ("$\Theta_{T/H}$") when Delay was 0.05 sec and a was reciprocal 250 msec. Bottom trace is the same as the middle trace, except that vision was blanked for 100 msec beginning just prior to saccade onsets to simulate the effect of saccadic suppression. Time begins on the left for all traces and lengths of vertical bars correspond to rotations of 40 deg. arc in any trace.

begins making saccades the object should appear to be constantly changing position.[4] This does not seem to happen in ordinary viewing and our problem is to explain why.

Erdmann and Dodge (1898) noticed that objects that could be clearly seen when the eye was fixating could not be seen during saccades. Since then many investigations have been aimed at understanding the magnitude and mechanisms

---

[4]Failure of the model in Fig. 5 to predict veridical space perception is not restricted to saccadic eye movements. In fact, the model predicts that perception will be inaccurate whenever the eye changes position. For example, if the subject smoothly pursued a target moving sinusoidally, the model predicts that perceived target motion will be 90 degrees out of phase with target motion at all frequencies below $1/2\pi$ times the reciprocal of the time constant (a) and 180 degrees out of phase for all motions at higher frequencies.

involved in the modest suppression of vision during saccades (see Matin, 1974; 1976 for reviews). Many investigators (e.g., Matin, 1972; Matin, 1974) have noted that suppression would help explain perceived stability. They are correct. The bottom trace in Fig. 6 shows the consequence of blanking vision completely for the time course of saccadic suppression, that is, for a time interval of 100 msec beginning just prior to saccade onset. The result removes large apparent shifts in the scene casued by the saccades themselves, but what remains is clearly not a perceptually stable visual world. Other known visual phenomena like backward lateral inhibition or *metacontrast* are functionally similar to saccadic suppression and would help that mechanism approximate the complete blanking shown during saccades in Fig. 6.

The question remains: What mechanism allows us to see a perceptually stable and accurately mapped world in the interval between saccades? Clear as this problem is, the answer is not so clear. The only possibility is that retinal information about eye position is used to upgrade the eye position signals. Exactly why this would be needed is not clear because a very precise eye position signal is

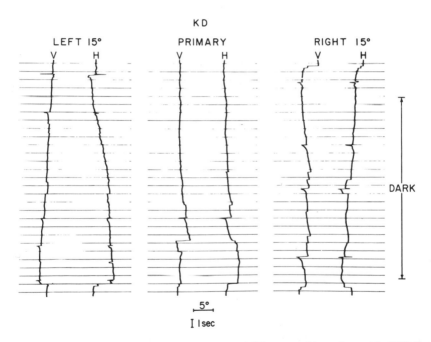

FIG. 7.   Recordings of horizontal (H) and vertical (V) eye position when subject KD first attempted to control eye position in the dark in the Primary position and 15 deg. arc to the Left and Right of primary position. Time begins at the top and repetitive horizontal lines show 1 sec intervals. The horizontal bar at the bottom corresponds to a 5 deg. arc rotation. Rightwards trace movements correspond to right in H and up in V. Position defining fixation targets were switched off during the interval indicated by the vertical bar labeled Dark. (From Hansen & Skavenski, 1977. Accuracy of eye position information for motor control. Copyright 1977 by Pergamon Press, Ltd. Reprinted by permission.)

now known to be present in the brain. To illustrate, in the last few years evidence has accumulated that the motor systems know where the eye is at all times. Merton (1961) used an afterimage mapping technique to show that the eye could be directed in total darkness as well as the arm, and he concluded that eye position was known to the central nervous system as accurately as arm position.

Stavenski and Steinman (1970) used an objective technique to record subjects' eye movements during attempts to maintain eye position in the dark. Recordings illustrating the good control they observed are reproduced in Fig. 7.

Actually, these records were made of experimentally naive subjects' first attempts to control eye position in the dark (Hansen & Skavenski, 1977). A magnetic field search-coil technique was used to record two-dimensional eye movements. The record made for primary position was one subject's very first attempt and shows that she never went further than about 4 deg. arc from the reference position before making a corrective saccade. Detailed statistical analyses of 14 trials like this, made at seven different reference positions, show that, on the average the eye was within 2 deg. arc of the reference position over a 25-sec dark interval. A second naive subject performed in the same way. Thus Hansen and Skavenski concluded that reasonably accurate *eye position information* was readily available *for oculomotor control*. Experimentally naive subjects needed no special training or experience to permit them to use this information to control eye position in the dark.

The oculomotor system also has this eye position information available for all types of eye movements. In the records shown here, drift eye movements tended to carry the eye away from the reference position. All of our subjects can detect errors introduced by these slow eye movements and correct them with saccades. Becker and Fuchs (1969) have noted the same behavior in all of their subjects.

Figure 8 illustrates that subjects can also readily correct errors in eye position caused by saccades or the slow phase of vestibular nystagmus in the dark.

In this experiment, trials began with about 5 sec of fixation of a visible target in one of seven positions equally spaced on a 50 deg. arc horizontal arc. The target was switched off, placing the subject in total darkness. Then, on half of the trials, the subject rotated so that the slow phase of vestibular nystagmus drove the eye out of the reference position in the head defined by the fixation target when it was visible. On remaining trials subjects were instructed to saccade away from this reference position. Five seconds after the onset of these movements, subjects were instructed to return their eyes to the position in the head defined by the fixation target. Records reproduced in Fig. 8 show that the subject could return to the reference position equally well in both cases. In fact, over a large number of trials like this, two subjects returned their eyes within about 2 deg. arc of the reference position in the head regardless of the type of movement used to drive the eye away from this position. Combined with the prior observation, these data suggest that accurate eye position information is available for oculomotor control following slow and fast *smooth* eye movements *and* very rapid saccades as well.

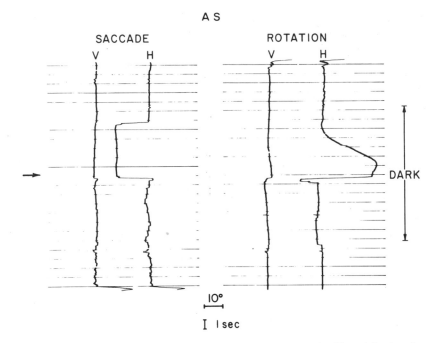

FIG. 8.   Representative horizontal and vertical eye records of subject AS when he attempted to return his eye to the reference position in total darkness (at the time indicated by the arrow on the left) following errors in eye position caused by Saccades or the slow phase of vestibular nystagmus (Rotation). Other features are the same as those in Fig. 7. (From Hansen & Skavenski, 1977. Accuracy of eye position information for motor control. Copyright 1977 by Pergamon Press Ltd. Reprinted by permission.)

Eye movement control experiments also indicate that the eye position information is closely time-locked to movements. Hansen and Skavenski (1977) carefully examined how accurately subjects could return their eye to a reference position as a function of the time elapsed after a saccade away from that position. Trials were similar to the saccade experiment shown in the left panel of Fig. 8, except that the time interval between saccades was varied between 0.25 sec and 2 sec. In this experiment the amplitude and the direction of return saccades can be programmed only on the basis of nonvisual eye position information.[5] If

---

[5]The possibility that subjects memorized the amplitude and direction of the saccade made away from the reference position and programmed return saccades on the basis of this remembered trajectory was eliminated by the following control experiment. Subjects' eyes were moved out of the reference position in the dark by requiring them to make about 20 saccades paced by a metronome whose beat was varied between 0.25 and 2.0 sec. Subjects' accuracy in saccading back to the reference position did not vary with the time between saccades or with the pattern of movements they made. Consequently, they must have based their return saccades on eye position information because it was very unlikely they could have memorized the trajectory of every saccade that they made and used this remembered scanpath to look back to the reference position.

the position signals followed saccades sluggishly they would have underestimated the distance of the eye from the reference position by an amount that decreased with time since the eye moved away. Consequently, return saccades should have fallen short of the goal by an amount inversely related to the time since making a saccade away. This did not happen. Data shown in Fig. 9 indicate that two subjects could accurately look back to the reference target regardless of the time between saccades.

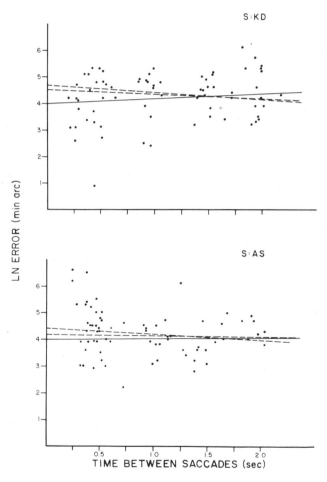

FIG. 9.   The natural logarithm of error (LN ERROR) for subjects KD and AS when they attempted to return their eyes to a reference position in total darkness at various times after they made a saccade away from that position (Time Between Saccades). Data points are all return errors for each subject's first session and the solid lines are "best fit" regression lines to these points. Dashed lines are regression lines for two other sessions. (From Hansen & Skavenski, 1977. Accuracy of eye position information for motor control. Copyright 1977 by Pergamon Press Ltd. Reprinted by permission.)

In Fig. 9 the natural logarithm of return error has been plotted as a function of time between saccades. Data points show all of the return errors for each subject's first session. The solid line is the linear regression line fitted to these points and has an intercept of about 4, which corresponds to an error of 0.9 deg. arc. Dashed lines are regression lines for two other sessions. For both subjects slopes of regression lines were not significantly different from zero. This means that the eye position signals had completed their change within 200 msec after a saccade and were uniform thereafter. In other words, the eye position signals had to follow eye position with a time constant of less than 70 msec. It should be noted that this time constant is very much shorter than that obtained in Matin's (1972) perception experiments as noted earlier. In fact, this time constant may be nearly zero given Hallet and Lightstone's (1976 a, b) report that subjects could make goal-directed saccades to targets which were briefly flashed on at various times during a preceding saccadic eye movement. These corrective movements could not be based solely on the position of the target image with respect to the fovea because the flashed targets were seen with the moving eye and the eye was in a different position when the first saccade ended. A strategy that would work is for the oculomotor system to use eye position information to determine where the flashed target was located with respect to the head and then make a saccade to that place! If the task was accomplished in this way, then an extremely accurate eye position signal must have been available at all times during a saccade.

Taken together, these data lead to the conclusion that the oculomotor "engineer" in our brains, the "person" who computes the motor commands for positioning the eyes, has accurate eye position information at all times and for all eye movement types. Virtually all of our attempts at burdening this engineer have fallen short. It can be forced to generate all manners of eye spins, pauses, and flicks, in any pattern, at any pace, in any direction, and it still knows where

TABLE 1
Accuracy of Target Localization During Fixation[a]

Subject	Light		Dark	
JC	10.9	(22)	0.8	(24)
KD	6.3	(31)	3.5	(53)
HR	0.3	(31	2.6	(52)
AS	3.0	(54)	4.7	(58)
Overall Mean	5.1	(37)	2.9	(50)

[a]Distances (in min arc) of the mean position of 175 hammer blows from targets on the horizontal meridian and standard deviations in parentheses when subjects viewed targets in full room illumination (Light) or in total darkness (Dark).

the eye is. Perhaps this is not surprising. What about the other motor engineers in our brains? Does the engineer who controls our arms also have access to precise eye position information? The next experiment shows that it does.

Hansen and Skavenski (1977) began by asking whether ballistic arm movements (like driving a nail with a hammer) were sufficiently accurate to serve as a sensitive index of the accuracy of eye position signals. Data shown in Table 1 indicates that they are. Table 1 shows mean errors and standard deviations when four subjects used a pointed hammer to hit targets randomly selected from a 70 deg. arc horizontal array. Each mean error is the distance of the mean position of 175 blows from the target on the horizontal meridian. Data for the light condition were collected with the entire visual scene well lighted so visual cues could potentially help subjects localize targets. Although these errors are small (and consequently accuracy was good) they are not surprising because Howarth, Beggs, and Bowden (1971) have observed comparable accuracy in a similar task and it is virtually common knowledge in the manual arts and sports that ballistic limb movements can be executed with great accuracy. What is surprising is the precision of the blows struck in the dark where the subject saw only the target in an otherwise totally dark room. Here great care was taken to insure that subjects had no visual cue to target location, so blows could be guided only on the basis of eye position information. The fact that the mean position of the blow was within five minutes of arc of the target indicates that there is a very accurate *eye position signal for motor control* when the eye is reasonably stationary. So the limb engineer, like our sensory homonculus, has a precise eye position signal when the eye is fairly stable. What happens when the eye moves?

We examined the dynamics of the eye position signal for limb movement control by asking subjects to hit targets they could see only during saccades. The subject sat in a large magnetic-field generating system that permitted recording rotations of the eye independently of head translations. Potentials induced in a search-coil attached to a contact lens worn on the right eye were used to detect saccades. Ear phones presented loud white noise to prevent auditory cues from helping them localize targets. They attempted to strike the targets with the round end of a ballpeen hammer as in the prior experiment. In the experiment the subject was placed in total darkness and an anvil holding the target was placed in a position selected at random from an array of 8 positions equally spaced on a 20 deg. arc to the right of the subject's straight-ahead position. This somewhat restricted range of target positions was adopted to insure that target images fell no further than about 15 deg. arc in peripheral retina. When ready, the subject pressed a button which initiated a trial composed of the sequence of events shown in Fig. 10.

Two seconds later a tone signalled the subject to make a rightwards saccade of from 5 to 15 deg. arc amplitude. When eye velocity exceeded a criterion of about 150 deg. arc sec a pulse of current caused a bulb to illuminate the target for a period of 25 msec. This means that the target came on when the eye was

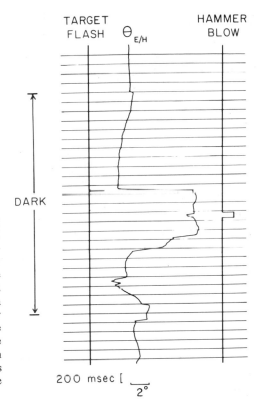

FIG. 10   Recording illustrating the timing of Target Flashes and Hammer Blows when subjects attempted to strike targets seen only during horizontal saccadic eye movements ($\Theta_{E/H}$). Rightward trace movements indicate when the light came on, when the blow was struck, and rightward eye movements. Other features of the record are the same as those in Fig. 7, except calibration marks correspond to 200 msec in time and rotations of 2 deg. arc.

about a third of the way into the saccade and went off just before the saccade was over. The subject hit the target about 0.5 sec later. Subjects were never given feedback about their performance. There were no visual cues to the target position. Targets could be localized only on the basis of eye position information. If that information followed eye position slugglishly (as in Fig. 4C) it would have indicated the eye was to the left of its actual position and all hammer blows based on this signal would have been to the left of actual target position regardless of the position of the retinal image of that target. The results summarized in Table 2 show that this did not happen.

Table 2 shows that the mean position of the blow was within 15 min arc of the target for this and two other subjects for rightward moving saccades. Comparable accuracy was observed for all three subjects for leftward saccades in a second experiment. All of these means are closer to the target by more than one order of magnitude than would be predicted if the eye position signals followed eye position with a time constant of 200 msec or longer. In fact, the only way to explain the accuracy of these blows is to assume that the motor system has very elegant information about eye position at all times during a saccade.

TABLE 2
Accuracy of Localizing Targets Presented During Saccades[a]

Subject	Saccade Directions			
	Right		Left	
JC	−3	(67)	−11	(77)
RH	14	(64)	15	(65)
AS	−1	(81)	25	(81)

[a]Distances (in min arc) of the mean positions of 120 hammer blows from targets on the horizontal meridian and standard deviations in parentheses when targets were only flashed on during Right or Left going saccadic eye movements. (Negative signs signify means to the left of the target position.)

In summary, we now have strong evidence showing that accurate nonretinal *eye position information* is available for control of eye position when visual information is absent. This accurate information is also available *for limb movement control* because accurate manipulation of the environment is possible when localization is forced to depend on eye position information alone. In addition, the motor systems know where the eyes are during several types of eye movements, and that information is very closely time-locked to the eye movements. In short, our motor systems appear to always know what the eye is doing. This is indeed fortunate, it helps us to understand, among other things, how a basketball star can race down court dodging, cutting, and swerving among the other players to set up and sink a 20 foot turnaround jump shot; how Alice got to the Mad Hatter's tea party; and how we got to this symposium. However, it makes the perception data described earlier quite puzzling.

The contrast between what the perceptual and the motor systems can do with eye position information is striking. When the eye is fixating, where we see objects to be located depends critically on the nonvisual eye position information. These perceptions are quite accurate. On the other hand, virtually all of the data indicate that whenever the eye is in motion (which is to say all of the time) accurate information about eye position is not accessible to perception, although it is accessible to, and used by, all motor control systems. Consequently, localization, which depends on cruder eye-position signals, is inaccurate and the visual world is poorly stabilized. This raises an important question for which we have no answer. Why do we say we see a perceptually stable and accurately localized visual environment? Does our sensory homunculus use *visual* information to determine eye position and, if so, what sort of visual information, and what is the advantage of doing so instead of using the accurate eye position information known to be present in the brain? Alternatively, have we set up our perceptual experiments in a way that *precludes* the use of nonvisual eye position signals? Until we gain some insight into this problem we must face the possibility that a perceptually stable visual world in which objects *appear* accurately localized is perhaps itself almost an illusion arising from the fact that our motor systems know where our body is.

DISCUSSION

LEISMAN: If eye position information is necessary for perception of visual direction, does that mean that individuals with an opthalmoplegia or lateralized third nerve palsy would be expected to experience distortions of perceived visual direction?

SKAVENSKI: In the normal person, anything that causes eye position to differ from the commands sent to the eye leads to mislocalizations that are systematically related to the discrepancy between eye position and the command, as in the experiments where we externally loaded the eye. Consequently, these disorders, which cause the oculomotor commands to fail to produce the desired eye position, might also yield perceptual distortion. However, I cannot answer your question with certainty because the neural structures serving as sources for the eye position information are not known. Certainly, if the source of the eye position information for perception of direction is central to the lesions in internuclear opthalmoplegia, then perceptual mislocalization might result.

MATIN: Needless to say I share your feeling that not everything has been explained about the stability of the visual world, but I wondered if you weren't overstating the case a bit about how bad the perception is relative to motor behavior. Most studies of oculomotor control based on non-visual eye position signals showed errors on the order of 2 deg. arc. We would have called this sloppy control, whereas you call it incredibly accurate, and I think it's more a semantic difference than a substantive one.

In your ballistic arm movement experiment, targets were flashed on when velocity was 150 deg/sec for 5 deg saccades. This must mean that the target was on when the saccade was over, and the subject could have localized it them. In other words, I don't think we are forced to conclude that the subject has extremely accurate information about where his eye is at any moment during the saccade. Finally, in your experiment and those of Hallet and Lightstone (1976a, b) the conclusion was that the motor behavior is very much more accurate than anything we would expect from perceptual behavior. Hallett and Lightstone (1976 a) quote an unpublished study by Templeton and Anstis in which they found errors in pointing accuracy similar to the kinds we found in the perceptual experiments. I wondered what differences there were between your experiment and theirs, because it may hold an important clue to the difference between the results of motor control and perception experiments.

SKAVENSKI: First, I agree that the control of eye position in the dark is not incredibly accurate, but it is not fair to say that the eye position information is as poor as the errors of approximately 2 deg. arc would indicate. Such large errors are due largely to the fact that the subjects were forced to keep their eyes in or return their eyes to a remembered target position in space. Most of us would agree that spatial memories are not perfect, and that it is very unlikely that a subject could remember with great accuracy where this target was located. Consequently, the oculomotor measure of the accuracy of the eye position information is contaminated by the subject's poor memory for the reference position. This conclusion is further reinforced by the result of the ballistic arm movements which do not rely on the subjects spatial memory and which do show that there is very precise eye position information for motor control.

Second, it was possible in the ballistic arm movement experiment that the target was visible for a few milliseconds at the end of the 5 deg saccades, which have a mean duration of about 40 msec in the dark. However, these small amplitude saccades comprised only a small fraction of those studies in the experiment. Most of the saccades studies were much larger (mean amplitudes ranged from 7 to 12 deg for the various subjects) with durations greater than 50 msec so that the targets were not illuminated when the saccade ended. Thus, for nearly all of the saccades studied, accurate localization was possible only if subjects had access to precise eye position information during the saccade.

I.3

Central and Peripheral Determinants of Saccadic Suppression[1]

Frances C. Volkmann
Smith College

Lorrin A. Riggs
Robert K. Moore
Brown University

Keith D. White
*University of Florida,
Gainesville*

Human visual perception occurs within the context of saccadic eye movements. Our behavior in the visual world is characterized by our ability (a) to detect potentially salient stimuli in the peripheral fields and bring them, rapidly and accurately, to the fovea, and (b) to inspect these stimuli in a succession of fixational pauses that permit foveal scrutiny of each of their fine details. Our visual systems are highly specialized for these adaptive behavioral sequences, and the eye movements that characterize them occur with a frequency of more than one per second for most of our waking lives.

Recent research has contributed much to our understanding of the neural bases of these behavioral sequences. Two-stage models of vision have been developed based on (1) a transient or ambient visual system, and (2) a sustained or focal visual system, located in the mammalian retina and its central projections (Cleland, Dubin, & Levick, 1971; Enroth—Cugell & Robson, 1966; Fukada, 1971; Trevarthen, 1968; see Breitmeyer & Ganz, 1976, for a comprehensive summary and analysis). The transient system may be characterized as a "where is it?" system (Schneider, 1969) which is particularly adapted to the rapid detection of large or moving stimuli that fall on the peripheral retina. The sustained system is a "what is it?" system, adapted for the slow, careful inspection of fine detail of a stimulus, which must be brought to focus on the fovea in order for this system to operate at maximal efficiency.

[1]Our work was supported by Grants No. 41103 and BNS 76-01450 from the National Science Foundation to Frances C. Volkmann and Lorrin A. Riggs. We wish to express our thanks to John Volkmann, Thomas Butler, Ann Fuehrer, Jillian van Nostrand, Delores Mel, Jerrilynn Peters, Martha Romeskie, and Carol Whitbeck for their contributions to the research.

It is easy to see that the smooth coordination of these two highly specialized visual systems requires the concurrent evolution of an eye movement control system that proceeds from the transient to the sustained mode of analysis, and then guides the accurate inspection of stimulus detail (see also Walls, 1962). In order to be most adaptive, the control system should operate in such a way as to favor (1) rapid positioning of the stimulus on the fovea, (2) accurate positioning of the stimulus on the fovea, and (3) clear foveal vision of the stimulus at the end of the eye movement. In addition, this eye movement system should work in conjunction with other control systems to (4) localize the salient stimulus within the framework of a stable visual world.

The saccadic system is, of course, the control system most directly related to these accomplishments in human subjects. The speed and accuracy of the system are impressive (Fuchs, 1971; Robinson, 1964) but do not directly concern us here. We are concerned, rather, with questions related to the accomplishment of clear foveal vision of the salient stimulus at the end of a saccade. The maintenance of a stable visual world within the context of eye and stimulus motion has been approached experimentally in a variety of ways (see, for example, Bridgeman, Hendry, & Stark, 1975; Hallet & Lightstone, 1976a, 1976b; Mack, 1970; MacKay, 1973; Matin, 1972; Stark, Kong, Schwartz, Hendry, & Bridgeman, 1976) but will be of interest to us only as it is directly related to vision at times during and closely surrounding saccades.

Early investigators (Dodge, 1900, 1905; Holt, 1903; Woodworth, 1906) pointed out that with every saccade, the visual scene is swept across the retina as a smeared streak in which all detail must be lost. Yet vision seems to be phenomenally clear during each fixational pause, and the visual background remains perceptually stable and unmoved. The system, apparently, does not notice the smeared stimulus that occurs during each saccade under the usual range of conditions of normal vision. This phenomenon of decreased visual sensitivity to stimuli which occur during or within about 100 msec of a saccade was first unequivocally demonstrated when stroboscopic means became available to present a flash with negligible retinal smear (Latour, 1962; Ditchburn, 1955; Volkmann, 1962). The phenomenon has come to be called almost universally *saccadic suppression* (Matin, 1974; Zuber, Crider, & Stark, 1964).

Explanations of saccadic suppression rest on one of two major classes of variables, or on their combination. In the early days, Holt (1903) believed that vision is "blanked out" during saccades by a neural discharge from the extraocular muscles which somehow interrupts transmission in the visual system. This "inflow theory" has more recently been replaced by the notion of a central corollary discharge or "feedforward loop" which accompanies the neural signal to the eye muscles to execute a saccade, and which acts to inhibit or decrease vision for a brief time related to the occurrence of the saccade. This efferent, or "outflow" model has drawn upon the ideas of Helmholtz (1909/1962) dating back to 1867, Sperry (1950), and von Holst (1954) (see also MacKay, 1973).

Other investigators, including Dodge (1900, 1905) concluded that saccadic suppression can be explained entirely by events originating at the level of the receptors (i.e., peripheral events) and thus not requiring any neural inhibition from higher visual centers. Prominent among these peripheral events is the "smear" of the image on the retina; during a saccade, each element of the stimulus image produces a decreased photochemical effect on each receptor because it is whisked so rapidly across it. Another prominent event that originates in the retina is the masking of a smeared image by the clear image which follows it at the end of a saccade. Several papers are now available (Cumming, 1976; Matin, 1974; Volkmann, 1976) that summarize a variety of experiments designed to separate the central from the peripheral variables in saccadic suppression; the results have led investigators to attribute suppression to one or the other type of variable (Brooks & Fuchs, 1975; Campbell & Wurtz, in press), or to their combination (Breitmeyer & Ganz, 1976; Bridgeman, Hendry, & Stark, 1975; Riggs, Merton, & Morton, 1974; Stark, Michael, & Zuber, 1969).

We address ourselves to recent experiments in which we have explored the effects of saccadic eye movements on a basic visual discrimination, that of contrast sensitivity to sinusoidal gratings. One purpose of these experiments is to differentiate some major retinal and central determinants of saccadic suppression. Since our experimental arrangement permits us to minimize contour in the stimulus field, the research also aims to supply information on the role of contour masking in suppression by investigating suppression in the absence of such masking.

EXPERIMENT 1: CONTRAST SENSITIVITY OF THE FIXATING AND THE SACCADING EYE

Method

The observer sat in a Ganzfeld of about 30 Ft L luminance. Her left eye was covered with a patch. With her right eye she viewed two fixation marks located 6° apart in a 9.5° square field of the same luminance as the Ganzfeld (Fig. 1). The observer fixated the blank area within one of the sets of vertical marks; this gap subtended 1° 30 min of arc. The edges of the Ganzfeld were not ordinarily visible; they blurred into the fixation field. These features were designed to minimize contour in the field, and the possible masking effects that might result from such contour.

The observer began each trial by fixating the designated (left or right) fixation gap. Then, on signal, she looked quickly to the other gap, and on another signal

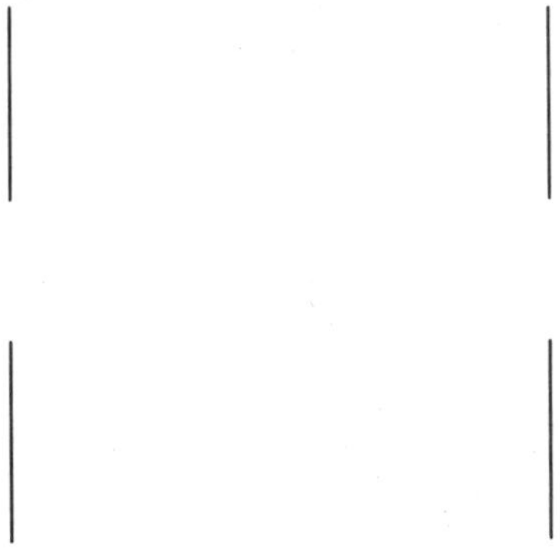

FIG. 1.   Fixation guides used in the present experiments. Observers fixated in the middle of the gap between one pair of vertical lines and executed horizontal saccades to the middle of the gap between the other set, over a distance of 6° of visual angle.

about 1 sec later, looked back again to the first gap. Before, during, or after one saccade of the pair a low-contrast sinusoidal grating having a spatial frequency of .65 c/deg replaced the fixation field for an exposure duration of 10 msec.[2] In the same temporal relation to the other saccade of the pair, a blank field of equal space—average luminance replaced the fixation field, also in a 10-msec exposure. The order of presentation of grating and blank was randomized, and the observer was instructed to make a temporal forced-choice judgment of which saccade within each pair was accompanied by exposure of the grating.

Figure 2 shows the experimental arrangements for presenting the blank field or grating stimuli, and for recording the observer's eye movements and the temporal relation of the stimuli to the eye movements. The observer's electro-oculogram (EOG), after appropriate amplification, activated a trigger circuit which, in turn, could be set to activate the timing circuit of an Iconix three-channel tachistoscope. By varying the delay set into the circuit, the experimenter could present the 10-msec stimulus at various times during or after a saccade. To present the stimulus before a saccade, the experimenter triggered it manually, just before the observer started a saccade from one fixation gap to the other.

The right-hand side of Fig. 2 shows how the three tachistoscope channels worked together to present the steady fixation field, and to replace it briefly with the blank or grating stimulus field. The space—average luminance of channels 2 and 3 together always matched the luminance of channel 1. Under these conditions of constant luminance, grating contrast was varied by rotating the two neutral density wedges in channels 2 and 3 so that a larger or smaller proportion of the light came through the grating.

An optical system focused the fixation marks or the stimulus field on the observer's eye at an accommodative distance of about 1 m, and filled the entire

---

[2]Contrast is defined as $(L_{max} - L_{min})/(L_{max} + L_{min})$, where L_{max} and L_{min} are the bright and dark extremes of luminance in the grating. Gratings were photographically produced transparencies provided to us by Dr. Charles Stromeyer. Transmission approximates a sinusoidal function, and maximum contrast is 60%.

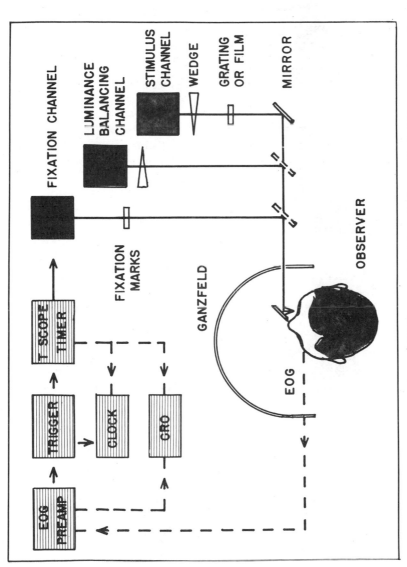

FIG. 2   Block diagram of apparatus. The electrooculogram (EOG) was used to trigger the lamps of a tachistoscope at one of a number of pre-determined times in relation to a saccade (upper left). The tachistoscope exposed either a sinusoidal grating of variable contrast or a blank field of equal space-average luminance (upper right). The stimulus could be made to move by reflecting it off a mirror galvanometer (lower right). For further explanation see text.

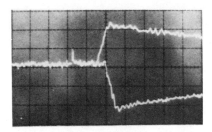

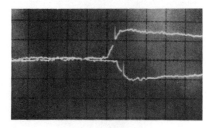

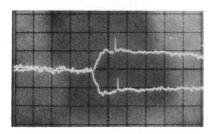

FIG. 3.   Photographs of storage oscilloscope display showing three examples of pairs of saccades that constituted a trial. In the top photograph, the stimuli (vertical blips) arrived before the saccades; in the middle photograph, during the saccades; and in the bottom photograph, after the saccades. One exposure of each pair exposed the grating stimulus, the other, a blank field.

9.5° square field with either the grating or with the blank film when the stimulus was presented. Thus, the fovea was always well within the stimulus field, no matter where the eye might be directed when the stimulus arrived.

The time relation between each saccade and each stimulus exposure was displayed on a storage oscilloscope, as shown in Fig. 3. It was also checked on a digital clock, which was activated by either the saccade or the stimulus, whichever came first, and stopped by the second of these events, thus giving in msec the relation between the stimulus and the onset of the saccade. In each trial, the observer judged which of the two exposures contained the grating rather than the homogeneous film, and the experimenter noted her response. The stimuli were presented in a range of contrasts, using a forced-choice, constant stimulus method with each of three optically corrected observers.

The grating in this experiment was always oriented horizontally, to minimize the effects of smear on the retina of the horizontally moving eye. Moreover, the low spatial frequency of the grating (.65 c/deg) served to minimize effects of possible changes in accommodation or deviations from a horizontal path in the course of the saccades.

To summarize, this experiment provides an assessment of contrast sensitivity to sinusoidal gratings under conditions that minimize both retinal smear and possible masking effects of contour in the visual field, when the grating is presented at times during, just preceding, or just following saccadic eye movements.

Results

In general, this experiment yielded results consistent with those of earlier studies that compared detection, recognition, or acuity thresholds when stimuli are flashed to the moving eye and when they are flashed to the fixating eye (for summaries, see Matin, 1974; Volkmann, 1976). We fitted curves by the method of least squares to our data of percentage correct responses as a function of grating contrast. From these we calculated contrast thresholds for each of three

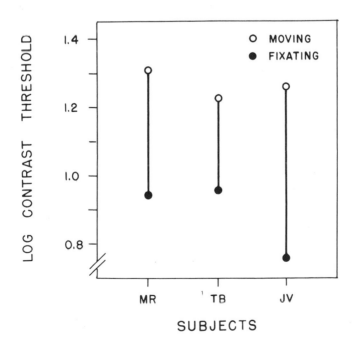

FIG. 4.   Log contrast thresholds for three subjects (MR, TB, and JV) for gratings presented during steady fixation and during 6° saccades in a Ganzfeld.

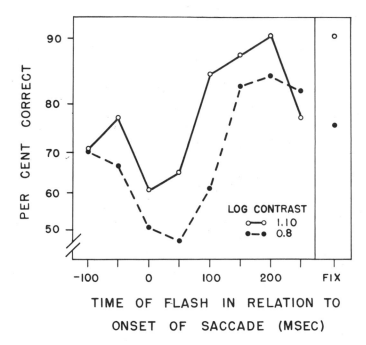

FIG. 5.   Percentage of correct forced-choice responses (probability coordinates) as a function of the time of the stimulus in relation to the onset of a saccade. Each curve represents a single value of stimulus contrast for the combined data of the three subjects. For further explanation see text.

observers for 10-msec stimuli occurring (a) in an interval 0–50 msec after the onset of a saccade, and (b) at times during which the eye was steadily fixating. Figure 4 shows these two sets of thresholds for each of the three observers. In each case the moving eye required between 0.3 and 0.5 log unit of additional contrast over that required by the fixating eye in order to see the stimulus 75% of the time in the forced-choice situation.

Figure 5 presents examples of the time course of the threshold elevation in this experiment for each of two stimulus contrasts. Since the three subjects produced similar results, the graphs show group data in which each point on the abscissa represents the midpoint of a 100-msec interval, though samples were taken every 50 msec on a sliding scale to help counteract the effects of small numbers of observations in some of the time bins. With this procedure the numbers of judgments ranged between 30 and 90 per plotted point.

The curves in Fig. 5 confirm, for contrast sensitivity, a time course of suppression similar to many that have been reported previously for other stimulus parameters. For both contrasts, we see that gratings are progressively less well identified as the time of their presentation approaches the time of the saccade. The time course of correct responding after the saccade is dependent upon the contrast of the stimulus, with suppression lasting longer for the lower contrast stimulus. There is a suggestion, particularly in the lower contrast data, of an oscillation in sensitivity as a function of time after the eye movement; at times of stimulation around 200 msec after the onset of a saccade, a period of unusually clear vision is indicated, in which correct responding is even higher than it is to stimuli presented to the steadily fixating eye (Volkmann & Riggs, 1975). We are currently undertaking experiments to investigate this possible effect more thoroughly.

The results of this experiment show, then, that saccadic suppression of contrast sensitivity to low frequency sinusoidal gratings occurs with a magnitude and time course similar to those measured previously for other stimuli. Of special relevance here is the finding of suppression under experimental conditions designed to minimize both possible masking effects of contour in the field, and effects of smear of the stimulus on the retina of the moving eye.

EXPERIMENT 2: EFFECTS OF RETINAL SMEAR ON CONTRAST SENSITIVITY OF THE FIXATING AND THE SACCADING EYE

Method

Although the experimental arrangements for this study were in general the same as for Experiment 1, three changes were made which permitted us to present controlled amounts of smear of the stimulus on the retina whether the eye was moving or stationary.

1. the orientation of the .65 c/deg sinusoidal grating was changed from horizontal to vertical, so that smear could be produced by moving either the grating or the eye horizontally;

2. the stimulus exposure time was reduced to 5 msec in order to produce the desired amounts of smear without changing the spatial frequency of our stimulus;

3. the mirror in the lower right hand optical path of Fig. 2 was replaced by a high speed mirror galvanometer. This galvanometer system could be triggered by the EOG to produce a horizontal excursion of the stimulus on a ramp which was linear over a substantial portion of its midrange. The moving mirror system was calibrated by comparing the excursion of a beam of light reflected from the moving mirror with the input signal to the galvanometer driver. The ramp speed, or time over which the mirror moved through a given angular excursion, was variable, and could be set by the experimenter prior to each trial. Figure 6 shows examples of three ramp speeds in relation to saccades (see figure legend for description). In each example, the 5-msec stimulus flash, indicated by a gap in the traces, occured during the midrange of the excursion of the eye and the mirror.

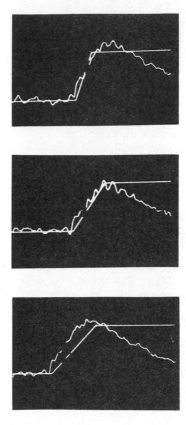

FIG. 6.   Photographs of storage oscilloscope display showing three examples of saccades (traces containing some noise) and mirror ramp velocities (smooth traces) used to produce stimulus motion. The time of occurrence of the 5-msec stimulus exposure is indicated by a gap in the traces. In the top photograph, the stimulus moves faster than the eye; in the middle photograph, the stimulus and the eye move at approximately equal peak velocities; in the bottom photograph, the eye moves faster than the stimulus. The apparent return of the eye movement trace toward its starting position at the end of the saccade is due to AC coupling of the EOG recording system.

Calibration of retinal smear.   We wished to produce specified amounts of smear of the stimulus across the retina ranging in amplitude from zero to half a cycle of the grating. Since the exposure time, the angular extent of the mirror excursion, and the spatial frequency of the grating were all known, the ramp speed required to smear the stimulus by any given amount on the fixating eye was directly calculable.

In order to determine the appropriate ramp speeds required to produce specific amounts of smear on the retina during a saccade, it was necessary to find the ramp speed at which the angular velocity of the mirror matched that of the saccading eye near the midpoint of its excursion (when stimulation occurred) and thus to approximate a "stabilized image" condition of zero smear. Since we found that the temporal characteristics of an observer's saccades of a given angular size were highly repeatable, as reported by Robinson (1964), Fuchs (1971), and Hendry (1975), we determined a psychophysical "tuning function" for each of our observers: that is, the function relating the percentage of correct judgments to mirror speed. To determine this tuning function, the vertical grating and a blank film were presented during pairs of saccades, and the observer indicated in a temporal forced-choiced, as described in Experiment 1, which saccade she judged to be accompanied by the grating rather than the blank. With contrast constant, mirror ramp speeds were varied systematically according to a constant stimulus method. Figure 7 shows examples of "tuning functions" obtained in this way for the two observers. Zero smear of the grating on the moving retina was taken to be the ramp speed that was located at the midpoint

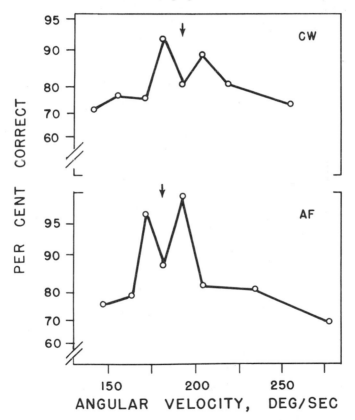

FIG. 7.   Tuning functions for two subjects (CW and AF). Percentages of correct forced-choice responses to stimuli presented during saccades (probability coordinates) are plotted in relation to the angular velocity of the stimulus in deg/sec. Arrows indicate the estimated zero-smear condition, or the stimulus velocity which most nearly matches the velocity of the eye.

of the range of speed over which contrast sensitivity was maximal. For subject CW this occurred at an angular velocity of 192°/sec; for AF, at 181°/sec. Once zero smear had been specified in this way, values of smear could be calculated as they were for the fixating eye condition.

The tuning functions shown in Fig. 7 are characteristic of many that we have obtained. They are consistent in showing slightly better vision with small but measurable amounts of smear than with the least amount of smear that we are able to produce. We are currently investigating more thoroughly this intriguing finding.

In Experiment 2, contrast thresholds were obtained under four conditions of retinal smear (0, .17, .33 and .5 cycles) for both the moving and the fixating eye. All conditions were run concurrently, with blocks of trials for the fixating and the moving eye alternated within each experimental session.

Results

The experiment yielded data relating correctness of forced-choice responses to stimulus contrast for each amount of smear for the moving and for the fixating eye. The results show a progressive decrease in contrast sensitivity with increas-

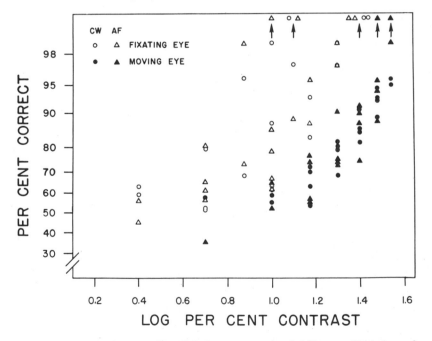

FIG. 8.   Percentages of correct forced-choice responses (probability coordinates) as a function of stimulus contrast (logarithmic coordinates) for two subjects. Open symbols show data for conditions of stimulus smear ranging between 0 and .5 cycle of the stimulus grating when it was presented to the fixating eye. Closed symbols show the same conditions of stimulus smear when the grating was presented to the eye during a saccade. N = 72 judgments per plotted point.

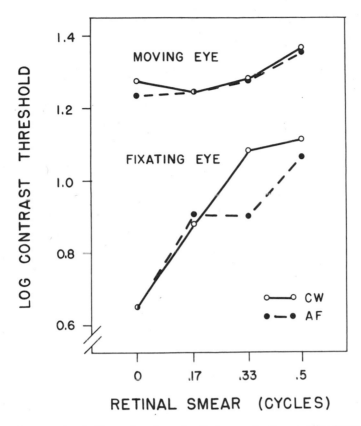

RETINAL SMEAR (CYCLES)

FIG. 9.   Contrast threshold as a function of retinal smear in the saccading (upper curves) and fixating (lower curves) eye conditions. The figure shows the data of two subjects (CW and AF) indicating log percentage contrast required for detection of vertical gratings smeared horizontally through various proportions of a cycle.

ing amounts of smear on the retina, together with a separable decrease in contrast sensitivity attributable to the saccade itself. In Fig. 8, the data from both subjects for all smear conditions are plotted to show the effects attributable to saccades. Under the conditions of our experiment, even a smear of .5 cycle of the grating on the fixating retina does not decrease vision as much as the saccade itself does in the presence of the least amount of smear that we were able to produce on the moving retina.

We used least squares fits of the individual sets of data to estimate the contrast threshold for each condition. Figure 9 shows thresholds as a function of retinal smear for the moving eye and for the fixating eye for each observer. In general, the curves show the expected increase in contrast thresholds with increased smear for both the moving and fixating eye. The possible reversal of this trend from the zero smear condition to .17 cycle of smear for the moving eye may be interpreted as showing a slightly inaccurate calculation of the mirror velocity required to produce zero smear on the moving retina. Alternatively, it may be related to the inversion in the tuning functions mentioned above. The curves of Fig. 9 also show the effects of saccades on contrast thresholds, independent of retinal smear up to .5 cycle. It is important to remember that these effects are produced in an experimental situation designed to ensure foveal stimulation of the moving eye, to minimize contour in the field, and to foster vision during saccades by using a target for which precise accommodation is not required. We cannot say, of course, that all of these conditions have been ideally produced, but we can say that they have been very closely approximated. We interpret the results shown in Fig. 9 as showing that both efferent neural suppression and peripheral (retinal) smear produced significant decrements of contrast sensitivity during saccades.

DISCUSSION

At the previous Eye Movement Symposium in 1974, we reviewed briefly four major types of variables that might play a role in saccadic suppression. Three of these were based on events originating in the periphery: retinal smear, visual masking, and shearing forces on the retina. The fourth, neural inhibition, was based on centrally originating events (Volkmann, 1976; see also Matin, 1974). Now we would like to offer some suggestions, based primarily on recent psychophysical work from our laboratory and others, about ways in which some of these variables might combine to foster maximally clear vision with minimum time delay at the end of each saccade.

Evidence for Suppressive Effects that Originate in the Retina

There is substantial agreement that *visual masking effects* operate to decrease vision during saccades in a lighted, contoured environment, and that under these viewing conditions masking effects are of perhaps primary importance in preparing the eye for optimal vision at the end of a saccade (Alpern, 1969; Breitmeyer & Ganz, 1976; Brooks & Fuchs, 1975; MacKay, 1970; Mateeff, Yakimoff, & Mitrani, 1976; Matin, Clymer, & Matin, 1972; Matin, 1974; Mitrani, Mateeff, & Yakimoff, 1971; Mitrani, Yakimoff, & Mateeff, 1973; Mitrani, Radil-Weiss, Yakimoff, Mateeff, & Božkov, 1975).

According to the review and analysis of Breitmeyer and Ganz (1976), masking effects such as metacontrast (or perhaps backward masking by noise or structure, depending on the stimulus situation) prevent masking by integration, or the interference of stimulation occuring during the fixation preceding the saccade with vision of the stimulus fixated immediately at the end of the saccade. Neurophysiologically, sustained visual channels are seen by these authors to be inhibited by the activity of transient channels.

Brooks and Fuchs (1975) supplied quantitative data on visual masking during saccades. They studied effects of background contour and luminance on visual sensitivity to 10-μsec flashes presented (a) during saccades executed between small fixation points located 20° apart, (b) during steady fixation on a dark point, and (c) during saccade-like jumps of the background field (see also Brooks, in preparation). They measured detection of 1° diameter (spot) test flashes located at least 15° from the fovea, and of diffuse "full field" flashes. Stimulus flashes were presented according to a variant of a psychophysical method of limits, and subjects indicated whether they had detected the stimulus by a yes/ no response. A major finding was that the threshold for detection of the spot rose by more than 2 log units when it was flashed during saccades over a highly contoured (checkered or striped) background, but that the visual effects of displacing the background field across the retina were highly similar to the effects of moving the eye across the field. Brooks and Fuchs (1975) conclude that "The comparable consequences of eye movement and background displacement severely challenge the necessity of a 'corollary discharge' or other central mechanism with *inhibitory properties* ... [p. 1397]." Rather, they support an interpretation based on masking of the stimulus by the motion of contours across the retina.

Brooks and Fuchs (1975) also found that background conditions have a different effect on sensitivity to diffuse flashes than they have on sensitivity to small, well-focused spots: during saccades made over contour-free backgrounds, thresholds for diffuse flashes were raised more than were thresholds for spot stimuli. Contour in the background, on the other hand, raised saccadic thresholds for punctate stimuli more than those for diffuse flashes. They suggest that separate mechanisms may be operating in these two situations (related, perhaps, to sustained and transient systems), and conclude that the important variables in saccadic suppression include (a) overall background luminance, (b) test stimulus size and possibly focused edges, and (c) possible interference on the retina of the contours of the test stimulus and contours or luminance shifts produced by the movement of the eye over the background field.

In another recent study, Campbell and Wurtz (in press) investigated the variable of *retinal smear* under conditions that in some ways approximated viewing in the normal visual environment (see also Mitrani et al. 1970a, 1970b). In one experiment, trains of very brief, high frequency flashes were delivered to the eye during horizontal saccades made between two light-emitting diodes located 20–30° apart. The duration of the train of flashes was variable; sometimes it was briefer than the duration of a saccade, at other times it outlasted the saccade by up to 150 msec. The flash stimuli illuminated a bank of relay racks and electronic equipment located in the laboratory, at a single value of illumination, and the subject was required to judge after each eye movement whether the scene was clear or smeared. In another experiment, a row of three Snellen Charts replaced the laboratory equipment in the visual scene, and subjects located the row of letters that was just visible during saccades. In yet another experiment, sequences of clear and blank stimuli were flashed to the fixating eye in various time relations, in an attempt to simulate stimulus events occurring during saccades.

Campbell and Wurtz conclude from their experiments that (a) smear is visible during saccades, under conditions in which the scene is illuminated only during the saccade, and (b) a clear static image either immediately before or after an eye movement obscures the smear occurring during the eye movement, even though the smear is still present. In interpreting their findings, they write:

> Our experiments rule out any corollary discharge or central anaesthesia as the primary mechanism for eliminating vision during eye movements for the following reasons: First, we have demonstrated that the smeared retinal image can be seen during an eye movement under certain conditions and, of course, brief stimuli falling on the retina can be seen. A potent corollary discharge should eliminate any such perception. Second, this perception of the smear can be eliminated by simply extending the vision beyond the beginning or the end of the eye movement. This is a temporal visual manipulation, and any corollary discharge should be equally active in both the case where the smear is seen and the case where it is not.

They interpret their findings in terms of visual masking, and suggest, as Matin had suggested earlier, (Matin, Clymer, & Matin, 1972; Matin, 1974; see also Breitmeyer & Ganz, 1976) that visual masking may exist primarily to obscure or suppress the smear occurring during saccades.

In the present experiments, the effects of smear and those of masking have been in large degree separated by the introduction of specified amounts of smear under conditions of minimal masking. We see under these conditions that smear alone is important in raising the threshold of vision to stimuli presented either during saccades or during steady fixation. The effects of small amounts of smear alone, however, are not large (see Fig. 9). We would agree with the interpretation that under normal conditions of viewing in a contoured environment, visual masking is a most pronounced source of suppression. Under such conditions, stimulus smear would presumably act in conjunction with backward masking to foster clear vision at the final fixation, by decreasing the duration of stimulation and thus the photochemical effect of stimulation at each receptor, and thus making the smeared stimulus easier to mask.

Under conditions of optimal masking, the effects of a relatively small efferent neural signal may well be lost. In fact, as we have seen, the failure to find compelling evidence for a substantial neural effect under *some* conditions has led a number of investigators to conclude that the notion of a neural effect is unnecessary under *all* conditions. We believe that consideration of other rather different viewing conditions leads to a different interpretation, however.

Evidence for a Centrally Originating Effect

In psychophysical studies of saccadic suppression we are obliged to approach a neural effect "through the back door." If we can essentially eliminate all other probable sources of suppression and still find a residual effect, we suppose that it is neural. Thus the design of experiments that favor the finding of a neural effect is difficult, especially if the magnitude of the effect is not large. A few experiments have taken pains to minimize the effects of such variables as masking and retinal smear. Some of these experiments are conducted in the dark, others at photopic levels in a Ganzfeld.

Vision in the dark. In normal scotopic viewing, dim objects are typically observed against a dim background. Masking effects that depend on a contoured visual field must be minimal. Saccadic suppression that occurs under scotopic conditions cannot therefore be attributed to masking effects that are dependent upon the perception of crisp contours or edges. The variable of stimulus smear on the moving retina may be important in diminishing vision of the smeared stimulus, as described above, if the duration of the stimulus is relatively long. If visual thresholds are raised to very brief flashes presented during saccades in darkness, however, smear, like masking, cannot play a prominent role; suppression observed under these conditions thus presents compelling evidence for neural suppression.

A number of experimenters have investigated saccadic suppression of stimuli presented in darkness (Brooks & Fuchs, 1975; Krauskopf, Graf, & Gaarder, 1966; Latour, 1962, 1966; Richards, 1969; Riggs, Merton, & Morton, 1974; Zuber, Crider, & Stark, 1964; Zuber & Stark, 1966), but a number of the experiments used light fixation marks to direct the eye movements, thus making it impossible to rule out some masking effects. Two recent studies, however, speak directly to this question, those of Brooks and Fuchs (1975) and Riggs et al. (1974).

Brooks and Fuchs (1975) found a nonsignificant elevation of visual threshold of less than .1 log unit to flashes delivered in intervals extending from 100 msec before saccades to 100 msec following them. Saccades were executed over dark backgrounds without fixation points, and thresholds were determined by a yes/ no response to spot stimuli or to diffuse flashes, as described above. These investigators interpret their results as obviating the notion of a neural suppressive effect. Riggs et al. (1974), on the other hand, found a significant loss of visual sensitivity to electrically produced phosphenes during saccades in total darkness, using a forced-choice technique. By psychophysical comparison of phosphene current and real light, these investigators were able to express the amounts of suppression in terms of light, and they reported values of suppression equivalent to .36—.47 log unit of luminance for three subjects. They interpret their results as showing that "a substantial portion of saccadic suppression is neural rather than optical in its origin [p. 997]." As Matin (1974) points out, the differences in magnitude of effect obtained in these two experiments may be attributable to the psychophysical method employed: criterion-free forced-choice methods tend to yield larger values of suppression (Pearce & Porter, 1970). The weight of the evidence seems to us to lead to the view that a small but consistent decrease in sensitivity occurs during saccades in total darkness — a decrease not attributable to the effects of visual masking or optical smear, but rather one which represents a neural suppression.

Vision in a Ganzfeld.   Additional evidence for neural suppression comes from experiments conducted under photopic conditions in which masking effects are minimized by (a) use of a large, homogeneously lighted background, and (b) use of fixation marks that are designed to minimize masking (see, for example, Fig. 1), and in which retinal smear is minimized by presenting the stimuli in very brief flashes. In our earliest work, conducted under conditions approximating these, we found that the threshold for detection of a flash of added brightness superposed on a steady light background was raised by the equivalent of about .5 log unit of relative luminance for the eye executing a 6° saccade as opposed to that for the fixating eye (Volkmann, 1962). We interpreted these and subsequent results as indicating that (a) vision is not "blanked out" during saccades, but that (b) the threefold increase in threshold is substantial enough to mean that stimuli can be chosen such that they are seen almost all of the time with the fixating eye but almost never during a saccade (Volkmann et al. 1968).

The recent work of Brooks and Fuchs (1975) provides additional information on this point. They found that visual thresholds for detection of small stimulus spots flashed during 20° saccades made over a noncontoured background were raised by about .4–.5 log unit. Thresholds for the detection of diffuse full-field flashes under these conditions were raised by about 1.3 log units of luminance. With both conditions of stimulation, they found that the difference between thresholds with the eyes fixating and the eyes saccading increased with increased luminance in the contour-free Ganzfeld. Their additional finding that these effects could be mimicked by displacing the background instead of the eye are difficult to interpret since there should be *no* visual effect of moving a Ganzfeld across the retina.

CONCLUSION

In agreement with earlier results in the luminance domain, our present research shows that contrast sensitivity thresholds exhibit a rise of .3–.5 log unit when low spatial frequency sinusoidal gratings are flashed during saccades in a Ganzfeld, in comparison to the same gratings flashed to the fixating eye.

We interpret the evidence on saccadic suppression to date as indicating that central and retinal factors work together to optimize clear vision in a stable visual world at the end of each saccade.

Under conditions of normal viewing in a lighted, contoured environment, the contribution of visual backward masking may well be most prominent, with factors such as retinal smear and central inhibition working to support the adaptive outcome without playing a major role in it. We would agree with the general interpretation of Matin (1974), Breitmeyer and Ganz (1976), and Campbell and Wurtz (in press) in which masking is said to function to suppress vision during saccades; we would emphasize a slightly different aspect of the interpretation, however, by suggesting that masking has the effect of preparing the system for clear vision at the end of saccades.

Under conditions of decreased contour or contrast (precisely those conditions in which masking is least effective), the small but consistent contribution of central inhibition becomes most significant.

The effects of stimulus smear on the moving retina must vary widely with such parameters as stimulus size, configuration, luminance, and the velocity of the saccade. Nevertheless, it must be the case that whatever smear is present can only decrease the effectiveness of the smeared image on the retinal receptors. Thus, smear must combine with other factors to diminish the total visual effect.

Our present interpretation is based on findings from a number of laboratories over the past 15 years or so, and we think we can all take a certain pride in the recent progress that has been made in the analysis of this very old problem. Additional important results, of which we have not been able to speak here, are coming from the literature on neurophysiology and masking. See, for examples, the papers by Goldberg and Robinson in this volume; Davidson, Fox and Dick (1973), Bridgeman, Hendry, and Stark (1975), Matin (1975), Stevens, Emerson, Gerstein, Kallos, Neufeld, Nichols, and Rosenquist (1976), Vaughan (1973), White (1976).

Questions, of course, remain: What is the precise role of the luminance of a noncontoured background field in raising thresholds during saccades? Have masking effects really been eliminated in experiments in a Ganzfeld? Can the finding of significant saccadic suppression in complete darkness be replicated and extended? What are the roles of other possible variables such as retinal shearing forces? What is the mechanism of the central effect? What is the precise relation between saccadic suppression and other mechanisms for the maintenance of a stable visual world?

It is our opinion that this field has now reached a level of such sophistication that the answers to these and other related questions will come in large part not from experiments that are designed simply to illustrate an effect, but from systematic, painstaking, parametric work in which independent variables are varied under highly controlled conditions, and substantial numbers of judgments are obtained under appropriate psychophysical procedures from unbiased observers.

DISCUSSION

SKAVENSKI: I wonder if you can say, on the curves of your contrast sensitivity, where you got the decrease in threshold — at what retinal slip velocity did you see sensitivity actually increase?

VOLKMANN: Are you referring to our finding that, in the moving eye condition, vision seemed to be slightly better for very small slippage than it was for no slippage at all, insofar as we could produce this?

MOORE: We found the increase in sensitivity specifically while obtaining the tuning functions, and it occurred with about a 10 deg/per sec slippage relative to the saccading eye, but we were doing fairly coarse work. We have interpreted the result as showing slightly better vision with a small amount of slip than with, presumably, no slip at all.

KUNDEL: When you recorded your percentage of correct responses, did that include false positives? One of the things that concerns me whenever I see percentage correct responses is that experimenters haven't adjusted the responses for the decision-making criterion that the person may be using. In other words, with the stimulus moving on the retina the subject may be more uncertain and therefore may change the level of criterion that he's going to use to make the judgment. Did you measure the false positive responses or not?

VOLKMANN: We did use catch trials on occasion but, more important, we used a forced-choice rather than a yes—no type of judgment. The changes in criterion that might lead in a yes—no situation to the subject responding "I saw it," more often or less often generally don't apply in forced-choice situations. In our experiment, the two stimuli being compared are both coming under the same conditions, and the subjects always have to choose one of them as containing the grating. This procedure avoids the problems of criterion shift that may occur in the yes—no type of judgment.

I.4

Neurophysiological Mechanisms Underlying Metacontrast: Implications for the Coordination of Eye Movements and Perception

Leo Ganz
Stanford University

The coordination of vision and eye movements appears to involve masking: the reduction in visual sensitivity to light and to form by another briefly displayed light or pattern.

Masking phenomena have been divided into two classes (Kahneman, 1968). One type is called monotonic, or Type A. Here optimal masking occurs where Mask and Target are presented together, the effect diminishes as the stimulus onset asynchrony (SOA) increases, both in a positive direction (i.e., Mask follows Target) and in a negative direction (i.e., Mask precedes Target). Briefly, monotonic masking occurs where the Mask is a fairly homogeneous field, often much higher in intensity than the Target. The Target and Mask have to be presented to the same eye, that is, the effect is monoptic. Such masking is thought to occur largely at the retina; it is largely attributable to inhibitory interactions at the retina and possibly at the lateral geniculate nucleus (LGN).

Metacontrast, or Type B masking, is strongest when the Mask follows the Target by 60–100 msecs. The time of the peak effect at a substantially positive SOA comprises the defining characteristic of Metacontrast, and is the basis for an interesting theoretical question: Why should maximum interactions occur when effect appears to antedate cause by 100 msecs or more? I believe, the mechanism of Metacontrast involves the interaction of two branches of the visual system with interesting implications extending to the coordination of vision and eye movements. (Documentation, when not specifically cited here, can be found in a number of recent reviews: Alpern, 1953; Breitmeyer & Ganz, 1976; Lefton, 1973; Weisstein, 1972).

First, let us examine those conditions in which Metacontrast masking is obtained. The Target and Mask should be of comparable intensity or contrast and the contour of the Target must be near one of the contours of the Mask. In general, intercontour distance between Target and Mask must be kept small, preferably less than 1−2° to obtain strong Metacontrast masking. Moreover, the contour shapes of the adjoining Target and Mask should be *similar in orientation and form.* Metacontrast masking is obtained equally strongly monoptically and dichoptically; that is, Target and Mask can be presented to different eyes, and the effect is frequently obtained in full strength. The effect probably occurs at the visual cortex and not at the retina or LGN. Another important condition is the retinal position of the Target and Mask, for Metacontrast is best obtained when Target and Mask are not in the fovea.

One of the most interesting aspects of Metacontrast is that it affects only certain tasks, like the estimation of brightness and the recognition of form. Under optimal Metacontrast a letter is rendered totally unrecognizable, but the subject can still report that some stimulus was indeed shown, i.e., the subject's detection is unaffected (Fehrer & Biederman, 1962). Moreover, reaction time to the simple detection of the stimulus is unaffected, because it is equal to what he would have given had no Mask been presented (Fehrer & Raab, 1962). Also, the subject can report the position of the unrecognizable stimulus in a forced choice task. It follows that Metacontrast relates to part of the Two Visual System Hypothesis which separates Ambient Vision, which is concerned with the positions and motions of objects, from Focal Vision, which is concerned with the recognition of patterns. This dichotomy was already apparent to Max Wertheimer, following observations made during his classic stroboscopic illusion experiments. If two letters are presented successively at slightly different positions in space and at an asynchrony of about 100 msecs, subjects report a very powerful illusion of motion from the first stimulus to the second, although the first stimulus is frequently unrecognizable. Wertheimer called this "Optimal-Phi." In other words, Metacontrast is present during powerful motion perceptions when the shape of the first stimulus is unseen. In fact, the temporal properties of Metacontrast and the Stroboscopic Motion Illusion are strikingly similar.

NEUROPHYSIOLOGY OF PATTERN PERCEPTION

Organization of the Visual Pathways

There are two organizational features of the visual system that play a prominent role in its functioning. One involves antagonistic excitatory and inhibitory processes, and the other involves the hierarchical organization of the visual pathway.

At the retinal level of organization, the receptive fields of ganglion cells are characterized by circularly symmetric, antagonistically organized regions (Küffler, 1953). "On-center" cells have circular receptive field centers, which at light onset yield an increase in firing rate. The annular surround region yields an antagonistic effect, that is, a decrease in firing rate at light onset. "Off-center" cells are similarly organized. Space limitations prevent our discussing the finer details of LGN contribution to the hierarchical organization here. Cortical simple-cell receptive fields are characterized by two important features that differentiate them from subcortical receptive fields: (1) their antagonistic center-surround regions lie along an elongated axis with a particular orientation, and (b) in a cat, for the most part, they receive input from both eyes (Hubel & Wiesel, 1962). In a monkey there is a monocular stage converging on a binocular one at a subsequent level in the hierarchy (Hubel & Wiesel, 1968).

Transient and Sustained Visual Channels

To understand Metacontrast and other masking phenomena, one must appreciate the ways in which spatial and temporal resolutions interact. In this section I will describe low and high spatial frequency channels. The first term refers to neural elements in the visual system that are more sensitive to larger, homogeneous stimuli, but have low resolution for spatial detail; the second to high spatial frequency channels, that are more sensitive to small, discrete stimuli and are capable of high resolution. Recent psychophysical studies have shown that low spatial-frequency channels are particularly sensitive to transient stimulation produced by rapid motion and flicker (Breitmeyer, 1973; Breitmeyer & Julcsz, 1975; Keesey, 1972; Kulikowski & Tolhurst, 1973; Pantle, 1970; Tolhurst, 1973). Conversely, high spatial frequency channels seem more sensitive to slowly moving or stationary stimuli.

Kulikowski and Tolhurst (1973) showed subjects a grating of medium width (10 cycles/deg) that flickered in counterphase, that is, the bright and dark bands alternated. At high rates of flicker, when contrast was near threshold, the spatial properties of the grating were no longer visible, but the flicker was still evident. Conversely, very fine gratings were not visible at high flicker rates. These results suggest that form analyzers have a lower temporal resolution than do flicker detectors.

Another interpretation is that form detectors have a longer integration time than flicker detectors. It is as though our visual system were comprised of two types of channels: form detectors (along with stero-depth detectors), comprised of elements that integrate visual excitation over a long time, and transient or flicker detectors that integrate visual excitation over a comparatively short time. For instance, Kahneman (1964; Kahneman & Norman, 1964) found that the maximum duration or the *critical duration,* for Bloch's Law of time-intensity reciprocity was approximately 100 msec; however, for letter identification, or acuity tasks, the critical duration can range from 200–350 msecs. Also, Schober and Hilz (1965) have demonstrated that the detectability of fine square wave gratings benefits more from long exposure durations than the detectability of broad square wave gratings. Recently, Breitmeyer and Ganz (1977) have demonstrated that the critical duration increases from approximately 50 to 200 msec as the spatial frequency of a sinusoidal test grating increases from .5 to 16 cycles/deg.

Not only do the high resolution channels have a longer integration time, they also have a longer latency. Breitmeyer (1975) showed that the simple reaction time to sinusoidal gratings increased by 40—80 msec over spatial frequency ranging from .5 to 11.0 cycles/deg, even when the gratings were matched for subjective contrast. In other words, low resolution — low spatial frequency channels respond faster by several tens of msecs than high spatial frequency — high resolution channels.

All of these psychophysical responses have their neurophysiological correlates, as shown by single-cell studies of the mammalian visual system. Enroth-Cugell and Robson (1966) originally showed that a class of cat retinal ganglion cells, which they called Y cells, signal only the abrupt (transient) onsets and offsets of a grating, while another class, X cells, signalled the continued (sustained) presence of the stimulus. Moreover, the X cells responded much more linearly.

When the properties (Cleland, Dubin & Levick, 1971) of transient and sustained cells are compared, the functional aspects of this dichotomy become clear. Transient cells show more sensitivity to large patterns (low spatial frequencies), are not sensitive to retinal blur, and are very responsive to high frequency flicker or rapid motion. Sustained cells, on the other hand, respond better to small objects, high spatial frequencies, sharply focussed images, and to objects presented for long periods of time or at low temporal rates or low velocities. The X cells are found in highest proportions at the fovea (area centralis in the cat), and the Y cells are in higher proportions at the more peripheral regions of the retina. Both cell types are found at the retina, LGN, and visual cortex. Moreover, it has been shown that the dichotomies are maintained in the projections onto the visual cortex. Sustained retinal neurons project only to sustained LGN neurons, which in turn project onto sustained striate neurons, and similarly for transient cells. Therefore, the sustained-transient dichotomy is relayed in parallel channels from the retina, through the LGN to the visual cortex. The transient neurons, however, bifurcate and also project onto the superior colliculus.

Among retinal ganglion cells (Cleland, Levick, & Sanderson, 1973) the transient neuron has a shorter latency, reaches its peak response sooner, and decays more quickly than a sustained-response neuron.

These differences have been particularly well illustrated in neurons found in the monkey striate cortex (Dow, 1974), a structure very similar to the human visual cortex. Sustained-response cells responded in a sustained manner to stationary stimuli of proper orientation and dimension. Transient cells, on the other hand, responded to the onsets and offsets of the stimuli and were sensitive to rapid motion. The latter also had direction and orientation selectivity, though not as precisely as the sustained cells. Moreover, the response latencies of transient cells were on the order of 50 msec, whereas those of sustained cells were on the order of 100 msec and more.

One more fact is essential before we can proceed to an explanation of Meta-contrast: transient neurons inhibit sustained neurons at numerous locations within the visual system. That inhibition is substantially faster than the excitatory response of the sustained cells (Singer & Creutzfeldt, 1970).

THE MECHANISM OF METACONTRAST MASKING

Metacontrast Masking is an instance of interchannel inhibition (Breitmeyer & Ganz, 1976) involving the inhibition of sustained neurons by transient neurons. Consider a typical Metacontrast paradigm: a black Target letter is shown briefly and after 60–80 msecs is followed by adjoining black Mask contours, also briefly presented. The subject reports seeing something and can report its position, but cannot identify the stimulus and reports its contrast to be low. What happens, I believe, is that the Target letter elicits two processes, a transient one and a sustained one. The transient process is too fast to be masked by the Mask, and it proceeds, in part, to the superior colliculus, allowing the subject to report only the presence and position of the Target. Also, as in Feher's and Raab's experiment, subjects respond as quickly as if no Mask had been shown. The Target letter also initiates sustained neuron activity in the visual cortex, but this takes considerably more time. Meanwhile, the Mask is initiating fast, transient activity at the retina which reaches the visual cortex at the same time as the sustained activity initiated by the Target letter, and proceeds to mask that target letter with inhibitory processes generated at the visual cortex by the Mask's transient neurons. Moreover, because inhibition is always prolonged in cortical neurons, the Target's sustained neurons are inhibited for a substantial amount of time (a few hundred msecs), and this prevents the subject from recognizing the letter. The paradoxical, apparently retroactive, action of Metacontrast is thus explained; the processes are in fact interacting simultaneously at the Visual Cortex, even though the Mask is presented 60–100 msecs later. Several other aspects of Metacontrast masking are explained:

1. The fact that this masking is sensitive to the contour-orientation-similarity of Target and Mask is attributible entirely to the contour sensitive aspect of cortical inhibition, as demonstrated by Blakemore and Tobin (1972);

2. Metacontrast is dichoptic because, in humans, cortical neurons, at one stage beyond layer IV of the Visual Cortex, are indeed binocular;

3. Disinhibition can be obtained because the inhibition, itself prolonged in duration, can itself be inhibited by surrounding neurons. This aspect of the model remains to be worked out in detail, however;

4. Since transient neurons respond to black-on-grey stimuli as well as white-on-grey, we would predict that the contrast relationship of the Mask is not crucial, and indeed this is what Growney (1976) has found;

5. If the spatial frequencies of the Mask and Target are controlled, our model would predict that somewhat lower spatial frequencies would be effective for the Mask, relative to the Target. White and Lorber (1976) recently reported this in one of their experiments.

6. The fact that subjects report excellent stroboscopic movement between two successively presented stimuli at the same asynchrony at which the first is strongly masked is readily explained by a two channel model, since motion and form recognition are thought to be carried by different channels, motion by the transients and form by the sustained, to oversimplify a bit. Kolers (1972) has also concluded that these two aspects of perception, form and motion, are easily dissociated. The sustained-transient dichotomy addresses itself to this dissociation.

7. Similarly, the fact that the subject's reaction time to the Target stimulus is unaffected when its identity is masked is readily understood, since detection and position information are carried by the transient channels, either to Visual Cortex, or to Superior Colliculus.

Thus, the model explains the bulk of the Metacontrast phenomenon in a parsimonious manner.

A number of cognitive psychologists, among them Sperling, Haber, and Turvey (see Breitmeyer & Ganz, 1976, for references) have been impressed by the fact that Metacontrast Masking displays a very constant SOA maximum, under a wide variety of stimulus conditions, specifically a maximum at 60–100 msecs between Target and Mask. They conclude that this constant time is the duration needed to process iconic information before transferring it to its non-iconic code. We are convinced this is entirely fallacious. The maximum occurs at 60–100 msecs, we believe, entirely because this represents the retino-cortical latency difference between transient and sustained channels.

IMPLICATIONS OF THE SUSTAINED-TRANSIENT DICHOTOMY FOR SACCADIC SUPPRESSION

Whether reading or actively searching a visual scene, we observe the world by alternating periods of fixation of approximately 250 msecs with saccades lasting approximately 20–50 msecs, depending on the length of the traverse The reduction in visual sensitivity during the saccade, i.e., saccadic suppression, is known to start some 50 msecs before the beginning of the actual eye rotation, to continue during the saccade, and to outlast the saccade by 50 msecs after the eyes have reached their destination (e.g., Volkmann, 1962; Volkmann, Schick, & Riggs, 1968; for a review of saccadic suppression, see Matin, 1974). Matin (1974) distinguishes several causal components: (a) smearing of the retinal image during the rapid movement, (b) an afferent component attributed to backward masking, and (c) an efferent component, central inhibition, which is related to corollary discharges originating from the mother command (von Holst & Mittelstaedt, 1950).

MacKay (1970) has provided psychophysical evidence for the afferent component. A subject views a steady fixation point in order to eliminate corollary discharges from eye movement commands. The presentation of a Target is coupled with the rapid movement of a contoured field, resulting in a substantial reduction in sensitivity to the Target, beginning about 50 msec before the movement and lasting about 100 msec after the termination of the movement. Correlated suppression effects have been recorded in the lateral geniculate nucleus of the cat using macroelectrode techniques (Jeannerod & Chouvet, 1973). The neurophysiological suppression also begins some 50 msec before the displacement and extends some 100 msec after the eye movement has terminated. We attribute this component specifically to metacontrast initiated by the stimulation of transient channels at the beginning and at the end of the saccade (see also Matin, 1974). In light of our model, it is easy to see how the transient stimulation produced by the rapid movement of the retina during the saccade could generate inhibition of sustained channels which, as in metacontrast, would begin about 50 msecs prior to the saccade and last some 100 msecs or more after the saccade is completed.

I have described the long integration time of sustained channels and, more particularly, the increase in integration time in channels sensitive to high spatial frequencies (viz., channels mediating high spatial resolution). If sustained response channels integrate for 300—400 msecs or more, and if a saccade lasts only 20—50 msecs, then these channels will integrate visual stimulation across pairs of fixation. The channels that have been activated on Fixation 1 can continue to be activated on Fixation 2, and vice versa. It is also possible that the last 100 msec of a prior fixation interval could interfere, through integration, with the first 100 msec of the following fixation interval; this interference is called *proactive inhibition.* This interference would increase in severity as the spatial resolution demands of the task increased, since higher spatial frequencies are associated with longer integration times. Metacontrast acts to reduce this proactive effect by retrograde suppression.

However, the operation of this mechanism exacts a price — it requires that interfixation intervals not be too short. Tinker (1958) notes that under luminance conditions in which a 100-msec stimulus presentation results in a clear percept, 200-msec intersaccade fixation intervals are required to attain a clear percept from equivalent stimuli. The explanation of this effect is easily derived from the Breitmeyer-Ganz model of Metacontrast. During any fixation of high resolution material, an additional 100 msec is required at the end of the fixation to provide a temporal buffer for protection from the effects of a subsequent fixation. The buffer must attenuate the retrograde suppression of the pattern, processing in sustained channels activated during the initial 100 msecs. Thus, metacontrast sets a lower limit on intersaccade interval which is dependent on the spatial resolution requirements of the task and should increase as finer discriminations are required.

Evidence for a pure efferent component derives from a recent psychophysical experiment by Riggs, Merton, and Morton (1974). They showed that, in complete darkness, electrically induced visual phosphenes were suppressed during saccades. The degree of suppression was only about 0.15 log units contrasting with estimates of 0.5 log units or more obtained during saccades in a lighted structured environment (Volkmann, 1962) presumably involving summation of both afferent and efferent components. Recent neurophysiological recordings (Duffy & Burchfiel, 1975), from single neurons in monkey striate cortex, have also shown suppressive effects during saccades performed in total darkness. The Transient-Sustained Interchannel Inhibition Model of Metacontrast described here suggests that the afferent and efferent components of saccadic suppression are synchronized in a surprisingly elegant manner.

Part **II**

METHODS AND MODELS

II.1

Semiautomatic Eye Movement Data Analysis Techniques for Experiments with Varying Scenes

David Sheena
Gulf & Western Applied Science Laboratories

Barbara N. Flagg
Harvard University

INTRODUCTION

Although automatic eye movement data processing is straightforward for simple target tracking and reasonably easy for scan studies of fixed scenes, it constitutes a problem when the scene is continually changing, as in a TV presentation, an aircraft, a flight simulator, or an automobile. We have addressed this problem with the development of a semi-automatic digitizer system, which is used to manually track the x—y coordinates of those objects of particular interest in a changing TV or film sequence. When combined with digitized eye movement records, the system provides a record of eye fixation relative to these particular picture elements.

Most eye movement experiments may be categorized according to the role played by the scene presented to the subjects as: (1) static scenes such as slides, or (2) dynamic scenes like TV presentations, simulator displays, or the real world as viewed by a driver, a pilot, or a mobile subject operating some machinery or performing some task.

STATIC SCENE ANALYSIS

To answer most research questions posed in this category, it is necessary to relate the patterns of eye fixations to what was displayed before the subject at a particular time. We must know the history of what was viewed by the subject and be able to describe the stimulus in some form easily related to the eye movement data.

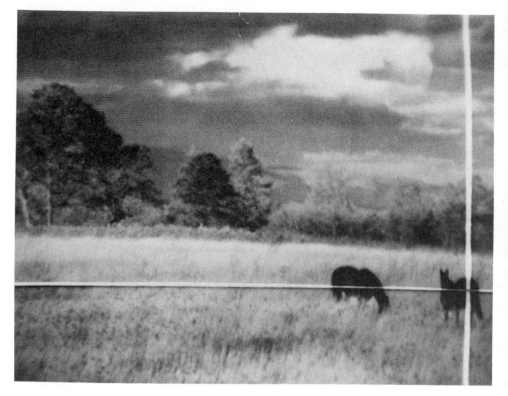

FIG. 1.   Positioning of crosshairs over a scene to obtain coordinates.

Analytic description of simple or constant scenes is obviously much easier than description of a continuously varying scene. It is straightforward if there is a computer or a signal generator that produces the display or drives a spot on a CRT monitor, or if the scene is some regularly moving object like a pendulum. In the case where the scene is a general static pictorial presentation, it becomes necessary to break it down into a number of elements. These elements might be uniform squares throughout the scene or coordinates of relevant parts of the scene. A common method of analysis is to use rectangles to cover nonblank parts of the scene in some logical fashion, and to define the scene with the coordinates of the corners or diagonals of these rectangles.

Figure 1 shows one technique for acquiring the coordinates. Crosshairs, which usually represent eye position, are artifically placed at the various points of interest, and the coordinates generated by the instrument representing that particular point are recorded for all the required elements.

VARYING SCENE ANALYSIS

This category of experiments is obviously the least amenable to quantitative or automatic analysis. Precise and automatic recording of eye position exists to relate, independently of head motion, points of fixation to the scene in any of a number of convenient formats. Nonetheless, if the scene is describable only in verbal and not in mathematical terms, analysis must be manual. Consequently, the experimenter must normally go over the data, which are usually recorded on videotape, on a field by field basis, and score and record the information by hand. Most people involved in this area are all too familiar with studies in which hours of work are necessary to reduce minutes or even seconds of actual data. This procedure is very prone to the introduction of human error, and if more than one person reduces the data, individual differences are a further confounding variable.

The problem is to devise a method that automatically provides a machine-readable quantification of the continuous visual scene information as well as quantification of the eye fixation position coordinates. In most practical experiments, the investigator is satisfied to relate the points of fixation to a limited and reasonable number of elements in the scene, thereby producing sufficient data to address particular experimental questions. While driving, for example, such elements might be the center of the road, the other vehicles in the scene, traffic lights, and road signs. In the case of operating equipment or machinery, the limited number of elements might be the various controls, the subject's own hands, or his tools. These will usually add up to a manageable, practical total number of scene elements. The analysis problem is, of course, that their positions or the positions of their outlines, vary from one instant of time to the next. One solution is to transduce the positions of these parts of the scene into numerical values in a way analogous to the transduction of eye geometry into fixation points.

GRAPHIC—TO—DIGITAL CONVERTERS

The conversion of a point in x—y space to numerical coordinates is feasible in any number of ways at the present time. Examples are light pens, standing wave devices, and resistive pads. Figure 2 shows our application of one such transducer, an acoustic position digitizer. Two microphone bars extend along the vertical and horizontal edges of the scene, and a stylus is placed over a point in that scene. The stylus generates an acoustical pulse which is sensed by the two microphone bars. The first instant of reception by the microphones fixes the time of transit from the stylus point to these edges. The computed times are directly proportional to the distances from the point in question to the two

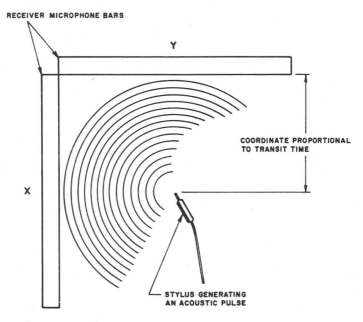

FIG. 2.   Acoustic position digitizer.

edges. This, then, determines the x–y coordinates of the actual position of the stylus point.

The rationale for the choice of an acoustic digitizer, as opposed to the other available transducers, is that such a device is most suited to the particular application. Light pens usually function with specific TV rasters and are tied to such systems, making them somewhat inflexible. They are certainly unusable for motion picture film, and might lead to problems with videotape sync because of the latter's instability. The acoustic transducer does not have this limitation.

The device used must also have a clear aperture for viewing a TV monitor; this clearly is obviously not the case with any transducer that requires some opaque base like a resistive pad. Our device has a resolution of 0.1 mm and an accuracy of 0.1%. This is generally more than is required by eye movement experiments and is certainly superior to the measurement capabilities of most eye movement devices. The only factor that may affect the accuracy of such a digitizer is a change in the speed of sound through air in the experimental environment, and this is sufficiently constant for most indoor conditions.

The digitizer may be operated in a manual mode so that it provides a pair of coordinates any time it is actuated by a foot switch or by a depression of the stylus, or it can provide information in a "line mode" yielding a set of coordinates at a preset rate. It may also be driven by an external signal such as a television sync pulse. The maximum data rate of this device is 140 samples/sec, a rate greater than real time television scan rate.

By its very nature, this is an extremely linear device with negligible cross coupling, since the microphones, as shown in Fig. 2, will respond to the first arrival of the radiating pulse from the point of the stylus. Ambient noise can be a problem if it confounds the microphone, and some television monitors were found to issue high pitched sounds that did interfere with the performance of the digitizer. In any case acoustic shielding procedures were sufficient to solve the problem.

SCENE DATA RECORDING

With the use of the acoustic x–y digitizer, the recording of scene element positions has been reduced to the placement of the stylus or pointer on an element as the element moves continuously with time, or as the scene frames advance one by one.

The output most often available from an eye movement instrument is a videotape or film, resembling that shown in Fig. 1, which presents the scene at an instant of time with a marker indicating the fixation point.

To reduce the elements of a scene to data, the experimenter runs through the videotape sequence at actual or reduced speed, once for each elements, and tracks the appropriate point of each videotape field with the stylus. The control system records these x–y coordinates, along with time information from a timer or a frame count, onto digital tape.

If the elements move too fast in real time for the operator to follow them with a stylus, they may be slowed down. When all elements have been recorded, the eye fixation position itself, usually available as a superimposed marker, may be treated like any other element and tracked with the same stylus for the duration of the experimental sequence. This last procedure is, of course, necessary only if the eye position is not available in quantitative form.

OVERALL DATA RECORDING SYSTEM AND ANALYSIS

The overall control system for producing the necessary recording is shown in Fig. 3. Here acoustic information from the digitizer microphones is converted into position data, x and y coordinates, by the digitizer computer. Timing information can be read from any number of sources; here it comes from a frame count reader that reads a frame number coded onto the videotape. This frame code may be on an audio channel or in the sync interval between the videotape fields. This frame count and the x–y output are fed into the digital tape recorder controller and formatter. The timer assures that all components of the system work synchronously. The controller and formatter format this information, along with manually entered data which denotes the element number, subject number, and other experimental information, and writes them on digital tape.

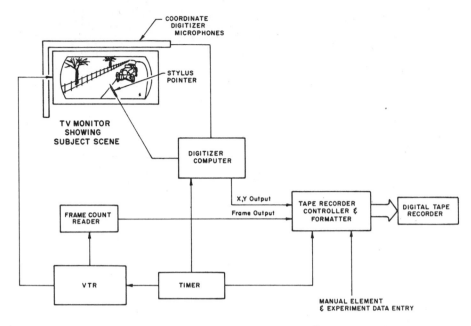

FIG. 3.   Overall scene digitizing and recording system.

Once the entire tape segment has ended, the codes on the controller and formatter are manually incremented to the next element number and the process
is repeated. After completion of all elements of the scene, the procedure is repeated for the eye position marker if that information is not available as an
electronic signal.

The resultant data on tape will appear in a format like this:

$$E1, x, y, T1/E1, x, y \; T2/ \; \ldots \; E1, x, y, Tn/E2, x, y, T1/\ldots$$

where E is the element number and x and y are the coordinates at time Ti. The
slashes delimit individual samples.

The eye movement information recorded on digital tape is now ready for
computer analysis. The programmer will have to specify the data processing
algorithms to obtain results of interest to him. In other words, he will have to
program the computer to tell what percentage of the time the driver, for example, is looking at the center of the road, or in what order the driver looks
at road signs and traffic signals.

We may still be quite far away from completely eliminating manual interaction and judgment, but our technique makes practical many experiments which
would otherwise be prohibitively difficult and time consuming. It requires little
subjective judgment, no manual scoring, reading of scales, or recording of numbers. It is also clearly less prone to all the errors such manual data reduction can
produce.

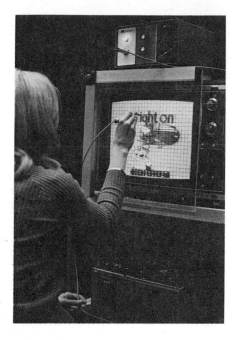

FIG. 4. Acoustic digitizer mounted for encoding of television image.

APPLICATION EXAMPLE

The Center for Research in Children's Television at Harvard University has developed an eye movement recording facility to study child and adult moment-to-moment visual response to television presentations. The information gained from eye movement recording has a direct impact on the production of children's television via our close association with the Children's Television Workshop (Flagg, Allen, Geer, & Scinto, 1976). In addition to our applied interests, our research deals with the basic psychological problems of information processing of dynamic displays by children and adults.

To record eye movements, we employ a Gulf & Western Applied Science Laboratories Monitor System[1] modified for use with television. The system produces a videotape of the scene with moving superimposed crosshairs on the scene showing the point of regard and a digital tape of the x–y coordinates of the crosshairs' intersection sampled every 30th of a second. Offline, the digital information is processed and edited into actual fixation coordinates.

One of the major problems we faced in developing the recording facility was that of relating the fixation coordinates to the visual scene that appeared on the TV screen at a particular time. For example, if we show a segment from *Sesame Street,* we may want to know how many subjects fixated a particular

---

[1]Formerly known as a Whittaker Eye View Monitor System.

target area (person, object, word, number, etc.) at different times during the segment. Previous methods of correlating the fixation patterns with the visual image have involved *static* presentations rather than *dynamic* images, which change thirty times a second. Applying these methods to each frame at thirty frames a second quickly mounts up to an astronomical and unacceptable amount of work.

Since our eye fixation data are easily handled by computer, the solution was a method that could quickly encode a limited amount of visual information appearing on the screen into a computer readable form. Ideally, this process should take place in a highly interactive computer graphic environment. However, our hardware was limited to a digital tape recorder.

The machine that allowed us to semiautomatically encode the video information was a Science Accessories Corporation acoustic digitizer. Figure 4 shows the digitizer microphones at the edges of a clear acrylic tablet mounted on a 17-inch TV monitor. The SAC controller is on top and displays the x—y coordinates of the stylus held by the operator. The television image is received from a Sony Model 3130 videotape recorder which provides slow-motion and still-frame capabilities. The still-frame image in Fig. 4 is from *The Electric Company:* the numbers at the bottom of the screen indicate the frame-code — hour 99, minute 32, second 11, frame 27. This frame-code matches a code on the digital eye fixation tape and permits an exact time correlation between the eye position coordinates and the digitized visual target areas.

We are presently investigating several encoding schemes. One simple scheme is shown in Fig. 4 and requires the touching of the stylus to each and every grid cell that covers a particular visual target area (e.g., "right" or "on" or, if desired, each letter individually).

By assigning specific meanings — alphanumeric characters, programming commands, element descriptors — to specific grid cells below the actual TV screen area, we can enter onto the digital tape more information than the target grid areas alone. For example, a grid "menu" for *The Electric Company* might look like this:

CLL	CLC	FCB	FCE						
0	1	2	3	4	5	6	7	8	9
CG	p	Mup	A	C	TG	S	Wd	Mor	L/N
OG									

where CLL and CLC are editing codes for Clear Line and Clear Character; FCB and FCE mark the beginning and ending of Frame-Code numbers entered with the alphanumeric symbols; CG stands for Character Group, of which P is a Person, Mup is a Muppet, A is an Animal, and C is a Cartoon character; TG stands for Text Group, of which S is a Sentence, Wd a word, M or a Morpheme, and L/N a letter or number; OG indicates a target area that is part of an Object Group.

In application, if we wanted to encode the words "right on" from *The Electric Company* show, the stylus coordinate data on the digital tape might appear in the following format:

FCB, 1, 00 32 11 27, TG, Wd, 1, grid cell coordinates for the word "right", TG, Wd, 2, grid cell coordinates for the word "on"/

The operator then advances the videotape frame-by-frame until the words change position or disappear from the screen, at which point the ending frame code is entered for target area "1":

FCE, 1, 00 32 13 08/

It is not necessary to enter the frame-code manually, since a frame-code reader automatically reads the frame-code off the audio track of the videotape and translates it into binary form for the digital tape recorder.

The use of the acoustic digitizer is certainly not limited to this encoding scheme. For example, it is possible to set the stylus on "LINE MODE" so that when activated, it outputs x–y coordinates at a continuous preset rate. One can then quickly outline target areas of interest or follow targets on a display shown at normal or slow motion speeds. Interactive computer equipment facilitates this kind of digitizing procedure by providing the operator with real time visual feedback of elements being acquired.

The complete scene transducer system allows the production, semiautomatically, of a digital tape consisting of the x–y coordinates of points representing visual elements in the television picture. With this information, we can now take the final step of performing a linked interrogation of the eye position and target area data sets to answer our visual scanning research questions.

DISCUSSION

RUSSO: The efficiency of the system you have just illustrated depends heavily on uniformity across frames, that is, the scene changes slowly enough that a particular letter or point of interest can be coded and then kept there for a fairly long sequence of frames. Suppose you wanted to follow eye movements on a very fast moving scene, for example, a violent interchange between two people, wouldn't it take a fair amount of time to break down an entire scene into various interesting areas and do a frame-by-frame decoding analysis?

FLAGG: Yes. Usually the areas of interest in educational television shows such as *Sesame Street* and *The Electric Company* do not change position quickly, and these are the stimuli that we deal with most of the time. Nevertheless, even with complicated scenes, the technique works, although it is tedious. In comparison with the usual hand-scoring procedure, the digitizing technique is still more efficient in the case of a complex scene because you only have to go through the stimulus *once* for however many subjects there are, rather than once for *each* subject.

SHEENA: There's another thing you can do for a complicated scene. Instead of progressing frame by frame, you can go at quarter speed or fifth speed or half speed, depending on what's going on and on the speed at which you can accurately track the elements. You can synchronize the entry of the data automatically, so the speed does not matter. Obviously, it will take you 10 to 20 times the real-time run, but it's still reasonable. The digitizer can operate up to 140 coordinates per second so the machine itself is not the limiting factor.

ROTHKOPF: Could you give me an illustration of some practical use that you put this to? What kind of things do you examine with eye movement recording and what do you do with your findings?

FLAGG: In effect, we do two kinds of research. First, we are involved in basic testing of hypotheses about visual information processing of the television medium. Second, we perform formative research studies for the Children's Television Workshop, which means that we provide feedback to the producers relevant to the actual program design of *Sesame Street* and *The Electric Company*. Producers rely on their intuition to guide their productions, usually without viewer feedback. We try, with our eye movement data, to provide precise information about viewers' attention and comprehension of program segments. The producers can then manipulate properties of the television display to improve both the educational and entertainment qualities of the show. For example, if we want poor readers to learn from *The Electric Company* program, what is the best way to attract attention to print material? Where do you put a letter or a word on the screen? How long do you keep it on? How large should it be? How much distracting material can be present? Should the letter/word be static or move? And, finally, how do all these variables interact with each other in drawing the poor reader's visual attention?

WALLER: I would suggest that you consider using computer-generated letters and mix them with your ordinary video raster scene. With the computer-generated image you always know where each part of the scene is, because it's stored in the computer. It would speed up your analysis process by taking the man out of the loop and making this a wholly automated process.

SHEENA: What you're saying is very true and that's obviously a very practical thing to do, but it's a question of whether the tail wags the dog or the dog wags the tail. Until they make *Sesame Street* by computer, the visual coding process will have to be done somewhat in the manner which we have described. Similarly, if we were dealing with real driving as the problem, we wouldn't have the choice of computer-generated stimuli.

SIMMONS: How do you deal with the problem of the viewer's looking at one object when another object is at the same location on the screen?

FLAGG: That is a problem we haven't solved yet. The real question is how do you decide which of the elements the viewer is looking at — the foreground or the background object. If the scene shows Cookie Monster behind the letter F, it is easy enough to encode the outside area as Cookie Monster and the inside overlapping area as the letter F. However, it's the interpretation of which element the eye is focusing on that we have difficulty with. Unless I can trust my four-year-old to say that she was looking at Cookie Monster or the F, then I don't really have the answer.

SIMMONS: I sort of hoped you did have the answer. I work with visual performance in helicopters and we have continually changing scenes. Unfortunately, right now the only method we have of scoring is simply to sit down with a keyboard of 13 keys and prescore the film, dividing it into 12 major areas plus "all other." If the percentage in area 13 is low, then obviously we've gotten the main part of the material looked at. We can do this at no more than one quarter real-time, so I was looking for a more automated system that would be faster than that.

ROSEN: I was wondering why you have the scorer marking off each successive square. Couldn't you just have the scorer outline the area?

FLAGG: Yes, we could. As I have said, this scheme is just one of many that could be used. We thought of using a number of different area shapes; squares were handy for computer programming. We could also just digitize two points for each of the corners of a rectangular area. Other digitizing schemes are certainly possible and in many cases others are more appropriate.

II.2

Dynamic Interactions in Binocular Vision

Michael R. Clark
Hewitt D. Crane
Stanford Research Institute

INTRODUCTION

Although there is a voluminous literature reporting the responses of the versional and vergence systems and a lesser one touching on accommodation, very few researchers have been able to monitor the responses of these systems simultaneously in both eyes (Campbell, 1960; Goodwin & Fender, 1973; St. Cyr & Fender, 1969, a, b, c) and none reported the state of accommodation and eye position simultaneously during eye movements. Because of inadequate instrumentation most conclusions about the interactions of accommodation and eye movements have been reached solely by inference. Recently, we have developed a vision facility capable of stimulating and monitoring both eye position and accomodation simultaneously in both eyes.

EYE MONITORING FACILITY

The monitoring of horizontal and vertical eye position is achieved by tracking the first and fourth Purkinje images with a closed-loop electro-optical servosystem (Cornsweet & Crane, 1973). The first Purkinje image is the image reflected from the frontal surface of the cornea. The fourth Purkinje image is produced from the very dim reflection from the back surface of the eye lens. The change in separation of the first and fourth Purkinje images gives a measure of true horizontal and

---

[1]This work was supported by NIH Grant No. EY 01031, from the Department of Health, Education, and Welfare.

vertical eye rotation without the usual translation artifact that seriously limits the accuracy of corneal or limbus eyetrackers. This method requires no attachment to the eye and operates invisibly in the infrared. It has a resolution, noise level, and repeatability of about 1 min/arc rms and a bandwidth of 300 Hz. The instrument can track eye movements over a field 25 deg in diameter. The measurement of accommodation is accomplished with an optometer (Cornsweet & Crane, 1970) which also operates in the infrared and utilizes a modified Scheiner principle. It has a resolution of about 0.1 diopter over a 20-diopter range.

These two instruments, the eyetracker and the optometer, are integrated in such a way that the optometer views a partially stabilized eye by using the servo-tracking of the first Purkinje image. It is this technique (Crane & Steele, 1978) that allows the optometer to operate in the presence of large eye movements.

Two eyetracker—optometer instruments, one for each eye, are used in the binocular visual monitoring system. This monitoring facility has been combined with a binocular three-dimensional visual stimulator (Crane & Clark, 1978), that is capable of moving an arbitrary visual field (25° in diameter) ±5 unit 12° horizontally and vertically while varying the apparent distance of the target from beyond infinity to 6 cm without changing its size or brightness. The stimulator has a bandwidth of 200 Hz for horizontal and vertical movement, and a

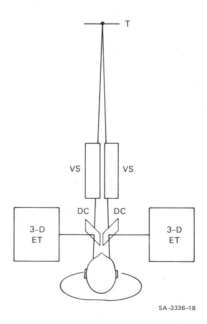

SA-3336-18

FIG. 1.   Subject configuration for stimulating and recording three-dimensional eye movements: 3D-ET, three dimensional eye-tracker, which includes dichroic mirror DC; VS, 3-D visual stimulator; T, target.

slewing rate of 40 diopter/sec for changes in distance. Figure 1 depicts the binocular visual monitoring facility.

SEPARATE MEASUREMENT OF THE TRANSLATIONAL
AND ROTATIONAL MOTIONS OF THE EYE

Corneal and limbus eyetrackers can record very small eye movements, but they cannot separate translational from rotational components. An eye rotation of 1° results in approximately 0.1-mm (100-μm) lateral shift of the corneal image. An eye translation motion of the same magnitude therefore causes a 1° artifact signal in the eye rotation record from a corneal reflection or limbus eyetracker. However, the effects of eye translation on image location on the retina are drastically different than the effects of eye rotation.

The double-Purkinje-image eyetracker eliminates the translation artifact from the eye rotation measurement. It is based on the use of a pair of reflections from optical surfaces of the eye. These reflections move by the same amout with eye translation but differentially with eye rotation. By monitoring the spatial separation of these two images (henceforth called double Purkinje measurement) eye rotation is measured accurately independently of translation. Similarly, eye translation can be measured accurately independently of eye rotation.

Figure 2 shows the horizontal motion of the eye while fixating a target. The top record is the horizontal motion of the first Purkinje (i.e., corneal) image alone. The bottom record is the horizontal rotation derived from the double Purkinje measurement. Note that the first Purkinje record has a wandering baseline, typical of corneal (or limbus) eyetrackers, which results from translation-induced errors.

For the record of Fig. 2, a tight-fitting dental plate (biteboard) was used. During Period A the subject was asked to lean to the left in the biteboard, and during Period B to lean to the right. Note that the lower record is immune to such movement, although the upper record shows an output variation of almost ± 2 degrees, indicating a movement of the head with respect to the biteboard of approximately ± 0.2 mm. During Period D the subject's head was translated approximately 0.3 mm to the left (with respect to the instrument) and then returned to its original position. Note the 3° output variation in the upper record and again the stability of the lower record. During Periods C and E the subject made voluntary eye movements of 5° amplitude, indicating the ability of both systems to record actual rotation movements of the eye.

Figure 2 indicates the difference, then, between sensitivity and accuracy. A corneal, or limbus, tracker can detect very small eye movements, but its accuracy, or repeatability, cannot be better than the eye movement effects induced by any translation movements of the eye relative to the recording instru-

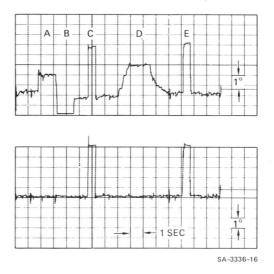

SA-3336-16

FIG. 2.   Upper: horizontal eye movements recorded from first Purkinje image output while the subject fixates a target at infinity. Lower: simultaneous record from the double Purkinje image output. The upper track shows the wandering baseline, typical of corneal image trackers. During Periods A and B, the subject leaned first one way and then the other way in the biteboard. During Period D, the biteboard was translated laterally by ≈ 0.3 mm, and then returned to its original position. Note the stability of the lower record during each of these intervals. During Intervals C and E, the subject made voluntary eye movements of 5°.

ment. We have recorded drifts, that is, artifacts, of 1 −2° during a recording span of less than 1 min, even with the head held rigidly by a tight-fitting dental-impression plate with the extra support of a forehead reset. In this case, translation-induced effects must be principally attributable to movements of the eye within its socket.

The usefulness of the double-Purkinje tracker in detecting translation movements of the eye (separate from rotation movements) is indicated in Fig. 3 by the translation fluctuations of the globe in response to the heartbeat. Part (a) of the figure illustrates axial eye motions (recorded from an axial position sensor within the instrument). A simultaneous EKG recording, Fig. 3(b), verifies that the repetitive pattern is that of the heartbeat. Figure 3 (c) shows a recording from the first Purkinje (horizontal) channel, with the subject relaxed to infinity and voluntarily suppressing saccades. The heartbeat pattern does not show in the simultaneous double Purkinje record (not shown), indicating that the heartbeat record is a pure translation motion of the eye (of approximately 30 μm), or a rotation component that is too small to be seen in the double Purkinje record. After vigorous exercise, both the rate and the amplitude of these eye translation motions increase, as shown in Fig. 3 (d).

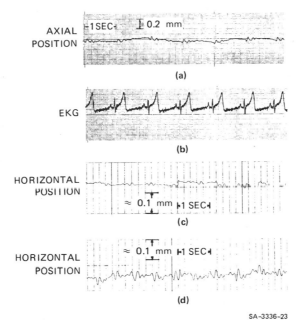

AXIAL POSITION

⊢1SEC⊣   ⊥ 0.2 mm

(a)

EKG

(b)

HORIZONTAL POSITION

≈ 0.1 mm ⊢1 SEC⊣

(c)

HORIZONTAL POSITION

≈ 0.1 mm ⊢1 SEC⊣

(d)

SA-3336-23

FIG. 3.   Eye movements in response to heartbeat. These illustrate the sensitivity of the instrument in detecting three-dimensional translational as well as rotational motions of the globe. (a,b) Axial eye motion and simultaneous EKG; horizontal eye motion (c) before and (d) after exercise.

Figure 4 is a record of square-wave diagonal tracking. The upper portion of Fig. 4 (a), a recording of the First Purkinje image from the eyetracker, contains both translational and rotational components; the lower portion, which is from the normal, double Purkinje output of the instrument, is a measure of the rotational component only. Another example of what might be translational artifact is seen in the upper record. The approximately 200-msec, 0.5° "glide" to final state following a left-directed saccade, in the upper record of Fig. 4 (a), does not appear in the lower record (the large overshoot in the lower record is discussed below), implying that the slow movement is a translational rather than rotational motion of the eye. It is certainly not surprising to find a small translational component of motion accompanying any large saccade. Recall that translational motion of only 50 μm would generate a 0.5° artifact signal in the rotation record.

Unless these translation components and fluctuations are recognized as such in any eye movement record derived from a corneal tracker, they might easily be misinterpreted as rotational components of eye motion and lead to confusion among eye-movement researchers, who try to account for every detail of the response in their controller and plant dynamics models.

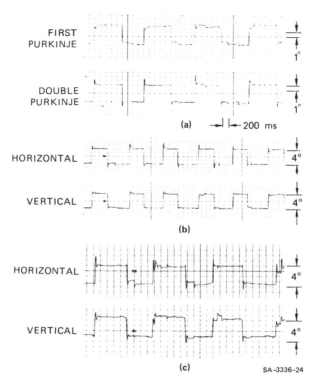

FIRST PURKINJE

DOUBLE PURKINJE

(a)   200 ms

HORIZONTAL   4°

VERTICAL   4°

(b)

HORIZONTAL   4°

VERTICAL   4°

(c)   SA-3336-24

FIG. 4.   Overshoots in the eye movement records during saccades. As discussed in the text, these seem to be caused by lateral motions of the eyelens within the globe. (a) Simultaneous records from the first and double Purkinje image output signals. Note the small overshoots in the first Purkinje record and the large (and inconsistent) overshoots in the double Purkinje record. The 100- to 200-msec "drift" in the first Purkinje record, following each saccade, may be caused by a translation motion of the eye, inasmuch as a similar component is not seen in the double Purkinje record; (b,c) comparison of simultaneous horizontal and vertical overshoot components in the double Purkinje records with the subject relaxed to infinity and accommodated to 4 diopters. Note the large increase in overshoots at 4 diopters.

DYNAMIC OVERSHOOT AND MOTIONS OF THE LENS WITHIN THE GLOBE

While a type of dynamic overshoot, that is, the transient movement of the eye past the final resting position, followed by a return to this position, has been reported before with contact lenses (Ditchburn, 1973) and corneal, EOG, and limbus techniques (Bahill, Clark, & Stark, 1975; Weber & Daroff, 1971 a, b), we have discovered a fundamentally different kind of overshoot that seems to be related to lateral motion of the lens within the globe. To reiterate, the rotational component of eye motion is derived by measuring the separation between the first and fourth Purkinje images, and any movement of the lens that changes the separation will therefore be measured.

The overshoots we refer to can be seen at the end of the saccades in the lower record of Fig. 4 (a). The source of these overshoots appears to be relative lateral motion of the lens within the globe, inasmuch as similar motions do not appear at all, or are much smaller, in the corneal image movements. If this is the correct explanation, we might expect the size of the overshoots to vary with accommodation level (i.e., with changes in the physical configuration of the eye lens). That this is the case can be seen from Fig. 4 (b, c), which shows the simultaneous horizontal and vertical eye movement components of response to the diagonal tracking target. In Fig. 4 (b), the eye was relaxed to infinity, and in Fig. 4 (c), the eye was accommodated to 4 diopters. At 4 diopters of accommodation, there is a large increase in the size and time constant of the overshoots in both the horizontal and the vertical channels, as compared with relaxed accommodation. Note that the overshoots may vary from saccade to saccade, between the two eyes, and that temporal saccades (i.e., movements to the right in the right eye, and to the left in the left eye), seem to have more overshoot than nasal saccades and vertical saccades seem to have less overshoot than horizontal saccades.

If overshoots derive from lateral motion of the lens within the globe, they provide a potentially useful method of measuring the effects of this motion. Any such motion causes a shift in the visual axis of the eye and, therefore, a shift in the retinal image. We estimate that overshoots in the double Purkinje record are approximately ten times as large as the actual shift in the visual axis; that is, a lateral shift of the lens large enough to cause a 1° overshoot in the fourth Purkinje record would actually represent about a 6-min shift in the visual axis of the eye. If the magnitude of the overshoot could be scaled properly with respect to tracking image position on the retina rather than of the globe as a whole, the double-Purkinje tracker, offers the advantage of potentially greater eyetracking accuracy than contact lens methods that are completely insensitive to movements of the eye lens.

BINOCULAR STIMULI AND RESPONSES

Asymmetrical Responses

With our binocular monitoring capability, we can monitor the responses of both eyes simultaneously and compare them, noting especially any differences in response. Cases have been observed where accommodation, vergence, and version were unequal in both tracking and fixational tasks. Figure 5 depicts an eye movement response to a target that is moved in depth along the midline axis between the two eyes. Note the unequal versional and vergence responses in this divergence movement, in violation of Hering's Law. The horizontal saccades in the left eye at Instants A and B are much larger than those in the right eye (and

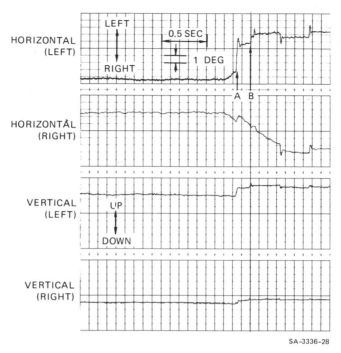

SA-3336-28

FIG. 5.   Binocular responses to a target that moved in depth along the midline axis between the eyes. Note the unequal horizontal and vertical saccades in the two eyes, as well as the dissimilar vergence movements.

also have more overshoot); the vertical saccade at Instant A is much larger in the left than in the right eye; and the long-lasting vergence response in the right eye has a much smaller and shorter-lasting counterpart in the left eye. Such responses, which can be measured only with a binocular eyetracker, force us to question the well-accepted descriptions of vergence and version as being simply highly yoked responses.

Binocular Accommodation Stimulus

We have performed a number of experiments that stimulate the systems of vergence and accommodation while monitoring responses in both eyes in monocular and binocular situations. Some of these experiments produce conflicting clues to the systems. Figure 6 is a record of step stimulation of accommodation to both eyes (without the usual vergence stimulus), viewed binocularly and monocularly. One can observe the well-known accommodative—vergence response with one eye occluded (right hand half of the record, marked "right eye occluded"), but what is especially interesting is the response when there is no change in target position in either eye (first half of the record). It might be expected that (1) the eyes would transiently converge due to the accommodative—

convergence system, or (2) a yoked saccade might occur (controlled by the dominant eye?), as in the well-known binocular response to step-target movement along the axis of one eye. Since neither response takes place, it seems, at the very least, that the disparity—vergence system is able to override the accommodative—convergence system.

The record also shows that the accommodative response in the binocular presentation (first half of record) is often of smaller magnitude than the response when the stimulation is monocular (second half of record) with the occluded eye converging. It is as though the lack of convergence eliminates a normally present input signal to the convergence—accommodation system.

Monocular Vergence Stimulus

We can also easily cause the target to move in one eye only, while keeping the target presented to the other eye fixed (target distance maintained constant in both eyes). It is not clear which visual system should respond to this type of

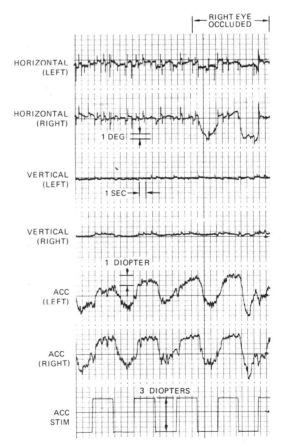

FIG. 6. Binocular responses to simultaneous target movement along the axis of each eye, without any change in the lateral position of the target in each eye (i.e., no change in target vergence). Note the accommodative responses, without any vergence response, in the left-hand half of the record and the accommodative vergence responses in the right-hand half of the record when one eye is occluded.

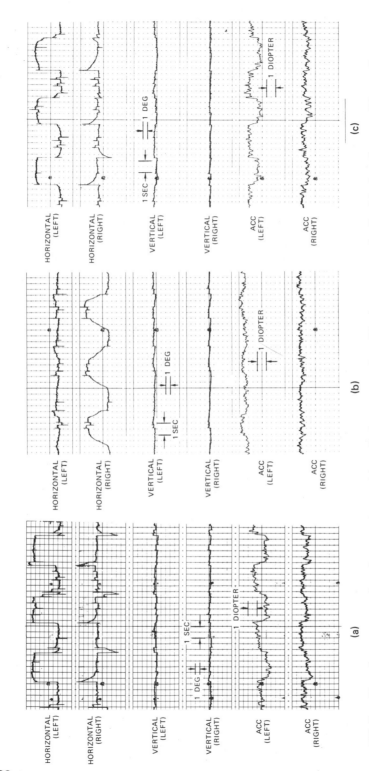

FIG. 7. Binocular responses when the target is moved laterally in one eye only, while the target remains fixed in the other eye. (Observe the nonfunctional accommodative responses.) (a) Moving target in the left eye; attention to the target with both eyes equally; (b) moving target in the right eye; attempt to suppress any movement of the (dominant) left eye which has a steady target; (c) moving target in the left eye; attempt to suppress any movement of the (nondominant) right eye which has a steady target.

86

stimulus in which one eye sees a moving target that looks like a versional stimulus and the other eye sees no movement; the retinal disparity between the two eyes should elicit a disparity vergence response.

Figure 7 (a) illustrates this experiment, in which the stimulus is a horizontal square-wave movement of the target in the left eye; observe the change in accommodation in both eyes to the "vergence movement," even though the target does not change its distance in either eye. (With pinhole pupils, that is, with open-loop accommodation, this nonfunctional accommodative response is even larger.) The target is a high contrast ring surrounding an X.

Although it is well known that disparity vergence can induce a change in accommodation (i.e., vergence accommodation), this is the first record to depict, simultaneously and in both eyes, changes in accommodation and eye position in response to a pure vergence stimulus. In response to a square wave of target movement in one eye only, this eye moves primarily in a saccadic response, while the eye that sees no target change has the well-known yoked saccade (which is nonfunctional, since it takes this eye away from the target) and a "vergence" movement that is not present in the other eye. It is questionable whether this should be called a vergence or smooth pursuit movement, since both eyes are neither converging nor engaged in pursuit.

Although the typical response in the experiment described above (with a step-target movement in one eye) is depicted in Fig. 7 (a), the response can be changed by consciously attending to the stimulus in one eye only. Figure 7 (b) shows a response when the square wave of target movement is in the right eye and the subject is instructed to hold the left eye still. Note that the eyes do not exhibit the saccade, and the right eye shows only a slow tracking movement that serves to bring the two images once again to fusion. In Fig. 7 (c), the moving target is back in the left eye, and the subject is again instructed to hold the (nondominant) eye, which now has the steady target still. Note that the subject can suppress saccades in one direction and then not perfectly. These records are from a highly trained subject; we have not yet explored their generality.

DISCUSSION

The double-Purkinje-image eyetracker can measure the rotational and translational components of eye movements separately. With this new capability, we have demonstrated (1) axial and lateral translational movements of the globe, in synchronism with the blood pulse; (2) translational components of motion accompanying saccades.

The Purkinje eyetracker is also sensitive to relative motion of the eye lens within the globe. With this capability, we have demonstrated movement of the eye lens within the globe during saccades.

The translational components of motion can cause serious artifact signals in records from corneal or limbus eyetrackers. Because movement of the lens within the globe causes a shift in the retinal image, the availability of signals that reflect such movement makes the Purkinje eyetracker potentially more accurate than contact lens methods.

Each of these components of motion may also be useful in its own right. The ability to detect the blood pulse in eye movements may have clinical use. Scott (personal communication) suggested that overshoots resulting from lateral motion of the lens in the globe during a saccade may prove useful in the study of certain visual problems associated with the lens, such as in Marfan's ("loose lens") syndrome, where the lens detaches itself from the supporting tissue, or for exploration of the stability of a new lens following lens removal for cataract and replacement by plastic. An understanding of the translational motions of the globe that accompany rotational motions of the eye may be useful in defining more precisely how the extraocular muscles attach to the globe and how they exert their force.

Interesting features of monocular and binocular vision become evident when it is possible to monitor the visual responses of the extraocular and accommodative systems simultaneously in both eyes. Accommodative, versional, and vergence responses can be unequal in the two eyes, in violation of Hering's Law. In particular, we have shown (1) binocular accommodation without vergence; (2) a large saccade in one eye with only a very small one in the other; (3) a large, long-lasting vergence movement in one eye with a small and much shorter-lasting vergence movement in the other eye; and (4) a difference in response depending on whether the subject concentrates with his dominant or nondominant eye.

We are confident that many other interrelationships will become evident and more clearly defined with more extended use of binocular, three-dimensional eyetracking capability.

II.3

Adaptation of Cognitive Processes to the Eye Movement System[1]

J. Edward Russo[2]
Carnegie-Mellon University

Higher cognitive processes require the continuous input of information. If that information is to be obtained visually, eye movements are needed. Although eye movements are relatively quick, an ongoing cognitive process still experiences a noticeable lag between the request for new information and its actual arrival. The purpose of this chapter is to analyze the impact on cognitive processes of the lag in information delivery by an eye movement. In all that follows, eye movement refers exclusively to the voluntary saccadic eye movements that are initiated by cognitive processes. The class of involuntary eye movements is not considered.

THE USE OF EYE MOVEMENTS BY THE COGNITIVE SYSTEM

Cognitive processing can be divided into two phases: the computation performed on available information and the acquisition of new information. The computational function and the control of the acquisition function are executed by some central mechanism(s) that will be referred to as the cognitive system.

The essential components of this system are a memory and an active processor. The active processor has limited resources, often identified with the concept of limited *attention*. Information is stored in *long-term memory* (LTM) and thought of as a network of associated concepts, whereas the execution of cognitive

---

[1]The author thanks Larry Rosen for extensive discussions of these and related eye movement issues, and Patricia Carpenter for a discussion of the material in this chapter.

[2]Currently at the University of Chicago, Graduate School of Business.

operations takes place in a temporarily activated, task-relevant portion of LTM called the *workspace*. *Short-term memory* (STM) is that portion of the work-space that has received attention so recently that each concept in it can be directly reported. (For extended treatments of the cognitive system the reader is referred to Bower, 1975; Newell & Simon, 1972; Norman, 1976.)

Eye Movements versus Alternative Information Acquisition Behaviors

Eye movements are one of many means for acquiring information. Processing efficiency dictates that an eye movement will be used when it is less costly than other acquisition behaviors. This section compares the effort required by an eye movement to that required by alternative behaviors.

All sources of information are subject to a twofold classification. Acquisition effort ranges from negligible to excessive, and the locus of information may be either internal (in memory) or external. This classification scheme forms the basis of Table 1.

Five acquisition (or retrieval) actions are listed. At one extreme, no action is required if the desired information is already in the locus of attention (STM). At the other extreme, a maximum effort general search strategy may be needed. General search strategies are open ended in that they guarantee neither success-

TABLE 1
Classification of Sources of Information

Acquisition Action	Location of Information		Effort Cost (Time)
	Internal	External (Visual Only)	
No action	Current locus of attention STM		Instantaneous
Attention shift	Currently active "workspace"	Current visual field, especially foveal area	Tens of msec
Single acquisition operation	Directly addressable LTM	Visual field accessible via an eye movement	Hundreds of msec
Fixed sequence of acquisition operations	Directly accessible LTM	Beyond immediate visual environment	Seconds
General search strategy	LTM	Beyond immediate visual environment	Tens of sec

ful retrieval nor known execution time. For our purposes, they will be arbitrarily limited to durations under one minute. Otherwise, the search process replaces the primary cognitive process it was called to serve.

For those readers unfamiliar with the terms used in Table 1, examples of the various information acquisition actions may help. A single retrieval operation (internal) might be the recall of your own telephone number. A fixed sequence of such operations (internal) is used if you employ a mnemonic to remember a friend's phone number, such as a seven-letter word that can be transformed into the seven-digit number. An external version of the fixed sequence is looking up the needed number in a telephone directory. A general search strategy (internal) is probably needed to recall the telephone number two residences prior to your present one. Alternatively, you could search your personal records for this number, which would require an external general search strategy. Finally, Kowler (1977) provides an example of an external attention shift by having subjects count objects in a visual display while their eyes were fixated.

An estimate of the time necessary for each action is shown in the rightmost column of Table 1. These estimates are given only within an order of magnitude. There is sufficient variability within each action to preclude precise estimates. Furthermore, there is certainly some overlap of the range of durations for adjacent actions. Thus, the longest attention shift may take longer than the shortest single acquisition operation, and so forth. Nonetheless, the time assignments can effectively distinguish the five types of action with respect to effort. This, in turn, provides a basis for aligning the external and internal actions. Thus, an eye movement is seen as roughly equivalent in effort to a direct (single operation) acquisition (or retrieval) from LTM.

The classification scheme of Table 1 emphasizes the function of an eye movement, as viewed by the cognitive system. This approach should be contrasted with the traditional structural comparison between internal and external information sources. Structurally, STM is the center of internal attention just as the foveal stimulus is the center of the visual world. Similarly, an internal shift in attention parallels an external eye movement. As shall be argued in the next section, however, it is the functional rather than structural characteristics of an eye movement that impact our cognitive processes.

A FUNCTIONAL ANALYSIS OF THE
EYE MOVEMENT SYSTEM

To analyze the function of the eye movement system (from the viewpoint of the cognitive system), the concept of an eye movement must be extended beyond the physical movement itself. A *complete eye movement cycle* is defined to begin immediately after the decision to acquire visual information and to end with the delivery of that information to the ongoing cognitive process. The actual movement of the eye forms only one part of the complete cycle. This cycle can be partitioned into the following component operations:

1. determine the location of the next fixation;
2. transmit the movement command to the motor system;
3. move the eye to the new position;
4. transmit the new visual stimulus to the cortex;
5. decode the received stimulus.

Independence of the Operations

The above partition is designed so that the several operations use separate systems. Operation 3 uses the motor system to redirect the eye. Operations 2 and 4 involve the neural transmission of information between the eye and cortex. Operations 1 and 5, location determination and stimulus decoding, are performed by the cognitive system.

The separation between Operations 2 and 3 and between Operations 3 and 4 is relatively clear both physiologically and behaviorally. It is assumed that location transmission (Operation 2) must be completed before movement (Operation 3) begins and movement must cease before stimulus perception (Operation 4) begins. A large body of data suggests that a saccadic eye movement is ballistic in nature. That is, once the next fixation position has been registered by the motor system, the movement is not capable of modification until it has been completed as originally programmed. This ballistic model of the saccadic system is not strictly true, as recently demonstrated by Becker and Jurgens (1975) and by Zee, Optican, Cook, Robinson, and Engel (1976). Nonetheless, it is probably a satisfactory description under typical conditions, including those obtained during the performance of cognitive tasks. Note that serial independence between the movement command and the movement itself is a unique property of the saccadic system. Modification during movement is characteristic of other muscular systems, including others for the eye (Westheimer, 1976).

The assumption that perception cannot begin until the eye arrives at the new fixation point is more problematic. First, the fact that the eye is moving complicates perception by "smearing" the stimulus across the retina (Uttal & Smith, 1968). Then the phenomenon of saccadic suppression elevates the intensity levels required for perception both during a saccade and also before and after movement (Volkman, 1976; see also Volkman, this volume). Finally, most of the stimulus during movement is in the periphery where acuity is reduced. These factors combine to make extremely difficult the perception of cognitive stimuli like words or pictorial patterns while the eye is moving. It is probably safe to assume that, in the face of such perceptual difficulties, subjects do not take in visual field information during the relatively brief time that the eye is in motion.

The separation of the first and last operations relies on their definition. Both operations are assumed to include everything that requires the participation of the cognitive system. Only straightforward neural transmission is assigned to Operations 2 and 4. This division of function is sufficient to insure independence between all contiguous operations of an eye movement cycle.

Typical Durations

The durations of the five component operations are either given or can be estimated from durations reported in the eye movement literature. Movement duration is a well known function of movement amplitude. A typical movement amplitude for cognitive tasks is assumed to be about 5°–6°, and requires about 30 msec to complete (Bahill & Stark, 1975). The time for efferent transmission of the signal to move the eyes can be estimated from cortical stimulation studies to be about 30 msec.[3]

Similarly, single cell recording techniques yield an estimate of 60 msec for the afferent transmission of a new stimulus to the cortex.[4] The difference between the 30 and 60 msec estimates reflects the longer time for the retinal processing of a stimulus relative to the time for contraction of the muscles that move the eye. These three estimates are collected in Table 2.

The durations of the two cognitive components of an eye movement cycle cannot be measured in isolation. They must be inferred from the durations of longer tasks. Consider the well-known latency of 200 msec to initiate a small movement (Fuchs, 1971). (This is only a consensus value; Westheimer, 1954, reports lower values while Leushina, 1965, reports higher values.) This latency is composed, in order, of Operations 4, 5, 1, and 2. Subtracting the previously given durations for Operations 2 (30 msec) and 4 (60 msec), the combined duration of both cognitive operations is estimated to be 110 msec.

The 200 msec latency just cited varies considerably across experimenters, and it is worth pausing a moment to consider why. Several researchers, notably

---

[3]Robinson (1972) reports 25–35 msec motor response latencies to stimulation of the frontal eye fields. Schiller (personal communication, 1977) estimates 25–30 msec motor response latency to stimulation of Area 17. This estimate is based on a 5–6 msec transmission duration from Area 17 to the superior colliculus (Finlay, Schiller & Volkman, 1976) and 20–25 msec for motor latencies to stimulation in the superior colliculus (Schiller & Stryker, 1972). The resulting overall estimate of typical efferent transmission duration is 30 msec. This value is considerably less than the 70 msec reported by Fuchs (1976). The difference may be due to a narrower definition of Operation 2 or to the use of more recent data.

[4]Wurtz and Mohler (1976a) report a 25–70 msec range of delays between the onset of a visual stimulus and the response of single cells in monkey striate cortex. Mohler, Goldberg, and Wurtz (1973) report 50–120 msec delays for response in the frontal eye fields. Slightly longer times are being recorded for latency to response in the parietal eye fields (Goldberg, personal communication, 1977). An estimate of 60 msec has been selected, somewhat arbitrarily. Again, this estimate is less than the one reported by Fuchs (1976), which is 80 msec.

TABLE 2
Functional Analysis of a Complete Eye Movement Cycle

Component Operation	Active System	Duration (msec) Typical	Minimal
1. Determine location of Fixation N + 1	Cognitive	50	0+
2. Transmit command	Efferent	30	25
3. Move eye	Motor	30	10
4. Transmit stimulus	Afferent	60	35
5. Decode stimulus	Cognitive	60	0+
Complete Eye Movement Cycle		230	70

Westheimer (1954), have reported values less than 200 msec, while greater values have also been observed (Leushina, 1965). It is disturbing to find such variation for an apparently simple and replicable experiment. The typical explanations offered are procedural variation and individual differences, including motivation. Another explanation is possible, one based on a speed—accuracy tradeoff. It is a familiar phenomenon of task performance that accuracy increases at the expense of speed and vice versa (Pachella, 1974). Indeed, Festinger (1971) reports that longer latencies in response to a test flash are found when the target must be fixated more accurately. If the subjects tested by different experimenters performed under different speed—accuracy instructions, whether communicated explicitly or implicitly, variation in the observed latencies would be expected. No experiment has systematically tested this explanation. Furthermore, the published studies seldom report either the accuracy of the saccades or the in-structions to the subjects concerning accuracy. The speed—accuracy explanation is appealing, however, and it deserves a rigorous experimental test.

Returning to the durations of operations, a final source of evidence is the long-standing estimate of between 100 msec and 150 msec for "cleared up percep-tion" following an eye movement. A tachistoscopic study by Dodge (1907) provided the initial basis for the estimate of a minimum of 100 msec for cleared up perception. This value is supported by recent studies using a sequence of tachistoscopically presented stimuli to simulate eye fixations (Potter, 1976; Sperling, Budiansky, Spivak, & Johnson, 1971; see also Loftus, 1976). Taking 120 msec as representative, the duration of stimulus decoding is estimated to be 60 msec. To estimate the last duration, that of location determination (Opera-tion 1), we subtract 60 msec from the total cognitive time of 110 msec to arrive at 50 msec. This calculation assumes, however, that in the task of moving to a test flash, the two cognitive operations are executed sequentially. To the extent that they overlap, 50 msec will underestimate the duration needed for location determination.[5] The duration estimates for the two cognitive operations are also summarized in Table 2.

---

[5]I thank Dr. Michael Goldberg for pointing this out following his reading of this paper.

The estimates presented above must be qualified in two ways. First, they are based on a personal evaluation of empirical results, some of which were not designed to provide estimates of durations. New, more pertinent experiments can be expected to provide revised estimates. Second, there is variability, often considerable, around each estimate. This variability is known with some precision for Operations 2, 3, and 4 (see the previously cited studies). Operation 5 (stimulus decoding) will vary with stimulus complexity and familiarity. The duration will be longer for complex or novel stimuli and shorter for simple, predictable, or familiar ones. The same flexibility holds for the determination of fixation location (Operation 1). This computation may vary from an almost automatic operation executed at a lower level of the control hierarchy (Thomas, 1969) to a complex, time-consuming subtask.

Minimum Durations

It is useful to consider the minimum possible time for a complete eye movement cycle. If we consider 1° to be the minimum movement, 10 msec is required to redirect the eye. From sources cited above, the minimum duration of Operation 2 is 25 msec and of Operation 4 is 35 msec. Finally, the two cognitive operations are considered, in the extreme, to be capable of complete automatization. If so automatized, they might require almost no execution time. Thus, a lower bound for the duration of a complete eye movement cycle is about 70 msec. This value is compatible with the briefest times reported in the literature (see Fuchs, 1976, p. 40).

Conclusion

One purpose of estimating durations is to contrast the time of a complete eye movement cycle, 230 msec, with the 30 msec required for the movement itself. The point is that the lag between the request and the delivery of information is many times longer than a relatively quick saccade. Like all other information acquisition actions, eye movements entail a noticeable delay; although fast, they are not instantaneous.

A second goal of the duration analysis is the partition of the total duration of an eye movement cycle into cognitive and peripheral components. The 110 msec duration required for the cognitive operations emphasizes the important role of the cognitive system in executing a saccade. Cognitive strategies are needed both to determine the location of the next fixation and to decode a new stimulus. On the other hand, the fact that the cognitive system is not needed for the remaining 120 msec poses an important question. Is the cognitive system idle during this period? If it is, an eye movement may be even more costly to cognitive processing than previously concluded. This issue is taken up in the next section.

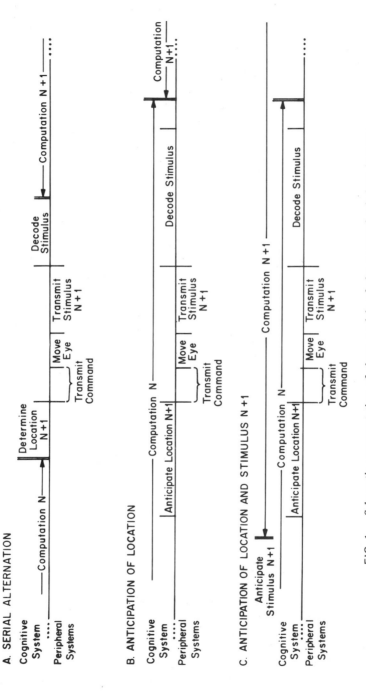

FIG. 1. Schematic representation of three models of the temporal relations between the component operations of an eye movement cycle and the cognitive system.

HOW COGNITIVE PROCESSES ADAPT TO THE
COST OF AN EYE MOVEMENT

Eye movements are inexpensive only in relation to other information acquisition behaviors. For any task that continually demands information acquisition, a significant proportion of processing time may be consumed by the eye movements. In tasks such as search, vigilance, and monitoring, the ratio of information acquisition to computation may be quite high. It is natural, therefore, for the cognitive system to adapt so as to minimize the cost of an eye movement. In this section we consider two adaptive procedures available to the cognitive system. The first is the anticipation of the time, location, and contents of the next fixation. The second, when possible, is the storage of part of the relevant information in memory.

Serial Alternation

Suppose that the acquisition of new information alternates with its computation — that is, that the termination of the one signals the initiation of the other. This view of the relation between the cognitive and eye movement systems is pictured in Fig. 1A. This model implies that the determination of the next fixation takes place at the *end* of the current fixation, an assertion frequently found in the literature (e.g., Loftus, 1976). The advantages of serial alternation are two-fold. The decision of *when* to begin the next eye movement cycle is greatly simplified, namely after all computation has been completed. The decision of *where* to fixate next can be based on information obtained from the completed processing of the current stimulus.

In spite of these advantages, the serial alternation model is untenable. The problem is that the cognitive system is forced to remain idle during the time that peripheral systems are in use. Based on the typical durations summarized in Table 2, this amounts to 120 msec of "idle time" for the cognitive system.

Anticipation of Fixation $N + 1$

The solution to this predicament is to initiate an eye movement before the computational processing has been completed. The cognitive system can then complete the remaining computation during the idle time (or extend it into the next processing unit). This overlap assumption is depicted in Fig. 1B. Note that Computation N must share cognitive resources with the two eye movement operations that require the cognitive system (Operations 1 and 5). As a result, these two operations take longer to execute. Computation N can end anywhere during the eye movement cycle or even after Computation $N + 1$ is ready to begin (as shown in Fig. 1B). When this is the case, Computation $N + 1$ is postponed, at some cost. This cost arises because of a presumed incompatibility between perceiving Stimulus $N + 1$ while computing Stimulus N.

An example will illustrate both the idle time entailed by the serial alternation model and also its reduction by the use of the processing scheme represented in Fig. 1B. Consider a search task in which the subject memorizes a standard pattern and then searches for an exact match among a series of similar patterns. Each new pattern requires an eye fixation. The testing strategy is a standard serial comparison process (Townsend, 1974). Assume five "features" per pattern, tested in sequence. All distractor patterns differ from the standard in only one randomly selected feature. The testing of each feature requires 60 msec, with an additional 60 msec verification operation if no mismatches are found. Perfect matches occur on 5% of the test stimuli. The test of a pattern terminates when any mismatched feature is identified, or when a match occurs. In accord with the simple serial alternation paradigm of Fig. 1A, assume that the eye movement cycle begins when the test is terminated. In this task, the location of the next fixation may be assumed to be known in advance. The subject's only decision is when to move, a decision which will be viewed as thoroughly automated and requiring no time. The time in peripheral systems (the idle time) is 120 msec, and the decoding time is 60 msec. These specifications complete the model.

Based on this model, the expected total processing time is 369 msec per stimulus. Of this, the cognitive system is active for 249 msec and idle for 120 msec. That is, for 33% of the total task time the cognitive system is not in use.

Consider instead the model described in Fig. 1B. The rule for deciding when to initiate the next eye movement is: move to Stimulus $N + 1$ after k operations have been performed ($k \leqslant 6$), or if a mismatch is detected before k operations have been completed. This departure rule requires the specification of one additional parameter. It is now possible to have arrived at Location $N + 1$ before Computation N has been completed. The incompatibility between the perception of Stimulus $N + 1$ and the computation of Stimulus N will be modeled as a doubling of the processing time remaining prior to Computation $N + 1$.

What is the optimal value of k? The earlier the eye movement cycle can be initiated, the more idle time can be eliminated. However, if it is initiated too soon, it is finished before the preceding computation has been completed, and the incompatibility (or overlap) penalty is incurred. These competing time costs are pictured and resolved in Fig. 2.

The maximum idle time of 120 msec occurs when $k = 6$, that is when the serial alternation model holds. It decreases to 11 msec when $k = 0$, that is, when Movement $N + 1$ and Computation N are initiated simultaneously. In contrast, cognitive processing time decreases as k increases, a direct result of a decreasing overlap penalty. The resolution of these two effects is shown in the plot of expected total time. The minimum occurs at $k = 3$. Thus, the optimal strategy is to make three feature comparisons and even if no mismatch has been detected, to depart for Location $N + 1$. The time saved is the difference between 369 msec at $k = 6$ and 335 msec at $k = 3$. This is 34 msec, or a 9% reduction. It is more appropriate, however, to evaluate the saving of 34 msec against the

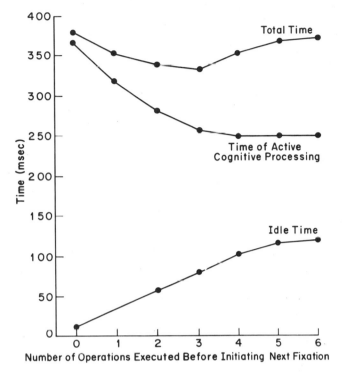

FIG. 2. Partitioning of total time per stimulus for a matching task. The serial alternation model is represented by an abscissa of six. Anticipation models are represented by values less than six.

maximum possible reduction. Note that the minimum execution time is 180 msec, namely the total time for Operations 2, 3, 4, and 5 (recall that to simplify the example, Operation 1 is assumed to have been automatized). Thus, the maximum possible reduction is 189 msec, so the 34 msec saved by the model in Fig. 1B corresponds to an 18% saving in execution time.

Anticipation Strategies

The more efficient use of processing time just illustrated is based on extending Computation N through the idle time associated with an eye fixation. Unfortunately, the decision of when and where to fixate next cannot be similarly extended. This decision must be made before Computation N is complete and, therefore, can no longer be based on the results of Computation N. Thus Fixation $N + 1$ must be partly *anticipated*. The need to anticipate the results of Computation N encourages the development of *anticipation strategies*. Such strategies provide information for the determination of Fixation $N + 1$, without benefit of the results of Computation N.

Let us consider exactly what must be anticipated. Most generally, there are three aspects of the next fixation that either can be determined from all possible information or can be anticipated from partial information. These are the initiation time of the eye movement cycle, the location of the next fixation, and the contents of the next fixation (Stimulus $N + 1$ itself). In the previous simplified example, only initiation time was a factor. Usually, however, location must be computed and anticipation of Stimulus $N + 1$ will also occur. When Stimulus $N + 1$ is anticipated Computation $N + 1$ can begin *prior* to Fixation $N + 1$ (although it can only be based on anticipated information). Figure 1C illustrates this situation, which is the most general form of overlap among computations and eye movement operations. The anticipation of Stimulus $N + 1$ can be considered the most sophisticated form of anticipation. Besides the advantage of reducing cognitive idle time, it may also shorten the eye movement cycle itself by decreasing the decoding time (Operation 5). Recognition of a stimulus is faster when the stimulus is expected.

Anticipation strategies are based on three sources of information: stored structures, completed computations, and peripheral perception. In some situations a stored structure, without any information from the current stimulus, may provide a sufficient basis for anticipation. A routinized monitoring order for a set of instrument dials is one example. Usually, however, anticipation relies on a combination of remembered structures and current stimulus information. The latter is derived either from the computation of stimulus components already perceived foveally, or from the (partial) computation of peripherally perceived areas. Highly developed anticipation strategies rely on both sources of stimulus information. In reading, the ability to anticipate the next words based on current text has long been appreciated (e.g., Gray, 1923), and recent studies have convincingly demonstrated the anticipatory value of peripherally perceived information (e.g., Rayner, 1975).

The need for an anticipation strategy depends on the nature of the task. The need is greatest when the ratio of computation-to-acquisition is low, that is, when the computation time per stimulus is relatively brief and a continual input of new information is necessary. Typical tasks are search (including pattern matching, inspection, monitoring, etc.) and reading. Tasks where the computation-to-acquisition ratio is high are intellective tasks like problem solving, decision making, and so on. The two types of tasks can be roughly distinguished by the length of an average fixation duration. The briefer the duration, the lower the computation-to-acquisition ratio, and the greater will be the need for anticipation strategies.

Just as greater need will encourage anticipation strategies, so will a greater supply of the information on which anticipation strategies are based. Specifically, where stored structures are readily available or where the next stimulus components can be peripherally perceived, anticipation is facilitated. In contrast, if the next fixation must be based on the computation of the current stimulus, anticipation is hindered. In general, therefore, anticipation strategies should develop for tasks with a low computation-to-acquisition ratio and for which sophisticated stored structures or adequate peripheral perception are available.

Finally, note that anticipation strategies are not as separate from regular computational strategies as they may appear. The same understanding of the task environment that leads to efficient anticipation strategies often leads to efficient computational strategies. Reading is a good example. Both the semantic and syntactic knowledge used to comprehend perceived text can be used to anticipate the next phrase. An important corollary is that the reduction of the idle time inherent in an eye movement may not be the only cause of anticipation strategies. As mentioned earlier, it is well-known that correct expectation facilitates stimulus decoding. More importantly, however, the ability to anticipate may be a natural concomitant of efficient computational strategies.

Memorization Strategies

A second way in which cognitive processes can adapt to the delay in information delivery by an eye movement is to rely on memorization of the needed information. This approach reduces the time cost of an eye movement cycle by completely eliminating the need for a new fixation.

Consider the task of typing. Novice typists must continually look from the text to the keyboard to retrieve the location of each key, the "hunt and peck" method. This method takes longer than skilled typing, which relies on memory of the keyboard. Notice, however, that memory-based typing is possible only because the keyboard arrangement is never changed. In contrast, the text to be typed is continually changing and must be continually looked at. Since most tasks require the continual acquisition of new information, a memorization strategy is only occasionally applicable. Though sometimes very useful, it is not nearly as general a solution to eye movement costs as an anticipation strategy.

The use of memorization to avoid an eye fixation has an unpleasant methodological consequence for researchers using eye fixations to trace a cognitive process. Reconsideration of stimulus elements is a natural part of many of these processes, including chess, problem solving, and so on. If the reconsideration is based on remembered information, then the acquisition action will not be observable and the trace of the process will be correspondingly impoverished. In a choice task, Russo and Dosher (1976) monitored eye fixations, while Jacoby and Chestnut (1977) used an "information display board" (see also Jacoby, Chestnut, Fisher, & Weigl, 1976). In the latter methodology subjects acquire stimulus information by reaching into one of a rectangular array of labeled pockets. Because a reaching response is considerably more expensive than an eye fixation, subjects are encouraged to memorize information rather than reacquire it. Russo and Dosher report that 75% of subjects' acquisitions (fixations) were reacquisitions (refixations), while Jacoby et al. report that a range of only

2% to 7% of reaching responses were used for the reacquisition of previously examined stimulus information. As might be expected, the two studies also reported very different conclusions about the structure of the choice process.

IMPLICATIONS OF ANTICIPATION STRATEGIES FOR THE INTERPRETATION OF EYE MOVEMENT DATA

The preceding analysis has implied that anticipation strategies ought to be a familiar aspect of cognitive processing. If people are using anticipation strategies, what effects should this have on their eye fixations? Or conversely, what phenomena of the eye fixation data indicate the use of anticipation strategies?

Manifestations of Anticipation Strategies

Overshoots. Subjects are sometimes reported to overshoot a target by one or more fixations and then to return to it. In a letter matching task, Gould (1973) reports overshoots on 27% of the trials, and Parker (1977) reports a 15% rate when subjects detected an alteration in a pictorial scene.

Overshoot fixations are usually considered indicative of poor performance and they are attributed to failures of attention or to inaccurate criteria for target recognition. However, the preceding analysis of anticipation strategies implies that overshoots should be expected. Efficient processing requires that sometimes the target will be detected only during the next fixation, that is, Computation N will be completed during Fixation $N + 1$. Thus, at least some overshoots may be caused by the use of sophisticated anticipation strategies, indicating skilled rather than inferior performance.

Regressions. Closely related to overshoots are so-called regressive fixations, or regressions, in reading (Tinker, 1958). When eye fixations are monitored during reading, subjects are often observed to return to a word just fixated. Taylor (1957) reports that an average of 15% of all fixations are regressions, although this value varies with reading skill. Regressions have traditionally been interpreted as a characteristic of poor reading. This unfortunate generalization persists (e.g., Norman, 1976), even though the necessity of regressions for skilled performance has been recognized for some time (e.g., Bayle, 1942). Because anticipation strategies are particularly well-developed in reading (Wisher, 1976a), we must expect some overshoots and corrective regressive fixations. It is not claimed that an individual regression is a good thing; it is not. Rather, for the most efficient performance, some regressions must be tolerated.

Not all regressions are caused by anticipation strategies. Many have been shown to be necessary for specific linguistic constructions. The identification of pronominal referents is one such situation (Carpenter & Just, 1977a). More generally, whenever there is a need to disambiguate present information based on (nonrecallable) past information, a regression may be required (Kaplan, 1974). In contrast to anticipation-based regressions, linguistic-based regressions depend directly on the text and probably are little influenced by subjects' strategies. Both types of regressions, however, are concomitants of skilled performance and imply that the optimal regression rate should exceed zero.

Overlap of Computation. If anticipation strategies are used, then overshoots and regressions are really the tip of an iceberg. These refixations represent the *unsuccessful* extension of Computation N into Fixation $N + 1$. However, assuming that anticipation is used effectively, there ought to be more successful than unsuccessful extensions of computation. If so, Duration $N + 1$ should reflect the extension of Computation N. Thus, wherever Computation N is likely to be longer than expected, the anticipation hypothesis predicts that both Duration N *and* Duration $N + 1$ will reflect this difficulty.

No studies have proposed and tested this hypothesis. However, at least two studies have examined situations where unexpected difficulty occurs and where eye fixations have been recorded. Rosen had subjects add a column of digits twice (Rosen, 1975, 1977). Memory for the digits obtained during the first addition provided a basis for anticipating the next digit during the second addition. Unknown to the subjects, the column was sometimes altered between additions. Two of these alterations produced significant disruptions and were followed by a nonaltered digit (enabling a test of the prolongation predicted by the anticipation hypothesis). Combining over both cases, Duration N was increased by 20 msec while Duration $N + 1$ was increased by 38 msec. Thus, the extra time required for Computation N was reflected in Duration $N + 1$, as predicted by anticipation. In a reading task, Just and Carpenter (Chapter IV.2 this volume) report a similar result. Target words required 100 msec more processing time and the following word required an additional 50 msec more than normal. The reported durations represent total fixation time, including refixations, but the effect would almost certainly appear for individual fixations as well. Thus, it appears that overlap of computation, an important prediction of the anticipation hypothesis, is confirmed in these two tasks.

Uniformity of Durations. A more subtle manifestation of anticipation strategies is a reduction in the variance of fixation durations. The use of anticipation accomplishes this by absorbing computation variability in the idle time and also by spreading out processing over more than one fixation. Consider the example of the pattern matching task used earlier. Without anticipation, mean duration is 369 msec with a standard deviation of 92 msec. With anticipation, the two values become 335 msec and 66 msec, respectively, a 28% decrease in variability. Unfortunately, the author knows of no experimental data that can be used to test the prediction of reduced variability of durations. The preceding prediction should be distinguished from the familiar finding that mean durations are remarkably uniform. For example, in a visual inspection task, Schoonard, Gould and Miller (1970) found wide individual differences in fixation frequency but no difference in mean duration. In a reading task, Morton (1964) varied the text's statistical approximation to English and found a significant effect on number of fixations, but constancy of mean fixation duration (240 msec). Gordon (1969) reports the same pattern of results in searching through a list of varying complexity. The prediction of the anticipation hypothesis for uniformity of duration is both within–subject and within–condition. (See Carpenter & Just, 1977 for a discussion of this issue in reading.) The findings of constant duration currently in the literature do not bear on the predictions of the anticipation hypothesis.

The Interpretation of Fixation Duration

A major implication of anticipation is that fixation duration may not be a valid measure of computation time. The equivalence of fixation duration and computation time is the fundamental assumption of all analyses of individual fixation durations. Failure of this assumption obviously calls these analyses into question. It has been argued above, however, that this assumption is not generally true. Computation can extend into the next fixation, as illustrated in Fig. 1B and demonstrated in the studies by Rosen (1977), and Just and Carpenter (Chapter IV.2, this volume). Moreover, computation may begin prior to the corresponding fixation, as illustrated in Fig. 1C. Thus, Fixation N and Computation N cannot, in general, be expected to be coterminous. A second cause of inequivalence of the fixation and computation durations is that part of the duration of Fixation N must be allotted to computing the location of the next fixation. If the determination of Location $N + 1$ is difficult, the extra time will appear as part of Duration N. In summary, besides Computation N, Fixation N may include Computation $N - 1$, Computation $N + 1$ and the determination (anticipated or otherwise) of Location $N + 1$. Thus, the natural tendency to equate the duration of Fixation N and Computation N is, at best, only an approximation.

How serious is the problem? In fact, relatively few studies have interpreted individual eye fixations, probably because there are so few theories that make predictions at this level of detail. Instead, most eye fixation research reports such summary statistics as the frequency, spatial distribution, direction, or duration of the observed fixations. Nonetheless, the inequality of the fixation and computation durations poses a serious barrier to any intended use of fixation duration. And it should be noted that even the considerable analytical power of mental chronometry, as developed by Sternberg (1969), cannot salvage a valid interpretation of fixation duration (Just & Carpenter, 1976a; Carpenter & Just, Chapter III.1, this volume).

The basic problem is a very general one: identifying and observing the appropriate cognitive unit. An eye fixation is a natural observable unit of behavior. Unfortunately, it may not correspond at all to the appropriate cognitive unit, and it corresponds only roughly to the underlying computational unit. Just and Carpenter (1976a) have argued for the total viewing time over one or more fixations, the "gaze time," as the appropriate unit of behavior. These authors report the successful interpretation of gaze times while individual durations were meaningless (also see Russo & Rosen, 1975). The value of gaze durations rests heavily on the ability to identify a group of fixations comprising a cognitive unit. If a cognitive unit has not been correctly isolated, the duration of a gaze unit will be no more meaningful than the duration of an individual fixation.

EXPERIMENTAL INTERVENTION IN THE EYE MOVEMENT CYCLE

The thesis of this chapter is that cognitive processes must adapt to fixed characteristics of the eye movement system. The ideal test of this thesis would be based on manipulation of the parameters of the eye movement system to produce predicted cognitive behavior. Of course, this is not possible (except for infrahuman subjects). However, manipulation of the relevant parameters can be simulated by several techniques, including stimulus control and use of a second task.

Varying the Duration of an Eye Movement Cycle

It has been argued that the time required for a complete eye movement cycle (typically, 230 msec) prompts the development of anticipation strategies. The crux of the problem is the 120 msec of the cycle during which the cognitive system is not used. If this idle time could be experimentally increased, then the use of anticipation strategies should also increase. Computer-controlled stimulus displays offer two ways of increasing the idle time. First, the stimulus could be defocused just as the eye arrives, and maintained out of focus for as long as desired. Periods from a few to several hundred msec could be used, although at long delays the subject may eliminate fixations entirely. A second procedure is to move the stimulus to a different but known location while the eye is moving. The first manipulation is the more promising because it permits continuous variation of the added delay in information acquisition. An experiment somewhat similar to this has been performed by Vaughan (Chapter III.2, this volume; Vaughan and Graefe, 1977). He concluded that subjects use a preprogramming strategy to anticipate the next fixation. Although not identical to any of the anticipation schemes described in Fig. 1, Vaughan's theory is analogous.

A manipulation similar to delayed perception occurs naturally in reading. The delay until perception of the next stimulus is always longer at the end of a line and at the end of a page. This suggests constructing textual displays that systematically manipulate the excursion distance. Computer-controlled displays are well suited to this manipulation. Furthermore, the use of naturally occurring line and page breaks permits this to be accomplished unobtrusively. Fixation durations are known to be shorter at the end and longer at the beginning of a line (Abrams & Zuber, 1972; Leisman, Chapter IV.4, this volume; Stern, Chapter IV.1, this volume). Varying excursion distance should not only test the anticipation hypothesis but should also help estimate how much of these differences in fixation duration are attributable to anticipation strategies.

A different approach to increasing the duration of an eye movement cycle is to substitute another acquisition response for the eye movement. This tactic involves several complications, however, and is less promising than the above suggestions. The dangers of a manual (reaching) response have already been illustrated above. The response that most nearly simulates an eye movement to acquire information is a head movement. These movements have been used with some success (Blair, 1958; Robinson, Erikson, Thurston, & Clark, 1972). However, head movements take much longer to execute than eye movements, and the two types of movements interact in complex ways (Bizzi, 1974; Mourant & Grimson, 1977). In general, using manual or head movements to lengthen the time for information acquisition runs the risk of altering the underlying process in important ways.

Varying the duration of an eye movement cycle should include its reduction as well as its prolongation. Unfortunately, these manipulations are difficult to contrive. For example, consider presenting the stimulus in a single fixed location, thereby saving Operations 2 and 3 of an eye movement cycle. How does the subject call for the next stimulus without introducing a delay as long or longer than that associated with an eye movement? Possibly an eyeblink response could be used. However, this would require training, especially to suppress disruptive intermediate blinks (and also to overcome the fairy tale atmosphere of blinking and seeing a changed visual scene). The difficulty of shortening the eye movement cycle evidences the unique speed of eye movements as information acquisition behaviors.

Manipulating Peripheral Cues

The use of anticipation strategies should depend on the availability of peripheral information, at least in some tasks. Many techniques are available for restricting this information, including computer-controlled displays (e.g., Just & Carpenter, 1976c; Rayner, 1975) and mechanical occluders (e.g., Farley, 1976; Poulton, 1962). By selectively eliminating peripheral cues, the basis of an anticipation strategy can be identified.

A few techniques might be employed to enhance peripheral information. For example, Williams (1966) and Luria and Strauss (1975) report that color can be an effective peripheral cue. Color can be used to identify the peripheral information on which anticipation is based. In reading, word length, initial and final letters, and various semantic information have been shown to be detected peripherally (Rayner, 1975). The differential information that these cues provide might be investigated by color-coding. For example, initial and final letters might be displayed in green, or red might be used for important words. Clearly a training procedure will be needed. If successful in an experimental context, this technique might even be used to teach reading. It would be especially valuable to remediate the failure to use one or more specific textual cues.

Second Task Techniques

Second task techniques are designed to use any cognitive processing resources not allocated to the primary task (Kantowitz, 1974; Norman & Bobrow, 1975). For example, a subject might be asked to remember a series of digits, the second task, while reading for a comprehension test, the primary task (Wisher, 1976b). As long as the primary task is dominant, performance on the second task can measure the allocation of resources during various stages of the primary task.

This technique might validate the view of the eye movement system described in Table 1. Do the three component operations involving neural transmission and motor functions use zero cognitive resources? If so, full processing capacity ought to be available for a second task. Similarly, this technique might identify the temporal dynamics of the shift from neural transmission of a new stimulus to the cognitive decoding of that stimulus. The cognitive aspects of an eye movement cycle have seldom been investigated. The 110 msec required to decode a stimulus and program a movement to it is the least understood part of an eye movement. What is being proposed here is the use of cognitive techniques to probe the cognitive component of an eye movement cycle.

CONCLUSION

I have tried to convey two main points. First, an eye movement, like all other information acquisition behaviors, entails real, measurable costs. Second, because almost all (saccadic) eye movements are directly controlled by cognitive processes, many aspects of eye movements can only be understood in the context of the cognitive system. Neither of these assertions is generally recognized in the eye movement literature. Instead, eye movements are considered impressively fast, with negligible execution cost. And cognitive processes serve only as a dim background for the explanation of eye movement behavior.

The Cost of an Eye Movement

A complete eye movement cycle includes the cognitive and neural activity that surrounds the relatively brief actual movement of the eye. For a typical eye movement, this nonmotor activity may add 200 msec to the 30 msec of observed movement. Thus, the delay in information delivery associated with a typical eye movement is 230 msec, not 30 msec.

This does not deny that eye movements are fast. On the contrary, they are the fastest of all information acquisition behaviors, with the exception of attention shifts (an internally controlled shift of attention within the current visual field; see Table 1.) But the preeminent speed of eye movements must not distract us from their cost. Recall the inefficiency of typewriting that included eye movements between the text and keyboard. Skilled typing is impossible without the elimination of these movements. An intriguing example of eliminating eye movements occurs in the landing of aircraft (Gerathewohl & Strughold, 1954; Thomas, 1963). During the 30 sec before landing, pilots increasingly tend to look ahead to the expected landing point, and there are almost no eye movements during the several seconds immediately prior to ground contact. Although other explanations have been offered, this behavior can be explained by a pilot's need to preserve continuous visual input. A change of fixation causes a "visual gap" that begins when the movement begins (even earlier if saccadic suppression is a factor) and ends when the new stimulus is perceived clearly. The typical duration of this gap is 150 msec (Operations 3, 4, and 5 in Table 2). The suppression of eye movements by pilots may be one of those rare natural situations where the cost of an eye movement is so great that information is obtained, instead, through an internally controlled attention shift. It would be interesting to know whether such attention shifts are reported by pilots during landing, or could be identified experimentally.

A final reason for emphasizing the cost of an eye movement is that this cost is unavoidable. The very fact that eye movements are uniquely fast (barring attention shifts) means that there is no substitute for them. Other systems must accept, and adapt, to the cost of an eye movement.

Recognition of the Role of the Cognitive System

The great majority of eye movements serve, and are controlled by, cognitive processes. It is these cognitive processes that must adapt to the relatively fixed parameters of the eye movement system. As we have argued above, and will not repeat here, this adaptation is accomplished primarily through the development of strategies for anticipation. The adoption of such strategies means that the cost of an eye movement is shifted to the cognitive system. That is, to reduce eye movement cost, it is the cognitive system that must develop anticipation strategies and allocate a portion of its limited processing resources to their execution.

Recognition of the control function of cognitive processes has an important implication for the interpretation of eye movement data. Eye fixations serve only to acquire the information needed to execute a given cognitive strategy. Therefore, "interpreting" eye fixations should imply identifying the underlying cognitive strategy. Instead, the use of eye movements to study cognitive processes has been characterized by sterile analyses based exclusively on summary statistics, such as fixation frequency, spatial distribution, and mean duration (e.g., Taylor, Frackenpohl, & Pettee, 1960). Rather, eye movements should be aggregated into meaningful cognitive units or examined for interpretable sequential patterns. Admittedly, identifying cognitive strategies is no simple matter, especially for processes as complex as reading or problem solving. However, because eye movements are always directed by the active cognitive process, an explanation of the eye movements must rely on an understanding of the controlling cognitive strategy. (For a similar argument made in engineering psychology, see Poulton, 1966, p. 192.)

Recognizing the intimate relation between cognition and eye movements may aid our investigation of the eye movement system itself. That is, application of the theoretical paradigm and experimental techniques of cognitive psychology may provide new insights into the nature of the eye movement system. Consider three specific applications. First, the cognitive demands of each of the five eye movement operations can be measured. Do neural transmission and motor action make zero demand on the cognitive system? Can we successfully automatize the two cognitive operations (location determination and stimulus decoding) to reduce their demand for cognitive resources? The second task technique can be used to answer both questions. The second application involves using the concept of a speed–accuracy tradeoff. This concept should guide the redesign of some classical but problematical experiments on the response latency of the saccadic system. Finally, the second task technique could be used to identify the boundaries between the cognitive operations and pure neural transmission. This should result in estimates of afferent and efferent transmission   times, derived through a cognitive rather than physiological methodology. Thus, recognition of the role of cognitive process in directing eye movements should improve our understanding of both the eye movement and cognitive systems.

DISCUSSION

LEISMAN: I probably misunderstood you, so maybe you can clarify a point. What exactly do you mean by idle time? Do you mean that nothing is happening, that there is no cognitive processing? If that's what you mean, I have a hard time buying it.

RUSSO: That's what I mean, and I'm sorry you have a hard time buying it.

LEISMAN: I'll tell you why I do. There is a good deal of data on something called contingent negative variation, which is a type of expectancy wave found in computer-averaged evoked potentials. It's related to cognitive types of activity. For example, if you set up a variable foreperiod reaction time experiment where the subject is presented with either regularly occurring light flashes or repeated clicks, he comes to anticipate what's going to happen next. Even if you omit a stimulus, the brain still responds. And this happens at times considerably beyond 400 msec. In other words, the latency of the CNV is considerably above 400 msec, and if you time that with the original stimulus, then I would imagine that it would have something to do with ongoing processing in times above that which is specified.

RUSSO: Is that your question? You want an explanation for that?

LEISMAN: Yes.

RUSSO: Well, let me say two things. First of all, I hardly mean to imply that during the three middle component operations of an eye movement cycle the brain is doing nothing. Second, the task that you've described is different from what I pictured here. Mainly, your subjects are executing something in the peripheral system after a computation has been completed. The subject has nothing to do but wait for the next stimulus. You are essentially inviting your subject to make that time useful. What subjects learn to do in such situations is to develop an expectation, or an anticipation strategy, or response preparation. Thus, my guess is that the cognitive activity represented by the CNV is response preparation. I think that this is different from the kind of ongoing alternation between acquisition and computation that I mean to describe in this time line [see Fig. 1].

STARK: I want to mention the Zuber effect. Abrams and Zuber (1972) studied reading latencies and found that the average latency when you are on a word was 255 msec. But if you were at the end of a line or making a corrective saccade, the average latency was only 180 msec. And if you put in blank spaces, when the eye got to a blank space it jumped on after 180 msec. This suggests that when the subject arrives at a fixation point he doesn't have to do cognitive processing or even very brief cognitive processing. He perceives that there's nothing there and goes on, saving 75 msec.

KOWLER: Might it also be possible that instead of programming one or two fixations, one could send off a chain of them? Thus, you would move your eye in a pattern, the way you use your fingers to type, for example. This might be more efficient because this way the little woman in the cortex would not have to have that much interaction with the little woman in the brain stem. (Applause) [In reading his paper the author referred to the little man in the brain. – Eds.]

RUSSO: What a good idea, not to mention an excellent editorial comment.

ROBINSON: This is somewhat tangential, but you mentioned overshooting. Since I don't know who else will mention it, I thought I would say this now. In wide-angle free fixation (which usually involves more than one saccade), I find no overshooting at all. One thing I'm doing is having the head move freely, a more natural kind of search than when the head is constrained. Perhaps some of the overshooting we've been seeing is bexause of an artificially constraincd head, which is causing some interference with the natural preprogramming package for this task.

RUSSO: That's an interesting point. I think the kind of overshooting that you're talking about is largely a function of the motor system that controls the eye movements. The kind that I was referring to is purely cognitive in nature. That is, it's a function of cognitive strategies for anticipation. What happens is that an anticipation strategy has you leaving a particular location earlier than you should. In many seaich tasks, the density of targets is quite low. You expect that you'll find nothing of interest at any given fixation location, so you keep on going rapidly from one fixation to the next not finding anything. Then suddenly you see the target, but meanwhile you have passed on, must stop and back up. It's this type of cognitively based overshoot that I was referring to, as distinct from the kind of overshoot which you so interestingly commented on.

STERN: Let me make a comment, not about overshoot, but undershoot. In examining the reading of competent readers, one often sees an undershoot as they shift from the end of one line to the beginning of a new line. Undershoot here means that they go back roughly seven-eighths of the way and then occasionally go back the other one-eighth. My interprctation of this is that readers usually have a good idea of what comes at the bcginning of the line. They can skip fixating that information, pick up information further in the line, and occasionally realize that they need that first bit of information and then go back. So here's an example of where obviously competent readers do a lot of anticipation of location.

RUSSO: That's very interesting. I hadn't thought of those data in this light. I would only add that I view the phenomenon you described as a kind of overshoot rather than undershoot. The person has gone past, has skipped over the entire first fixation, filling it in based on the anticipation or expectation developed during the time that he or she has to move the eye to the new line.

MOURANT: Gordon Robinson's recent work (Robinson, Koth, & Ringenback, 1976) has brought something to my mind. He has just published a paper on what he calls classical and predictive head movement. I have done some of those too (Mourant & Grimson, 1977). In classical eye—head coordination, the eye moves first and then is followed by the head with a latency of 50 msec. What he has found is that when the person has a central task, that is, he must continue to process centrally located information, then there sometimes occurs what is called the predictive head movement. The head will actually start first to move toward the peripheral point where the eyes have to go. This, then, is an anticipatory response. It would be interesting to reexamine the data and see what the duration of eye fixations is.

RUSSO: What this does is allow you to keep looking at and processing one stimulus (assuming you need to be processing it) but to begin that longer head movement to the next fixation location. A very interesting and efficient use of an anticipation strategy to acquire information.

Part **III**

COGNITIVE PROCESSES

III.1

Eye Fixations During Mental Rotation[1]

Patricia A. Carpenter
Marcel Adam Just
Carnegie-Mellon University

When a person mentally transforms a visual stimulus — for example, by imagining it rotating — his pattern of eye fixations reflects the underlying mental operations (Just & Carpenter, 1976a). In this paper, eye fixations will be used to trace the internal manipulation of spatial information and to derive a more precise characterization of the underlying psychological processes.

In the original "mental rotation" paradigm, Shepard and Metzler (1971) measured subjects' reaction time to judge whether two figures of different orientations, like those in Fig. 1, depicted identical or different objects. The reaction time results and the subjects' introspections suggested that the subjects mentally rotated internal representations of the figures. The duration of the rotation process, reflected in the response time for a Same judgment, was a linearly increasing function of the angular disparity between the orientations of the two figures. Similar data have been obtained using this paradigm with a number of different stimuli, such as three dimensional cube figures (Metzler & Shepard, 1974; Shepard & Metzler, 1971), alphanumeric characters (Cooper & Shepard, 1973), drawings of human hands (Cooper & Shepard, 1975) and two dimensional nonsense shapes (Cooper, 1975; Cooper & Podgorny, 1976). However, there are some differences among the pattern of response times for the various studies. While the rotation time usually increases with the amount of rotation, the estimated rotation rate varies considerably across studies. This result requires clarification if rotation is to be considered a basic mental operation.

The purpose of this research is to characterize the component processes underlying performance in rotation tasks by monitoring concomitant eye fixation

---

[1]The order of authors is arbitrary. This paper represents a collaborative effort. This research was supported in part by Grants MH-29617 and MH-07722 from the National Institute of Mental Health, and Grant NIE-77-0007 from the National Institute of Education, all of the U.S. Department of Health, Education, and Welfare.

behavior. In the first part of the paper, we will examine whether rotation rates do vary across tasks, comparing the duration of the rotation operations for two types of stimuli. The rotation rates will be estimated from the eye fixation behavior, providing a much finer measure than can be obtained from the total reaction times. Moreover, the eye fixation behavior will provide a detailed record of the sequence of processing stages. In the second part of the paper, we will examine eye fixations in another kind of rotation task, in which one representation is encoded from a visual display and the other is retrieved from memory. Finally, we will discuss the more general relation between eye fixations and spatial operations.

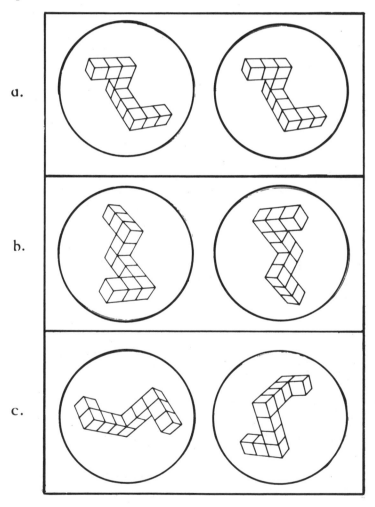

FIG. 1.   Complex three-dimensional stimulus figures: (a) a pair of Same figures with 0° disparity; (b) a pair of Same figures with 180° disparity; (c) a pair of Different figures with 120° "disparity." (From Just & Carpenter, 1976a.)

THE ROTATION OF CUBE FIGURES

In our previous research on mental rotation, we studied eye fixation performance when subjects were asked to judge whether or not two figures depict the same three-dimensional object (Just & Carpenter, 1976a). For example, Fig. 1a shows a Same trial, at 0° disparity; 1b shows a Same trial at 180° disparity; 1c shows a Different trial at 120° disparity. We were able to separate the processes in this task into three distinct stages called (1) search, (2) transformation and comparison, and (3) confirmation.

In the first stage, there is a search for segments of the two figures that superficially correspond to each other, such as the terminal segments that have three visible faces. The function of the search process is to select segments of the two figures that can potentially be transformed one into the other. During the next stage, transformation and comparison, the two chosen segments are rotated into each other. A transform-and-compare operation is applied stepwise to the representation of the two segments. Each step of the transformation may correspond to a rotation, so that at the end of the transformation the segment is represented at a new orientation. Each step of the transformation is followed by a comparison to determine whether the two orientations are now congruent. This stepwise transform-and-compare process continues until the necessary number of transformations have been made to make the internal representations of the segments sufficiently congruent in orientation. The third stage, confirmation, involves a check of whether the rotation that brought the two segments into

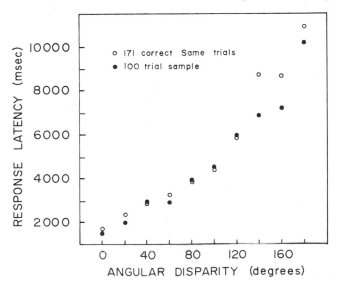

FIG. 2.   Mean response latency as a function of angular disparity for all correct Same trials and for 100 correct Same trials in which eye fixations were scored. The stimuli in this experiment were the complex three-dimensional figures. (From Just & Carpenter, 1976a.)

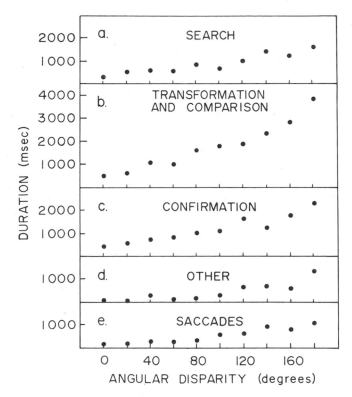

FIG. 3.   Mean duration of various processing stages in Same trials as a function of angular disparity, with complex three-dimensional stimuli. (From Just & Carpenter, 1976a.)

congruence will also bring other portions of the two figures in congruence.

The three stages were identified by the accompanying eye fixation behavior. For example, the transform-and-compare stage was identified by a pattern of repeated fixation between corresponding segments of the two figures. The search process was identified by the initial portion of the scan path that preceded transformation. Confirmation was often manifested as a comparison of the segments not fixated during the main transformation sequence. In other trials, confirmation appeared as a scan from the central point to an arm on one figure, followed by a similar scan on the other figure. Figure 2 shows the total reaction time for the Same trials. Figure 3 shows how the durations of the three stages in Same trials were affected by angular disparity. The bulk of the increase in total reaction time (as a function of angular disparity) was spent in transformation (Fig. 3b), increasing from about 500 msec at 0° to over 3500 msec at 180°. However, the search stage (Fig. 3a) and confirmation stage (Fig. 3c) also show an increase as angular disparity increases. Figure 3d presents fixations that could not be classified (about 4% of the total duration), while Fig. 3e presents the time spent in saccades (about 10% of the total duration).

HOW THE NATURE OF THE STIMULUS
AFFECTS THE ROTATION PROCESS

The three-dimensional cube figures used in the previous study of rotation are moderately complex (Just & Carpenter, 1976a; Shepard & Metzler, 1971). They are complex because they are three-dimensional, they possess four distinct segments, and the segments are not very discriminable. These complexities could affect any of the stages of processing described earlier. The next experiment examines the same rotation task, but with two-dimensional figures whose segments are more discriminable. The eye fixation behavior will be used to partition the processing into the three stages to examine the influence of stimulus complexity in rotation tasks.

Method

The task and procedure were very similar to that used in the preceding experiment. It was a Same—Different task in which the subject was timed, and her eye

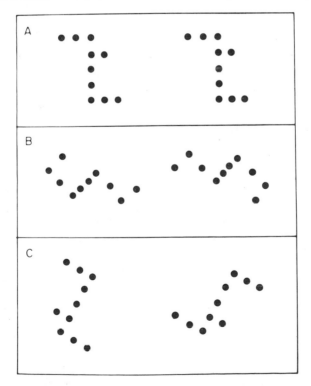

FIG. 4.   Simple two-dimensional stimulus figures: (a) a pair of Same figures with 0° disparity; (b) a pair of Same figures with 180° disparity; (c) a pair of Different figures with 0° "disparity."

fixations recorded, while she decided whether two figures depicted the same object or two objects that were mirror images of each other. The stimuli were two drawings shown in Fig. 4a and 4b plus their mirror images, for a total of four basic figures. The two figures were displayed side by side on a video monitor. The center-to-center distance between the figures was about 15° and each figure subtended about 9°. Figure 4a schematically shows a 0° Same pair; Fig. 4b shows a 180° Same pair. To construct a Different pair, the right-hand figure of a Same pair was replaced by its mirror image. Figure 4c shows a Different pair. There was a Same and a Different pair for four basic figures at each of 7 angular disparities for a total of 56 pairs of stimulus figures. Each subject had 15 practice trials and two blocks of 56 trials randomly ordered. The three paid subjects were right-handed females of college age with 20—20 corrected vision.

The locus of eye fixations was monitored by means of a corneal reflection eye-tracker that determined the coordinates of the eye spot 60 times per sec (Just & Carpenter, 1976b). Subjects initiated a trial by fixating a point that coincided with the center of the left-hand figure and pushing a "ready" button. The eye spot was calibrated with respect to this fixation point before each trial. After calibration the fixation point disappeared, and half a second later the stimulus appeared. The subject terminated a trial by responding Same or Different with the index and third finger of her dominant hand.

Results

The results for the Same trials reveal the usual increase in total response time with angular disparity, as shown in Fig. 5. The error rate was 14% for Same trials and increased with angular disparity. The error rate for Different trials was 7%.

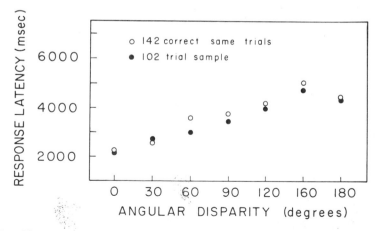

FIG. 5.   Mean response latency as a function of angular disparity for all correct Same trials and for the 102 correct Same trials in which eye fixations were scored. The stimuli in this experiment were the simpler two-dimensional figures.

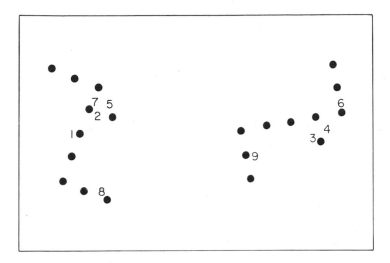

FIG. 6.   The numbers on the figure indicate the loci of successive fixations on a correct Same trial when the disparity was 60°. The subject's total response latency was 2704 msec, of which 12% had no visible eye spot. See Table 1 for the locus and duration of the fixations.

Figure 6 shows the sequence of fixations for a 60° Same trial. Fixations 2 to 7 would be classified as the transform-and-compare stage, identifiable by the sequence of repeated fixations on corresponding segments of the two figures. Fixation 1 is attributed to the initial search stage. Fixations 8 and 9 are classified as confirmation. This protocol is typical, except that most protocols showed no confirmation behavior.

The total reaction time function was decomposed into the three stages of processing, using the classification scheme outlined above. The time spent in each stage is shown in Fig. 7, for those 102 trials in which there were no head movements and the eye spot did not disappear due to apparatus failure. This

TABLE 1
Locus and Duration of the Fixations Shown in Fig. 6

Fixation	Figure	Location	Duration (msec)	
1.	Left	center	237	search
2.	Left	end with extra arm	236	
3.	Right	end with extra arm	186	
4.	Right	end with extra arm	169	transform
5.	Left	end with extra arm	388	and
6.	Right	end with extra arm	438	compare
7.	Left	end with extra arm	186	
8.	Left	end without arm	237	confirmation
9.	Right	end without arm	287	

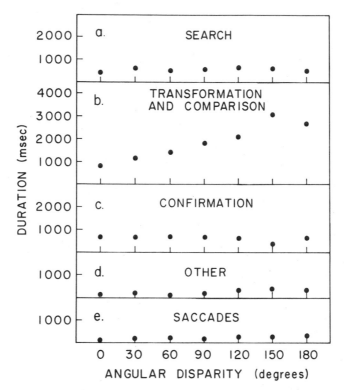

FIG. 7.   Mean duration of various processing stages in Same trials as a function of angular disparity, with two-dimensional figures.

figure indicates how increases in angular disparity affected each of the three stages. The most striking result is that the effect of angular disparity is selective and can be localized almost entirely to the transformation and comparison stage. The other two stages, initial search and confirmation, show almost no effect of angular disparity.

When the results of this analysis are compared to those in the previous experiment (Fig. 3), there is a striking difference and a striking similarity. The difference between the two patterns occurs in the search and confirmation stages. In the current task there is no effect of angular disparity, whereas in the previous study the durations of both of these stages increased with disparity. The similarity occurs in the transform-and-compare stage, where both experiments show similar increases. We will discuss the implications of both of these comparisons, beginning with an explanation for the differences in search and confirmation processes in the two experiments.

There are two procedural differences between the two experiments. One is that the current study included seven possible angular disparities spanning the 180° range, as opposed to ten in the first study. While this might affect certain aspects of the processing, it does not seem critical to the current point. The second difference, one that might be very important, is that the segments of the figures in the present study are more discriminable and are two-dimensional. These simpler figures may allow the subject, in the search and confirmation stages, to use heuristic processes whose durations are relatively insensitive to angular disparity.

When examining simpler figures, the subject quickly located a particular segment and proceeded to alternately fixate the corresponding segments on the two figures. By contrast, when examining the complex cube figures, subjects at times alternated fixations between two noncorresponding segments. This behavior increased as the angular disparity increased and was attributed to initial search. Simpler figures did not cause confusion between the segments, and hence there was no increase in initial search duration.

In addition, because the figures were treated strictly as two dimensional figures and because the two main segments of each figure were discriminable, the confirmation process was unnecessary. That is, after one segment was appropriately transformed, subjects rarely executed the confirmation process.

The comparison of this experiment and the previous one allows us to infer the effect of stimulus properties on the transform-and-compare stage. The reaction time results, and their decomposition into three stages, present a very telling story. First, it is clear that the total reaction time increases more with angular disparity for the more complex figures. The total increase, from 0° to 180°, is about 8 sec for complex figures, but only about 2.5 sec for the simple figures. However, this does not mean that with more discriminable segments, figures can be mentally rotated at a faster rate. The transformation-and-comparison functions have a very similar slope for the two kinds of stimuli. The total increase, from 0° to 180°, is about 2.2 sec for simple figures and about 3 sec for complex figures. If we consider only the range where reaction times are linear, namely between 0° and 100°, the functions are even more similar. Thus, the transformation-and-comparison stage is not greatly influenced by the complexity of the figures.

The eye fixations analysis suggests an answer to the question of why the reaction time slope is steeper when the segments of the stimulus figures are less discriminable. The fixation analysis suggests that the more complex figures do not take longer to rotate. However, the processes of selecting corresponding segments to transform, and finally confirming that the two figures are congruent after transformation, takes longer as the angular disparity increases. Thus, the durations of the search and confirmation stages increase with angular disparity for complex figures but not for simple ones. The total reaction-time slope, which is the sum of the component stage slopes, is thus steeper when the figures are complex. Of course, only three subjects were studied in each experiment, and only two types of figures were examined, so the generality of the results requires further confirmation. However, it is quite likely that figural complexity affects the stages that precede and follow the transformation-and-comparison stage, but the transformation-and-comparison rate itself is similar for the different types of figures.

Although the more complex figures produced a greater reaction-time slope, the effect could also be due to the relative discriminability of the figure segments, rather than to stimulus complexity per se. Cooper (1975) and Cooper and Podgorny (1976) examined the effects of polygon complexity on the total reaction time slope by varying the number of sides in the polygons from 6 to 24. The slopes were unaffected by this manipulation. The fact that stimulus complexity per se does not affect total reaction time slopes is compatible with the present framework. We have suggested that not necessarily all of the figure is mentally rotated; instead perhaps only one segment is selected for rotation and another for confirmation. If only one segment is selected from a figure, regardless of the figure's complexity, then rotation rates may indeed be unaffected. If the segment that distinguishes two figures from each other in a Different trial does not happen to be the one selected for transformation or confirmation, then an erroneous "Same" response should occur, as Cooper and Podgorny often found in some conditions. Perhaps an eye fixation analysis of the rotation of random polygons of varying complexity will provide a more detailed evaluation of the effect of stimulus complexity on the process of rotation.

Switches in Fixation

The transformation-and-comparison stage is identified by the alternate fixations between corresponding segments of the two stimulus figures. Therefore, the alternations themselves, or switches in fixation between the two figures, reveal some of the detail of the transformation process. In particular, each cycle of the transformation-and-comparison process may be accompanied by a switch in fixation. Table 2 shows that the mean number of switches during the transformation-and-comparison process increases with angular dispartiy. There appears to be one additional switch for each 41 or 42° in angular disparity.

The increase in switches is consistent with the processing model we have proposed for this task (Just & Carpenter, 1976a). According to the model, the transformation-and-comparison stage starts with a comparison of the orientations of the two segments. The comparison tests whether the two orientations are close enough to each other, where "close enough" is defined to be one-half of the transformation step size, or one half of 42° in this case. The 42° transformations are iteratively executed until the "close enough" test is satisfied. Thus, a 0° disparity requires no transformations and only one switch in fixation; 30° and 60° disparities require one transformation and two switches; a 90° disparity requires two transformations and three switches, and so on. The estimated and observed number of switches for each disparity is shown in Table. 2. The previous

TABLE 2
Distribution of Switches in 102 Trial Sample

| | | Mean Number of Switches During: | | |
| | | Transformation and Comparison | | |
Angular Disparity	Initial Search	Observed	Estimated[a]	Confirmation
0°	.4	1.3	1	1.4
30°	.6	1.7	2	1.2
60°	.5	2.4	2	1.2
90°	.4	3.0	3	1.2
120°	.8	3.8	4	.8
150°	1.0	5.8	5	.5
180°	.5	4.7	5	.8

[a]Estimates were derived by assuming one additional switch for every 42° in angular disparity.

research with cube-like figures showed an additional switch for every 50° in disparity. Thus, it is possible that rotation occurs in step sizes of around 40° to 50°. While the question of step size and its invariance over various experimental manipulations is still an open one, it is interesting that the two experiments yield similar estimates.

THE ROLE OF EXTERNAL STIMULI IN MENTAL ROTATION

In each of the previously described studies of mental rotation, subjects compared the representations of two objects while the figures depicting the objects were visually available. However, mental rotation can occur when one visually presented object is compared to a representation of a second object retrieved from memory. In a typical experiment of this latter type, subjects decide whether a figure depicts a normal character (such as an upper-case J) or its mirror image. The test figure is presented at one of several possible orientations. The reaction time (to decide whether the letter is normal or backward) increases monotonically as the orientation of the test figure departs from upright; decisions are fastest when the test figure is upright, and slowest when it is upside down (Cooper & Shepard, 1973).

These reaction time results can be explained in terms of mental rotation processes. To determine whether the test figure is Normal or Backward, it is necessary to compare it to a normal version of that character. The normal version is stored in memory in a canonical upright position. The test figure must be mentally rotated to that same upright orientation before the two representations can be compared. Hence, the reaction time function reflects the rotation process.

While this explanation is consistent with the reaction-time results, it leaves a number of questions unanswered. For example, is there some feature of the letter that is crucial to the rotation process, or is the entire letter transformed? In addition, it is possible to compare the processes in this task to the processes in rotation tasks where both figures are visually available. Are there distinct search, transformation, and confirmation stages when one of the figures is retrieved from semantic memory and the other is presented visually? If so, how are the various stages affected by the orientation of the test figure?

Method

Subjects were timed and their eye fixations monitored while they decided whether an alphabetic character (upper-case J, R, or L) was normal or backward. The letters appeared in one of six orientations: upright, 60° clockwise from upright, 120°, 180°, 240°, and 300°. The letter was presented either in its normal form or in a mirror image (backward) form. Thus there were 36 stimuli in total. The subjects received 15 practice trials and two test blocks of 36 trials each. The three paid subjects were right-handed females of college age with 20–20 corrected vision.

The letter was displayed on a standard video monitor and was composed of 8 to 17 asterisks that defined its contour. The major axis of the letters was 7 cm long, which subtended between 6.3° and 8.3° of visual angle, depending on the viewing distance. The procedure within a trial, and the method of monitoring eye fixations, was identical to that in the preceding experiment. Subjects initiated a trial by fixating a point that coincided with the center of the letter and pushing a "ready" button. When the eye spot was calibrated, the fixation point disappeared, and half a second later the stimulus appeared. The subject responded Normal or Backward by pressing one of two microswitches with the index and third finger of her dominant hand.

Results

The data reported are only for trials with the letter J, because a clearly localized critical feature, the curve at the base, distinguishes a normal from a backward J. (By contrast, the critical feature of the L, the stroke at the bottom, is not as localized since subjects must first compare the relative lengths of the stroke and stem.) The response latencies for all three subjects showed the usual orientation effect, so that latencies increased monotonically as the orientation of the stimulus letter departed from upright. Thus, the subjects showed the same reaction time pattern as Cooper and Shepard's (1973) subjects. The total response times for two subjects are labelled "control experiment" in Fig. 8.

The eye fixation data reveal a little more detail about what the subjects are doing. On 23% of the trials, there was only one fixation. The fixations were generally located at the center of the letter, approximately at the locus of the

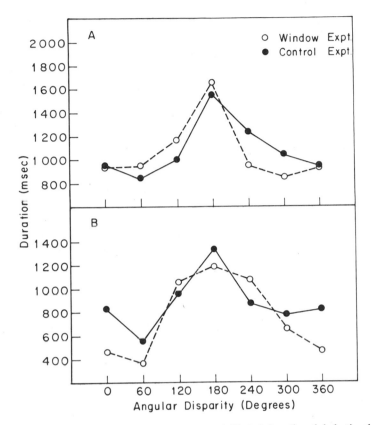

FIG. 8.   Mean duration for two subjects (A and B) judging the alphabetic character "J." The filled circles indicate the total response latency in the control experiment as a function of the test figure's angular departure from upright. The unfilled circles indicate the duration of gaze on the critical feature in the window experiment as a function of the test figure's angular departure from upright.

pretrial calibration point. Since subjects performed accurately, they must have been encoding the critical feature from about 3° or 4° away from the center of the fovea. On 68% of the trials there were two fixations, and on 9% of the trials there were more than two. On these trials, there was some tendency to directly fixate the critical feature. The eye fixation behavior is clear but, unfortunately, not rich enough to allow a decomposition of the performance into component stages. There appears to be little visual search or scanning behavior in this task. Most of the ongoing mental operations are executed in the absence of corresponding eye fixations.

The study replicates Cooper and Shepard's reaction time findings but, more importantly, it provides a baseline measure of the eye-fixation behavior. These baseline data provide a standard against which to compare the results of the next study in which subjects are forced to search for the critical feature. This next study will be called the window experiment, for reasons that will become clear.

Method

This experiment was like the previous one, except that the only asterisks that were displayed fit in a rectangular window that was 6 cm high and 4.5 cm wide whose center was the point of fixation. This window was small enough so that not all of the letter was visible even if the exact center of the letter was fixated. As the subject's point of fixation moved, the window moved with it arriving no later than 33 msec after the eye. The subjects were the same three as in the previous experiment. The order of conditions was balanced across subjects.

Results

The total reaction times in this condition were generally longer than in the previous experiment and showed no systematic relation to the orientation of the letter. However, the eye fixation protocols usually indicated two stages: a search for the critical feature, and then a prolonged fixation on that feature.

Perhaps the most important aspect of these data is the duration of fixation on the critical feature. This duration, unlike the total reaction time, increased monotonically with the letter's deviation from upright. The data for the forward J for two subjects are shown by the broken lines in Fig. 8. These are the same two subjects whose total reaction times were plotted in the previous control experiment. One of the three subjects, whose data are not shown, showed the usual results in the previous experiment but had difficulty in using the video window. Her total and component reaction times were extremely long and not systematically related to the orientation of the test figure. For the remaining two subjects, the duration of fixation on the critical feature was remarkably similar to the total reaction time function in the control experiment, as Fig. 8 indicates. The control and window experiments have a common transformation and comparison stage, and we suggest that it is this stage that shows the same temporal characteristics in both experiments.

In these experiments with alphabetic stimuli, two representations are compared: one is initially encoded from the visually presented letter, and the other is a canonical representation retrieved from memory. The transformation and comparison process may consist of transforming one or both representation(s), comparing them to determine if they are sufficiently congruent in orientation, and deciding whether the visually presented figure is normal or reversed. In other words, the same switching between two representations, demonstrated in the previous tasks, may also occur with alphabetic comparisons. However, the switches are entirely internal and are manifested by prolonged gaze on the critical feature of the visually presented letter. This transformation-and-comparison process appears to operate on the representation of the critical feature, and not on a representation of the entire letter. In the window experiment, the transformation stage did not start until the critical feature was located in the fovea.

In the control experiment, the critical feature was always within 3° of the center of the fovea, and parafoveal encoding seemed to provide sufficient information.

The window experiment had a measurable search stage that preceded the transformation-and-comparison stage. The search stage was identifiable by a visual search for the critical feature. The duration of the search stage depend on the location of the critical feature and the subject's scanning pattern. The location of the critical feature is letter-specific. For example, the feature that distinguishes a normal J from a backward one (Ⴑ) is at the base, but the critical feature for R is at the middle or top. Subjects tended to scan from top to bottom and, in general, the search for the critical features consumed as much time as it takes for the top-to-bottom scan to locate the feature. In the case of the J, the search is shortest when the critical feature is at the top, that is, when the figure is rotated 180° from upright. Thus, the duration of the search for the critical feature, and hence the time it takes to identify the letter, varies with the relative position of the critical feature in a top-to-bottom scan.

It is interesting to compare the current task involving one visual figure and one retrieved from memory to the preceding experiments that involved two visually presented figures. Both tasks involve a transformation-and-comparison operation whose duration increases monotonically with the amount of rotation. Both tasks may involve an initial search for a critical feature. However, when the entire letter can be encoded in foveal and parafoveal vision (as in the control experiment), the search stage is unnecessary or very short in duration. Finally, there was only some slight evidence of confirmation with alphabetic stimuli; one subject often rescanned the figure after gazing on the critical feature, but the other subject did not.

There were some notable differences between the results for the two kinds of tasks. First, the reaction time difference between 0° and 180° is much smaller in the alphabetic task, only about 600msec, compared to the estimated rotation time of about 2600 msec in the tasks with two visually presented stimuli. Second, the alphabetic task shows more curvilinearity, with very short rotation times at the smaller departures from upright. While the experiments do not allow strong conclusions about the reason for the discrepancies, several possibilities suggest themselves.

One possibility is that the rotate-and-compare operation is faster when the attention switches are totally internal, as in the task involving alphabetic comparisons, and slower when there are overt switches in eye fixation between two visual objects. Alternatively, it is possible that mental rotation is not a uniform phenomenon and that the rotation rates are influenced by factors such as the familiarity of the stimuli. A third possibility is that subjects do not always have to rotate a familiar figure to upright in order to judge whether it is a normal or mirror-image figure. Cooper & Shepard (1973) suggested that incomplete rotation would result in the marked curvilinearity observed with alphanumeric stimuli. It would also explain the attenuation in estimated rotation times, since the rotation function would include trials in which subjects were able to make a decision without performing a mental rotation but instead would use some orientation-invariant features. Thus, it would be extremely difficult to determine the precise rotation rate for alphabetic or familiar stimuli.

In summary, the processes underlying mental rotation can be studied in detail by examining the eye fixations that occur in performing the task. The fine structure of the performance changes is sensitive to task parameters like stimulus complexity. The nature of the modification of the process may not be revealed in the pattern of total reaction times, but can be examined by an analysis of the eye fixation behavior.

CORRELATIONS BETWEEN EYE FIXATIONS AND MENTAL OPERATIONS

Our analysis of eye fixations assumes that the eye tends to fixate the referent of the symbol being operated on. But what is the cause of this correspondence? Do the eye fixations play any functional role? To answer these questions, we will consider the possible functions of eye fixations in three categories of mental operations.

Encoding operations

Encoding refers to the process of generating an internal symbol or code for an external stimulus. Observers tend to fixate the object they are encoding. Such foveal fixations may allow more detail to be coded or allow the object to be discriminated and identified. The relation between eye fixations and encoding operations can be easily demonstrated and intuitively explained.

Retrieval Operations

Retrieval refers to the transfer of information from an internal memory system to short-term memory. Eye fixations often are associated with retrieval from long-term to short-term memory. For example, suppose a subject is shown a picture depicting a tree, a car, a person, and an airplane. If the subject is asked to name all the kinds of trees he knows, he will look at the tree while answering (Kahneman & Lass, 1971). More important, the subject will fixate that same location even if the pictures are removed prior to the question. Thus, the retrieval of information from long-term memory is accompanied by a fixation to a physical location that contains or contained an item associated with the information being retrieved.

Before discussing the role of such fixations, consider another situation where a retrieval operation between two other memory systems is accompanied by a seemingly functionless fixation. Suppose a 3 x 3 array of letters is briefly flashed onto a subject's retina, and a short time later the subject is signalled as to which row of letters to report, as in the Sperling (1960) partial report paradigm. Subjects tend to move their eyes in the direction of the cued row, even though the visual array is no longer present (Hall, 1974). As they attempt to retrieve information from iconic memory for transfer to short-term memory, they fixate the *former* spatial location of the to-be-retrieved row of letters.

In both of these situations, eye fixations are correlated with memory retrieval. The reason for this correlation may be that the spatial position of an element plays an organization role in visual tasks. The position of an element in space may be coded along with other attributes of the element, so that positional information may subsequently be used to index the element. Such spatial indexing is used in the mnemonic strategy called the method of loci. This mnemonic relies on the intentional association between an item and a spatial location; during recall, the location is accessed in order to retrieve the identity of the associated item. It appears that the spatial position information per se facilitates retrieval (Byrne, 1974). The method of loci is an extreme form of spatial organization, where the spatial index is coded intentionally. In tasks like those described here, the spatial location of an element may be coded incidentally. The eye fixations that accompany the retrieval of the information may reflect the internal indexing of that spatial information. This interpretation explains why subjects appear to be scanning an icon fixed on the retina, and why they look at the position of a previously shown picture. In both of these cases, the original information is apparently indexed by its spatial coordinates rather than its retinal position. The eye fixations reflect the fact that the subject is tapping the spatial organization of the original information when he is trying to retrieve the item.

This kind of spatial-index fixation appears to play no encoding role. In fact, when the retrieval function and encoding function are pitted against each other, the retrieval function sometimes dominates. For example, Rosen (1977) monitored the eye fixations of subjects doing the same simple addition problem twice. On some trials, one of the digits in the problem was altered without the subject's knowledge, so that the previous answer was no longer correct. The subject often reported the incorrect answer, even after directly fixating the changed digit. Thus, while fixating the changed digit, he must have been retrieving the value of the old digit rather than encoding the new digit. Memory retrieval dominated over encoding. The eye fixation at a given location was associated with retrieval of information indexed to that location. A goal for future research is to determine whether this indexing facilitates recall, and whether the eye fixations are necessary for spatial indexing or simply tend to be correlated with the indexing.

Transformation Operations

Transformation operations take as input spatial information and execute a spatial transformation, such as rotation or translation. The current research and some of our previous work (Carpenter & Just, 1976; Just & Carpenter, 1976a) suggests that eye fixations are correlated with these transformation operations. For example, in the rotation task involving alphabetic characters, the subject mentally rotated the critical feature of the J, and while he did this, he continued to fixate the critical feature. This is true even though the orientation of the visually presented J will not correspond to the orientation of his updated internal representation. Why are eye fixations correlated with the underlying spatial operations? One possible answer might be that an asynchrony between fixations and underlying operations would interfere with processing. For example, if the subject's gaze were to wander off, it might initiate some new encoding operation that would interrupt or slow down the priority processing. For that reason, there could be a general rule that the eye should continue to fixate the referent of the symbol that is operated upon. An alternative explanation for the correlation is that the eye fixations are controlled by a command to gather information. The mechanism that commands the eye may be occupied during a transformation, and hence issues no movement command. The absence of a command leaves the eye fixation at the position where the last encoded information is currently being transformed.

In the various situations cited, the relation between eye fixations and underlying mental processes may or may not be functional, but it appears that it does provide a valuable source of evidence for cognitive research. By optimizing certain task conditions — for example, by using speeded tasks and by minimizing peripheral encoding — the eye fixations can provide a useful trace of the underlying mental operations. In particular, fixations may provide a fruitful way to track spatial information processing.

DISCUSSION

COOPER: What criteria did you use to determine when search ends and transformation and comparison begins, and when confirmation begins?

JUST: A sequence of consecutive fixations between corresponding segments of the two figures was classified as transformation and comparison. The fixation before such a sequence was classified as initial search. Consecutive fixations on other segments were classified as confirmation. Some fixations could not be classified except as "other." With these criteria, it was relatively straightforward to analyze the sequence of fixations within a trial.

COOPER: Is it important that the transformation and comparison gaze time function be a linearly increasing function of angular disparity?

JUST: In terms of the general point that the eye fixations reflect the rotation process, the linearity does not have any special significance. The linearity or nonlinearity might influence the characteristics of the model of the rotation process.

COOPER: Is there much variation between subjects in the reaction time functions?

JUST: The individual reaction time results for the three subjects in the experiment with the complex figures are reported in Just and Carpenter (1976a). The functions for the three subjects are remarkably similar. Of course, these are data for only three subjects, and not all subjects can perform this mental rotation task.

MOORE: Is it possible that the mental rotation process is very quick, almost instantaneous, and that most of the transformation and comparison stage is taken up by looking back and forth?

JUST: The actual saccades, the movements back and forth between the two figures, take only a small proportion of the time, less than 10%. This saccade time is not part of the time labelled "transformation and comparison." However, it is true that the rotation process could be very quick and that the comparison process might consume much of the time labelled "transformation and comparison." With this technique, it is impossible to separate the transformation process and the comparison process.

VAUGHAN: Have you looked at the duration of individual fixations when a particular comparison is made, say, as a function of the stimulus complexity?

JUST: The durations of individual fixations appear to be weakly related to underlying mental processes. The average duration of a fixation increases with angular disparity, from about 200 msec at 0° to 320 msec at 180° disparity, but we found no other relation between durations of individual fixations and the concomitant mental processing. In general, I don't think that the durations of individual fixations map closely onto the cognitive processes analyzed with this model. Rather, it appears that gaze time is a more appropriate measure, and this does seem to be reliably related to the underlying processes.

ZIEDMAN: Have you looked at the eye movements of people who cannot perform this task to see if they differ from those who can and to try to train those who cannot?

JUST: We have not studied subjects who cannot perform the task. The reason is that it is difficult to do a precise analysis of the sequence of eye fixations when you don't know what the subjects are doing, as in the case for people who can't perform the task. If subjects were doing something systematic but incorrect, then there should be some potential for analyzing their eye fixation protocols.

III.2

Control of Visual Fixation Duration in Search[1]

Jonathan Vaughan
Hamilton College

When we read, search for a target, or simply look around the world, our visual input comes to us in discrete units. While the flow of visual information appears to us to be continuous, it is easy to show that people move their gaze from one place to another discontinuously. The experiments reported here are directed at the general question of how visual information processing is synchronized with this discontinuous visual input. More specifically, they have investigated how the duration of individual fixations is controlled during search. It is clear that two broad classes of factors affect fixation duration: both stimulus factors — for example, stimulus clarity, novelty, etc. — and oculomotor factors — for example, the minimum time it takes for a saccade to be initiated — will contribute to the control of the duration of fixations.

The experiments are aimed at dissociating stimulus and oculomotor factors by imposing a delay between the beginning of each fixation and the onset of the stimulus to be viewed during that fixation. The task that the subject has been given is simply to search between two stimulus alternatives, the letters X and O, with the O always the target stimulus. Obviously, the results will not be directly generalizeable to more complicated situations such as reading, but they may give us an indication of where to look in the reading situation in order to understand the control of fixation durations.

The general paradigm of the experiments is shown in the first figure. The subjects viewed a computer-controlled oscilloscope display about 38 cm away

---

[1]A brief version of this paper was read at the November, 1976, meetings of the Psychonomic Society in St. Louis. A number of my students have contributed to this research at its various stages. I thank Arthur A. Stone and Thomas M. Graefe, in particular, for their devotion to the project. The research reported here was supported by Grant MH 26303 from the National Institute of Mental Health.

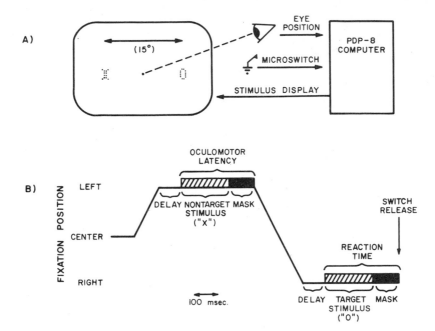

FIG. 1.   (A) The stimulus display (left) and apparatus used; (B) the sequence of stimuli presented in a typical trial. A fixation on a nontarget stimulus on the left was followed by a fixation on a target stimulus on the right. Stimulus onset delay was 90 msec and stimulus duration was 200 msec. Note that the oculomotor latency and reaction time are measured from stimulus onset and that oculomotor latency plus stimulus onset delay equals fixation duration.

while eye position was recorded using the electrooculogram. The stimuli were presented only when the subjects were looking at them (± 2.5 deg). Thus, there could be no contribution of peripheral cues to the detection of the stimulus or initiation of saccades. Stimuli were the characters X or O, generated in a 4 x 6 dot matrix subtending about 1 deg x ½ deg, and separated by 15 deg of visual angle.

The sequence of events in a trial was as follows: Subjects began by fixating on a center fixation point, giving the computer a calibration of the electrooculogram recording. Following calibration, fixation points appeared at the left and at the right fixation locations, and the subjects searched for the character O by alternately fixating those locations. On a typical trial a subject might have made 3 fixations in which the nontarget stimulus (the X) was seen, then on the fourth fixation the O appeared. When the target appeared the subject reported its presence by releasing a microswitch. Failure to report the target until after a fixation on the other side was considered an "overshoot" error. The number of Xs that preceded the target (O) stimulus varied from 0–6, randomly, from trial to trial.

The sequence of events during each fixation of a trial had three phases. First, from the beginning of the fixation for a time that was varied from 0–150 msec, the display was unchanged. Then the stimulus, X or O, was presented for 50–300 msec at the point of fixation, and was followed (in some experiments) by a masking pattern (random visual noise or a matrix of 24 dots) superimposed on the location of the stimulus. It should be noted that because the duration of the stimulus and the stimulus onset delay were varied from trial to trial or from fixation to fixation, the length of time (from the beginning of the fixation) that was required for detection and encoding of a particular stimulus varied from one fixation to another.

There were two dependent measures. The first, oculomotor latency, was simply the time between the onset of each of the *nontarget* stimuli and the beginning of the saccade away from it. Because of the stimulus onset delay imposed, the stimulus was not there for the whole duration of the fixation; so we measured oculomotor latency, instead of fixation duration.

The second dependent measure was reaction time, measured from the onset of the *target* stimulus until the instant that the subject released the microswitch. Each experiment used four or five subjects, with five sessions of about 150 trials each. The delay and stimulus duration were randomized either between or within trials, depending on the experiment. Practiced subjects easily maintained 90–95% accuracy levels.

There are two extreme strategies that subjects might follow for controlling the duration of their fixations in this situation. First, they might use a "sequential control" strategy, in which the duration of each fixation is determined by the time required to process the stimulus once it comes on. Having begun a fixation, subjects would wait out the delay and then continue to fixate for as long as necessary to process the stimulus. Oculomotor latency would then be constant for all stimulus onset delays.

Second, subjects might use a "preprogramming" strategy, in which the duration of fixations is controlled independently of the processing of the visual information. In this strategy subjects would preprogram a series of fixations of constant duration so that the duration would be long enough to process the stimulus no matter how long the delay was. In such a strategy the length of the delay would have no effect on fixation duration, and the slope of oculomotor latency as a function of stimulus onset delay would be -1.

Additionally, subjects might mix strategies, so that the duration of fixations would be preprogrammed at a value that was sufficient to process most of the stimuli. This would suffice unless the delay was particularly long or the stimulus was particularly difficult to process, in which case the subject would switch to the sequential control strategy.

There are advantages and disadvantages to both extreme strategies. The preprogramming strategy would waste time on all those fixations when the stimulus onset delay was short or when the stimulus was easy to process. On the other

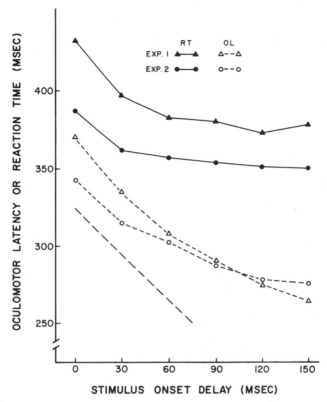

FIG. 2.   Reaction time and oculomotor latency at each stimulus onset delay, Experiments 1 and 2. The dashed line has a slope of -1.

hand, the sequential control strategy would impose on the observer the task of deciding, within each fixation, exactly how long to fixate. Thus, it would require an oculomotor reaction time during each fixation, an operation which might be relatively inefficient. A mixture of strategies may be viewed as a compromise or trade-off between these disadvantages.

Figure 2 shows the data for oculomotor latency and reaction time of two experiments in which stimulus onset delay was varied from 0 − 150 msec. Although the two experiments differed in several procedural details, these do not appear to have affected the results significantly. The most interesting result is the relatively steep slope of the oculomotor latency function. If the subjects were using a pure preprogramming strategy, the slope of the function ought to be −1 (indicated for comparison by the dashed line). It is clear that the oculomotor, but not the reaction time data, approach this slope at the shorter delays (0 − 90 msec). In a separate control experiment (Graefe & Vaughan, 1978) we compared the use of eye or finger movement as a target reporting responses and found no significant difference between the reaction time functions. While there is clear evidence that a warning stimulus foreperiod effect (Bertelson, 1967) and perhaps saccadic suppression (Volkmann, Schick, & Riggs, 1968) may have contributed to a decrease in both reaction time and oculomotor latencies at the very short stimulus onset delays (up to 30 msec), the steeper slope for oculomotor latency at longer delays cannot be accounted for by such factors (see Graefe & Vaughan, 1978; Vaughan & Graefe, 1977). The difference in slope between oculomotor latency and reaction time is most parsimoniously attributed, then, to the use of a preprogramming strategy for the control of fixation durations at delays up to 90 msec.

To examine strategies more closely, two manipulations are suggested that might lead to a flatter oculomotor latency function. The first comes from increasing the time required for processing the stimulus. Stimulus quality is impaired and processing time increased with a short stimulus duration (if it is followed by a mask). Furthermore, the time available for processing during a fixation of preprogrammed duration is less when the stimulus onset delay is greater. In either case, it is more likely that the information processing requirement will exceed a preprogrammed fixation duration. Thus, the slope of the oculomotor latency function ought to be flatter when stimulus duration is short, or the delay is long. Just these trends are evident in both experiments: short stimulus durations increase oculomotor latency only at the longer delays, and have no consistent effect at the shorter.

The second manipulation has to do with how stimulus onset delay is varied. If a subject using a preprogramming strategy could set the preprogrammed fixation duration more accurately in a situation where the stimulus onset delay was kept constant for a block of trials, we would expect a flatter oculomotor latency function. Recently, six subjects were presented with a single stimulus onset delay throughout some sessions, while stimulus onset delay was changed randomly from fixation to fixation during alternate sessions. All subjects showed nearly flat oculomotor latency functions in the constant stimulus onset delay sessions, while negative slopes (some approaching −1) were again observed in the variable stimulus onset delay sessions.

The preprogramming strategy would be of particular advantage to a subject in the situation where the time required to process each stimulus varied because of stimulus characteristics. It would not be of such great advantage if every stimulus required the same time to process, since, in the latter case, a saccade could be programmed to occur at a fixed time after stimulus onset. We have data that suggest that the more variable the stimulus processing time required (because of variable stimulus duration or masking conditions) the steeper the slope of the oculomotor latency function. When the stimulus is neither masked nor degraded, and stays on for the entire duration of the fixation, the function is flatter; while the steepest function (approaching a slope of −1) occurs when the stimulus duration is varied randomly (100–300 msec), and is followed by a noise mask for the remainder of the fixation.

Now let us turn to the implications of these results for performance in more complex tasks. Could subjects perform well in reading or search if the time of presentation of each stimulus were nearly constant because of preprogrammed fixation durations? Recently, a number of studies have demonstrated that the perception of visual material is not adversely impaired when the subject does not control the time of presentation of each stimulus. Bouma and deVoogd (1974), Kolers and Katzman (1966), Kolers and Lewis (1972), and Travers (1973, 1975) have each investigated situations in which a series of stimuli is presented in fixed temporal sequence at the same location on the retina, and each has found that performance is not impaired when the duration of each stimulus is constant (about 250 msec). For example, Bouma and deVoogd (1974) presented to the stationary eye a sequence of retinal stimuli that simulated those which occurred in normal reading. Part of a line of type was presented for a duration of 200–1300 msec; then the line was presented again, displaced laterally by the average distance of a saccade in normal reading. Comprehension was not found to be seriously affected over a wide range of presentation durations, so Bouma and deVoogd concluded that there is no need for precise programming of the duration of each fixation in normal reading. The present experiments show that, in fact, under some conditions, subjects may not exercise fixation-by-fixation control even when they do have the option to do so.

What might be the advantage of relinquishing fixation-by-fixation control of duration in reading? It might serve to avoid the complications of the psychological refractory period in this complex processing situation. Russo has elaborated on this in his theoretical discussion of the control of fixation duration elsewhere in this volume. If the duration of each fixation had to be determined after all the processing within that fixation, the reaction time for that determination might set an abnormally low upper limit on reading or search speed. Bouma and deVoogd (1974) have proposed a model that avoids this problem by using a buffer that is filled with only indirect regulation of its capacity. Visual information would be acquired to fill the buffer at a constant rate, while processing the information would occur at a variable rate. If the buffer could accommodate the information of at least a few fixations, the constant rate of information acquisition could be equated to the average rate at which the information was processed.

Similarly, in the model proposed here for search, the duration of fixations would be preprogrammed to accommodate the majority of stimuli to be processed. In this search task, unlike reading, there cannot be a buffer, so the duration of individual fixations would have to be lengthened when the information processing required exceeded the preprogrammed duration. The interpretation of the data is complicated by the possibility that at least three processes may contribute to the oculomotor latency function: warning stimulus foreperiod effects, saccadic suppression, and the strategy used. Overall, the results suggest that the duration of fixations in search may be in large part independent of the visual information presented in each of those fixations.

DISCUSSION

JUST: I don't think your citation of the Bouma and deVoogd (1974) results is accurate. You say that it was observed in their experiment that simulated saccadic duration and length did not adversely affect comprehension. First, they didn't administer comprehension tests. Secondly, and very importantly, they said that their subjects couldn't even do the task if they were told that a comprehension task would be administered. I interpret that as evidence that the procedure definitely did adversely affect comprehension.

So the issue is, does their experiment show that experimenter-controlled simulated saccadic durations and length did not affect comprehension?

VAUGHAN: I'll have to look at their discussion of comprehension again to answer that.

LOFTUS: I'd like to go back to a question I asked earlier about the probability of the target stimulus varying over the fixations. Did you look at the data as a function of where in the trial the target was presented?

VAUGHAN: One sort of data that I've been able to analyze in detail is the number of nontarget stimuli before the reported target on each trial. This varies between 2 and 6, and there were an equal number of trials with each number of nontarget stimuli, so the probability of a target is 0 on the first and second fixation (because there are always at least two nontargets), and then on the third fixation the probability of the target is .2 and it grows from there to be, after 6 fixations, 1.0. The oculomotor latency data show a shift in level as the probability of the stimulus varies, but there's no change in slope. The same with the manual reaction time data: the general shape of the curve is maintained over a wide range of stimulus probability.

RUSSO: Could you say something about the role of experience in preprogrammed strategy? Do the subjects get better at it — is it an automatic strategy or do they have to learn it in some sense?

VAUGHAN: Well, everybody who does eye movement research knows it is not easy to take a naive subject into the lab and get data the same day. All of the subjects that I've looked at have had at least four or five sessions before we've been able to get reliable data, and I have not gone through those sessions where the relatively low accuracy might affect the results.

RUSSO: By relatively low you mean the first session is low and the accuracy goes up?

VAUGHAN: The accuracy is 40% in the first session, then, 50, 70, and by session 5 or 6 they're all over 90%. Then we start getting data for the archives. So, I don't know what strictly naive subjects do, but these are still not highly practiced subjects. In the last study they were all serving in their first experiment, except for one subject who was in her second experiment.

Afterthoughts

VAUGHAN: Just was quite correct in his comment after my talk that Bouma and deVoogd (1974) administered no direct test of comprehension after this "linestep" reading task. Pilot experiments had shown that reading for comprehension interfered with keeping the eyes steady in the linestep reading condition. The evidence for comprehension is subjective: "The observers differed in their estimates of whether they had understood the meaning of the text in linestep reading. A difficulty is that attention is very much focused on keeping the eyes steady. Although this does not interfere with speed of reading, it is likely to interfere with memorizing. We have little doubt that some observers followed the general meaning of the text quite well." (Bouma & deVoodg, 1974, p. 278).

The data on the effect of target stimulus probability on oculomotor latency that Loftus asked about may be found in Vaughan and Graefe (1977).

Part IV

READING PROCESSES

IV.1

Eye Movements, Reading, and Cognition[1]

John A. Stern
Washington University

Our concern with the recording of eye movements during reading is based in part on the premise that such data can be used to make inferences about information processing strategies utilized during reading for specific purposes. Whereas a plethora of techniques for recording eye movements are available to the investigator, the techniques for data reduction are considerably less plentiful. Though many manufacturers of eye tracking equipment make claims for the ready translation of their signals into computer processable format, few if any offer more than pious platitudes when it comes to reducing the mountains of digitized data that are so readily collected.

Our research on visual search activity during reading was preceded by research in which eye movements of helicopter pilots were monitored. Those efforts in part determined our present data acquisition procedures. The single degree of control we generally exert is that the reading material is placed on a stand in front of the reader at a distance and angle selected by him. We choose electrooculography for the recording of eye movements since under "inclement" or "hostile" conditions such as recording on persons piloting helicopters (Stern & Bynum, 1970), this procedure, in our opinion, produced the least artifacts. Although in some eye movement research it is desirable to retain data that fall above 100 Hz, this is not absolutely necessary for analyses of saccadic eye movements during reading. Since, in most of our computer analyses we sample data at 10 msec intervals, and since at this sampling frequency one cannot faithfully represent sine waves exceeding 50 Hz, it seemed to us unnecessary to record data in excess of 100 Hz.

---

[1]This research supported in part by NSF Grant No. EPP75-15388 and NIAAA Research Grant No. 5 R01 AA00301.

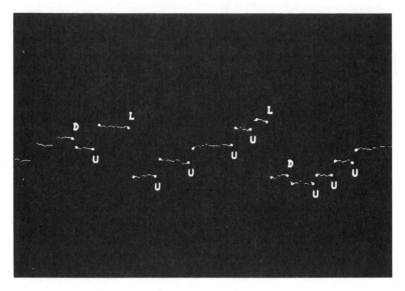

FIG. 1.   Digitized and computer labeled EOG during reading; L, D, and U refer to line change, regressive, and right-going saccades, respectively. Time is read from left to right.

Analog signals are digitized at 10 msec intervals. The program for the analysis of eye movements during reading performs the following operations:

1. Identification of saccades (a number of amplitude criteria can be applied for the defining of a saccade).
2. Identification of saccade direction (*R*ight; *L*eft).
3. Identification of left-going saccades associated with a line change.
4. Saccade amplitude determination.
5. Saccade duration determination.
6. Peak velocity of saccade determination.
7. Fixation pause duration (termination of one saccade to initiation of the next one).
8. Eye position "drift" between saccades.
9. Time to read a line.
10. A number of artifact detection routines.

Concurrently with data abstraction identified above, the computer displays the A–D converted signals on the oscilloscope display, and with a dot intensification program marks saccade onset and termination and labels saccade direction as shown in Fig. 1.

Upon completion of data processing the operator can call for a print-out of the raw data abstracted (Table 1 depicts a portion of the raw data print-out), and/or for a number of data reduction or summarization procedures (Table 2).

TABLE 1
Computer Generated Analysis of
Eye Movement Data During Reading

309	176							
REALTIME	TIMEFIX	DUR	DRIFT	AMPL	PEAK	OVF	PTRN	
0.62	0.62	0.05	0	662	370	#*$	R	
1.21	0.54	0.03	36	42	20	< R		
2.10	0.86	0.09	6	-266	-52		LINE	2.10	480
2.39	0.20	0.03	22	46	22		R	
2.64	0.22	0.02	14	40	22		R	
3.21	0.55	0.04	52	52	16		R	
3.70	0.45	0.06	14	-230	-48		LINE	1.60	10
4.81	1.05	0.04	34	58	18		R	
5.12	0.27	A 03	62	32	12		K	
5.50	0.35	0 03	28	44	20		R	
5.86	0.33	0 06	-18	-208	-46		LINE	2.16	32
6.15	0.23	0.03	-28	34	16		R	
6.46	0.28	0.02	-20	46	24		R	
6.76	0.28	0.03	-10	42	16		R	
7.64	0.85	0.06	36	-240	-56		LINE	1.78	-140
7.93	0.23	0.03	-18	38	16		R	
8.15	0.19	0.03	16	38	14		R	
8.32	0.14	0.07	-10	50	22		R	
8.64	0.25	0.03	-18	34	18		R	
9.13	0.46	0.03	-16	34	14		R	
9.37	0.21	0 03	-20	32	16		R	
9.90	0.50	0.06	20	-226	-50	< LINE	2.26	-46
10.13	0.17	0.03	-40	46	24		R	
11.54	1.38	0.07	88	60	18	< R		
12.18	0.57	0.06	4	-230	-58	< LINE	2.28	-72
12.47	0.23	0.03	16	38	16		R	
12.78	0.28	0.05	6	38	16		R	
13.04	0.21	0.03	-26	50	22		R	
13.91	0.84	0.04	26	42	14	< R		
14.20	0.25	0.03	-24	34	14		R	
14.65	0.42	0.07	26	-266	-54		LINE	2.47	-40
15.21	0.49	0.02	-2	32	20		R	
15.70	0.47	0.05	16	42	12		R	
16.11	0.36	0.05	-6	60	16		R	
16.43	0.27	0.04	-18	56	20	< R		
16.81	0.34	0.07	40	-242	-48	< LINE	2.16	-22

Rather than describe these procedures in detail, let me review some of our results which make use of these data reduction programs. Our first study (Hawley, Stern, & Chen, 1974) evaluated eye movement patterns in college students reading short stories for enjoyment. For any one subject, a minimum of 50 lines of reading were analyzed. We replicated some earlier findings (Huey, 1908) such as demonstrating that the first fixation pause on a line is significantly longer than any other fixation pause. We found that fixation pauses preceded and followed by right-going saccades (R-R fixation pauses) were considerably shorter than the averages identified by other researchers (Taylor, Frackenpohl, & Pettee, 1960; Tinker, 1951). Ours averaged 240 msec, with one of our competent readers utilizing fixation pauses averaging 150 msec, while theirs averaged around 250 msec. More novel findings were that fixation pauses preceding regressions (R–L) as well as those following regressive (L R) were significantly shorter than R–R fixation pauses.

TABLE 2
Data for Saccades Abstracted from Data
Shown in Table 1

TIME	LINES	PLINE	PLNC
105.05	46	33	42

A. 5ACCADS PER LINE

I	T:LN	L:LN	R:LN	PR:LN	L:LNC
00	0	33	0	0	42
01	2	8	2	2	4
02	4	4	4	4	0
03	9	0	12	9	0
04	13	1	13	12	0
05	8	0	7	5	0
06	3	0	2	1	0
07	1	0	2	0	0
08	1	0	2	0	0
09	2	0	1	0	0
10	2	0	1	0	0
11	0	0	0	0	0
12	0	0	0	0	0
13	0	0	0	0	0
14	1	0	0	0	0
15	0	0	0	0	0
	46	46	46	33	46

Our interpretation of these results, inferences drawn about information abstraction, are that these subjects abort information abstraction in the fixation pause preceding a regression because they realize that they have to regress to an earlier portion of the display to retrieve or reread some information. They apparently know exactly where this information is displayed, because most regressions are single regressive eye movements; they also must have a good idea as to what it is they are looking for, as this fixation pause also is significantly shorter than the "normal" R–R fixation pauses.

We were also concerned with time of day and time on task effects. Subjects came to the laboratory and read for 45 min on each of two occasions, the first during the morning hours (8–11 AM), and the second during the early evening (7–10 PM). Eye movement information was sampled during the first and last 5-min periods of each session over approximately 50 lines of text. A gross measure, like average time to read a line, showed no significant effect of time of day, but significant effects were evidenced as a function of time on task for the evening reading session. More time was required to read a line during the last 5 min of the evening reading session than either early in that session or in the comparable time (on task) period during the morning session. These results, shown in Fig. 2 suggest that measurable "fatigue" effects do occur.

A second series of studies examined the effects of psychoactive medication, such as diazepam (Valium) and alcohol, on aspects of eye movements during reading. Both drugs produced significant reduction in speed of saccadic eye movements. Because of our relatively slow sampling rate, we were able to evaluate duration and peak velocity only of large amplitude saccades, specifically those associated with the line change. Finding reductions in peak velocity is not unique to reading, but similar results were obtained when subjects "drove" our automobile simulator. Gentles & Llewellyn-Thomas (1971) obtained similar results under conditions where the subject was asked simply to shift eye position between two points approximately 20° apart. Interestingly, no change in cognitive information processing strategies as manifested in alterations in eye movement patterns were found with either of the drugs. It should be pointed out, however, that the alcohol dosage used was very low, 35 mgm%, and that the effect of diazepam was evaluated under "chronic" conditions.

Two studies dealing more specifically with information processing during reading will illustrate further efforts. A doctoral dissertation by Goltz (1975) evaluated how "competent" and "less competent" college students read historical texts when instructed to read for either general or detailed information. A number of significant effects were found. Competent readers, regardless of the instruction condition, utilized significantly shorter fixation pauses (R–R type)

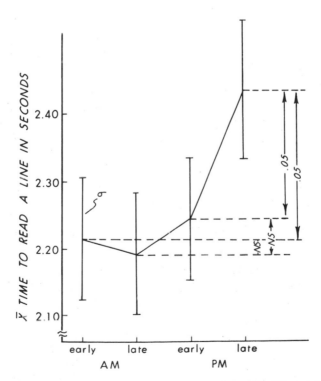

FIG. 2.   Average time to read a line of text, early (minutes 5–10) and late (minutes 40–45) in a session.

than their less competent colleagues. The effect of reading for general versus detailed information also produced differences. Competent readers demonstrated a small but highly significant increase in R–R fixation pause durations (190 to 200 msec) without a change in saccade amplitude. In other words, the effect of increasing information abstracting demands caused these readers to lengthen dwell time on "informational chunks" without altering the chunk size.

Less competent readers, on the other hand, manifested no change in fixation pause duration (240 msec under both instructional sets). However, they significantly reduced saccade amplitude, and, of course, increased the number of fixation pauses per line when reading for detail. They adjusted to the change in information processing demands by shifting to smaller informational chunks per fixation pause. Competent and less competent college age readers reading historical text thus use somewhat different strategies in abstracting information from the printed page. Whether these results can be generalized to the reading of other types of material, for different purposes, and to other age group readers remains to be seen. We suspect that such generalizing will be relatively limited.

What other differences in eye movements occurred that discriminated between groups? Looking at saccade amplitudes preceding regressive eye movements (R–R–L), we found differences between the two groups regardless of degree of information abstraction required. For less competent readers the average amplitude of right-going saccades preceding the regression was significantly larger than other R type saccades. We inferred from this that regressions for these readers occurred when they attempted to take in too large a chunk of information, one that they apparently could not abstract with one fixation pause. Our more competent readers, on the other hand, demonstrated regressive saccades when the prior two R saccades were significantly shorter than the subject's usual R type saccades. This suggests to us that the competent reader makes regressions when the material becomes more difficult for them. The greater difficulty is inferred from the smaller than usual informational chunks being abstracted prior to the regression. Thus, the inferred reasons for regressions are different for the more and less competent college age readers.

Since the written Chinese language uses symbols, or logographs, to represent words, rather than an alphabet, and the informational packing density of Chinese text per line is considerably greater than that of English text, we decided to evaluate eye movements during the reading of Chinese. Fortunately for us, modern Chinese is written from left to right, much like English text. One of our staff had Chinese as his first language and participated as a pilot subject. On many lines of text his eyes appeared to track smoothly from the beginning to the end of the line with relatively infrequent saccades and fixations. It appeared that the perception of the characters and access of meaning could be conducted at a speed that allowed for the use of pursuit rather than saccadic eye movements. With two student collaborators, V. Pollock and G. Feden, ten native Chinese readers, all undergraduate or graduate students at Washington Univeristy, were asked to read two short stories, one in Chinese and one in English. They were instructed to read for "pleasure" and told that they would not be tested for comprehension. Eye movements were recorded, but the pursuit pattern shown by our staff member was only infrequently found in this group of readers. Whether task difficulty, length of lines, reading skill level, anxiety about the testing situation or other factors accounted for the difference is not known.

We were struck by the fact that the incidence of saccades was large, not only in their reading of Chinese, but in their reading of English text as well. Although line width of text was identical in the two passages, information content per line was much greater in the Chinese than in the English passage. They averaged approximately ten saccades per line with approximately the same fixation durations.

Further, six additional students whose native language was Engligh read the English language short stories. This permitted us to evaluate the effects produced by knowledge of language, while studying the effect of initial training in reading a logographic written language on the reading of an orthographically written language. As expected, based on past research findings, our native English-speaking readers averaged approximately four saccades per line of print, compared to 10 saccades produced by our Chinese students. Fixation duration did not discriminate between groups. That comprehension of the English material was more difficult for our Chinese readers is shown by the finding that they made significantly more regressive eye movements than our American readers (X 1.9 per line for Chinese vs. 0.26 per line for American readers). Regardless of these and other differences between readers trained in a logographic versus orthographic representational system, our major interest focuses on the finding that our Chinese readers apparently apply the strategy that made them proficient readers of Chinese to the reading of English. This, of course, proved a most inefficient way to read English, or any other orthographically represented language. Our Chinese students had between 7–14 years of experience with English, and had relatively little difficulty in communicating in English. Thus, reading style appears to be persistent. Whether it is subject to retraining remains to be determined.

Our initial concern with "mechanical inefficiencies" focused on two other phenomena, namely, head movements associated with reading, and a variable we have labeled as "inefficient line return." We describe the procedures we have developed for evaluating and remediating such head movements. Because one of our rules is to give the reader as many degrees of freedom as possible in the reading situation, that is, to make it as "normal" a reading situation as possible, we needed a relatively unobtrusive procedure for recording head movements. We used a miniature accelerometer mounted on a set of headphones. The output of the accelerometer gives us information about the direction and peak velocity of head movement. The most readily detected head movement is that associated with the movement of the head from the right to the left side of the page as the reader returns to start a new line. There, of course, have to be movements to the right as well, but these are the smaller movements associated with changes in fixation. The computer program we have developed to record and evaluate head movements associated with the line change, shown in Table 3, does the following:

1. It utilizes eye movement data to identify the onset and termination of the line change saccade.
2. It generates a window 100 msec preceding onset and 100 msec following termination of the line change saccade.
3. It evaluates the output of the accelerometer, sampling the largest voltage during this period.
4. It samples an equivalent period starting 200 msec following the end of the line change saccade sample and identifies the largest voltage during this period.
5. It compares these two voltage levels.
6. If the voltage level is greater during the line changes saccade period, it suggests that it might be associated with a head movement.
7. If the incidence of such amplitude differences is in excess of 50%, they are most likely associated with head movements.

How does one remediate head movements that are minimally or not at all perceived by the reader? Our procedure was to reduce the number of characters per line of text until the incidence of head movement dropped to an acceptable level. To manipulate line width, we use a computer program that allowed us to store text in memory and call for the display of such text with any desired line width between 20 and 64 characters. The program also allowed us to specify the number of lines that were to be displayed at any one time.

Immediately after the subject read a "page" of text, the computer printed out the head movement information on the basis of which the operator decided whether to change the width of the displayed text. To date, seven high school students and five young adults who could be described as "head movers while

TABLE 3
Line Change Eye and Head Movement Data During Reading

REALTIME	TIMEFIX	DUR	DRIFT	AMPL	PEAK	OVF	PTRN		PKA	PKB	HEAD	INI
140	208											
11 48	0. 17	0. 03	32	70	28		R					
11 68	0. 17	0. 03	22	62	26		R		PKA	PKB	HEAD	INI
11 84	0. 13	0. 07	4	108	22		R					
11 96	0. 05	0. 08	-24	-582	-144	1. 14	LINE	-68				
12 12	0. 08	0. 07	36	-104	-40		L					
12 38	0. 19	0. 03	22	166	72		R					
12 72	0. 32	0. 08	36	216	68		R		1062	1064	0	0 09
12 94	0. 13	0. 07	-48	184	34		R					
12 28	0. 27	0. 10	40	-612	-152	1. 32	< LINE	-64				
12 63	0. 25	0. 04	-24	196	70		R					
12 91	0. 24	0. 07	32	-98	-32		L					
14 08	0. 10	0. 04	-2	140	50		R		1056	1056	0	-0. 07
14 25	0. 13	0. 06	32	218	60		R					
14 48	0. 17	0. 03	4	102	48		R					
14 61	0. 10	0. 08	22	-680	-134	1. 33	LINE	-58				
14 89	0. 20	0. 07	-22	236	80		R					
15 15	0. 19	0. 03	30	-84	-44		L					
15 33	0. 15	0. 07	18	324	86		R		1074	1062	+	0. 06

reading" have had their head movements significantly reduced by these procedures. Results like these could not have been achieved by repeated admonitions to hold the head still.

DISCUSSION

CARMODY: I have a question about the data coming from the evening sessions. I was wondering if either the material or the sessions were counter-balanced across trials.

STERN: The materials were short stories by Edgar Allen Poe, and there was no counterbalancing of material across sessions. The subjects simply read Edgar Allen Poe stories for 45 minutes in the morning and continued reading such stories for 45 minutes in the evening. So there is no counterbalancing at all, the presumption being that Edgar Allen Poe (A) and Edgar Allen Poe (B) short stories ought to be very similar in terms of reading difficulty.

ROSEN: Your first fixation data are interesting. I have data that show not only that the first fixation of a task is longer, but for some reason it is also much less variable. I noticed that in your data the first fixation was longer and *more* variable. Do the subjects perceive that they're spending longer on the first fixation? Why do you think it might be longer and more variable?

STERN: Well, I don't know what subjects perceive — I've not asked subjects, "Do you spend more time on the first fixation" because they are not aware of the fact that they're making fixations. With respect to the second question, what are possible reasons for longer fixations on the first informational chunk? I think there are a number of reasons. One is their vergence movements. That is, the eyes diverge and then have to reconverge at the beginning of a line that takes a unit of time; now, whether it is 20 msec or 30 msec, I don't know, we are currently looking at that. The second reason, I think, is that as a person looks at the first informational chunk, he also, in peripheral vision, abstracts some information a little bit further down the line, and that takes him some unit of time that he doesn't have to utilize when he gets to the second chunk. So there is some information already available to him when he gets to the second chunk that was less likely to have been available to him on that first informational chunk. We could speculate as to the reason for the longer fixation pauses, but it would be neater to develop experiments to test the hypothesis. I'm a hypothesis-generating organism (I think that's true of most of you) and the fun part is to test the hypotheses.

RUSSO: It seems that the effect of a line change might be even greater and therefore more easily observable when a page changes, that is, while switching from the bottom of one page to the top of the next page. Have you done this?

STERN: Sure, there all sorts of things that happen with a page change. For example, we know that our competent readers don't blink at all in reading a whole page of text when they are really interested in the material. They do all their blinking as they shift from one page to the next page. We find this a fascinating phenomenon. What else they do between page changes, I don't know. They may simply take some time out and sit there and rest and relax and recuperate. We usually delete the very first line of reading in our analyses. That's part of our editing function. We sit at the computer console and watch what the eyes are doing and edit out the data abstracted "between page changes" and as part of that we don't catch the person reading until he's in that first line and our editing procedure will pull that line out.

ANON: What is the relationship between head movements and multiple line change saccades, and do you believe subvocalization and vocalization are detrimental to reading?

STERN: Head movements and multiple regressive line change saccades are not mutually exclusive. Readers who make head movements also make multiple line change saccades. These are not statements of fact but inferences made from concurrent observations of EOGs and accelerometer output. Though some of the eye movements recorded under these conditions are secondary to head movements, that is, compensatory eye movements, it is our strong impression and conviction that both movements occur concurrently. We will, however, have to develop more sensitive head movement recording procedures and other techniques (photographic) for recording eye movements before we are convinced of this.

With respect to the issue of subvocalization and its relationship to information abstraction during reading, we believe that such vocalization may be necessary under conditions when the material is difficult for the reader. Such difficulty may be a function of such variables as lack of familiarity with the subject matter, complexity of sentence structure, and legibility of text. We believe that teaching readers to inhibit *all* subvocalization, as Hardyck and Petrinovich have done, is detrimental to the reader. As they have demonstrated, inhibiting subvocalization in readers who habitually subvocalize is readily managed with biofeedback procedures. Such inhibition speeds up reading; if the material is simple, it does so without affecting comprehension. If the material is difficult, it also speeds up reading, but comprehension is impaired. One has to be extremely careful with the kinds of remediation programs attempted; here is at least one example where biofeedback training has a detrimental effect!

FISHER: Could you speculate very briefly on the reason for the shorter fixation pauses associated with regressive movements?

STERN: I'll give you a rationalization for both of them. I think that the fixation pause preceding a regressive eye movement is shorter than normal R–R fixation pauses, because the reader realizes that he's not making sense out of the information that he is abstracting and aborts processing. Therefore, time spent on that informational chunk, that fixation pause, is shorter. What's interesting is that the fixation pause following the regression is also significantly shorter.

It appears to me that the reader knows exactly where to go to pick up that additional chunk of information that is missing, he goes back to it and picks it up. It is usually a smaller informational chunk than that which he normally takes in and it takes him less time to abstract that informational chunk.

ANON: Are there differences in slope between different types of saccadic eye movements, for example, those associated with left- and right-going saccades during reading?

STERN: I think that the saccades are under tight control of the "central processor," and that peripheral control is not terribly important when one looks at reading activity. I've always been surprised at the fact that one cannot discriminate between a saccade associated with a regressive eye movement and a saccade associated with a forward going eye movement on the basis of differences in slope. Though in one case the slope is negative and in the other positive, if one controls for saccade amplitude there is no difference in slope (i.e., peak velocity). Peak velocity is, of course, affected by saccade amplitude; the larger the amplitude the greater the peak velocity. Peak velocity is affected by "state" of the organism. When tranquilized with either alcohol, short-acting barbiturates, or "minor" tranquilizers such as diazepam, one finds significant reduction in peak velocity.

ANON: Can you say something about the distribution you obtain with fixation pause durations?

STERN: We normally utilize median fixation pause durations as the average across individuals since it is less influenced by extremely deviant fixation pauses (those shorter than 70–80 msec as well as those longer than 780 msec). These median fixation times are, of course, normally distributed. Within subject fixation, pause distributions are quite variable; however, for college student readers, roughly 40% of all fixation pauses preceded and followed by right-going saccades fall between 161–260 msec.

IV.2

Inference Processes During Reading: Reflections from Eye Fixations[1]

Marcel Adam Just
Patricia A. Carpenter
Carnegie-Mellon University

Since reading and understanding are moderately complex human activities, they are often studied and described from various perspectives. Our approach has focused on the mental processes that extract information from a text and combine those elements to construct a coherent internal representation of the text content (cf. Carpenter & Just, 1977a, 1977b). These processes are influenced by certain linguistic properties of the text, such as foregrounding, pronominal reference, and lexical entailments. We have examined the way in which these constructions initiate and guide comprehension processes. In this paper, we will describe our research on verb-based entailments.

Verb structures appear to play a central role in comprehension and inference-making (cf. Fillmore, 1968; Norman & Rumelhart, 1975; Schank, 1973). For example, the verb *to murder* entails an agent, a murderer. If a text contains the verb *murder,* followed at some point by the word *killer,* comprehension of the text involves computing the relation between the two words. The immediate object of this study is to learn how and when a reader computes that *killer* refers to the entailed agent of *murder*. The method includes the monitoring of eye fixations as subjects read and comprehend simple paragraphs. The general research goals are to both investigate the relation between eye fixations and comprehension processes, and to use it to develop aspects of a theory of comprehension.

---

[1]This research was a collaborative effort; the order of authorship is arbitrary. The research was supported in part by Grant MH-29617 from the National Institute of Mental Health and Grant NIE-77-0007 from the National Institute of Education.

SEMANTIC INFLUENCE ON EYE FIXATIONS

What determines where and how long a reader fixates while reading a text? In principle, the locus and duration of reading fixations could be controlled by visual information processes, oculomotor processes, and semantic processes (Carpenter & Just, 1977a; Haber, 1976; Kolers, 1976). It is clear that the fixation behavior is at least partially dependent on the processing of visual input from the text, such as where the lines of print begin and end. Visual (but nonsemantic) information, such as inter-word spaces, type-case, and punctuation marks also appear to have some effect (Fisher, 1976; McConkie, 1976). The current experiments will focus on more cognitive processes — semantic influences on eye fixations. We propose that the semantic processes that extract the meaning relations from the text can influence reading eye fixations. Although the degree of guidance and control remains to be fully specified, the experiments to be reported on lexically-based inferences reveal some of the temporal relations between semantic processing and eye fixations.

There are two major dimensions that must be specified when considering how semantic processes might influence reading fixations. First, they could influence either the duration or the location of reading fixations, or both. Second, they might influence the characteristics of the ongoing fixation, of subsequent fixations, or both. In other words, there could be some lag between the time semantic information is initially fixated and its manifestation in the reading eye fixations. Such a lag could reflect a delay between initial encoding and some subsequent semantic computation, or it could reflect a delay between the semantic computation and the manifestation in fixation behavior. The experiments to be reported explore issues of both dimensions.

FIXATION DURATION AND SEMANTIC PROCESSING

Historically, fixation duration has not been associated closely with semantic processing during reading. Fixation duration has been assumed to be an insensitive index of cognitive processing for a number of reasons. One is that fixation durations are erroneously assumed to be fairly constant, so there would be little variability to correlate with semantic processing. Perhaps the cause of this misconception is that mean fixation duration is fairly constant across subjects in simple reading tasks. The average duration is about 250 msec, and the standard deviation of subjects' average fixation durations is often as low as 25 msec (Tinker, 1951). However, this does not mean that one reader's fixations within one passage will all have the same duration. On the contrary, in an ordinary reading situation the variability of fixation durations for one subject is quite large, with a standard deviation of about 100 msec and a range of 150 to 375 msec (Walker, 1933). Because early researchers were attempting to account for the mean durations rather than individual durations, they had difficulty in relating the temporal characteristics of fixations to cognitive processes.

There are other indications that the duration of individual fixations may only weakly reflect cognitive processes. The mean duration is not strongly correlated with more global tests of comprehension performance ($r = .11$, Buswell, 1937; $r = -.05$, Anderson, 1937). Poor readers have mean fixation durations that are only 10–20% longer than those of good readers, for example, 295 msec versus 246 msec (Anderson, 1937; Buswell, 1937). Moreover, training in reading decreases the number of fixations a poor reader executes, but does not significantly decrease mean fixation duration (Buswell, 1937). Fixation duration does increase somewhat with the difficulty of the text or task but is not affected as much as the number of fixations (Tinker, 1951). One reason why fixation duration may be less flexible than the number of fixations is that there may be a lower bound set by physiological constraints and basic perceptual processes. While fixation duration may increase in response to task demands, decreases below some lower bound may be barred by these other constraints.

Perhaps the individual fixation is not the appropriate unit of analysis to relate to comprehension processes. An alternative measure of the temporal characteristics of fixation behavior is the total amount of time that a reader spends looking at a unit of text at any one time. This measure is called the *gaze*; it is simply the sum of the durations of the individual fixations that comprise a single inspection of a particular word, phrase, or sentence. The unit of analysis depends on the underlying theory. There is some evidence to suggest that gaze duration, rather than individual fixation duration, is closely related to comprehension processes. For example, it is known that text difficulty affects fixation behavior. As passages become increasingly difficult, some readers increase the number of fixations they make, some increase the duration of their fixations, whereas others increase both the number and duration of fixations (Walker, 1933). Thus, the gaze duration may be the measure that covaries most closely with text difficulty. Moreover, there is a high correlation between comprehension scores and the total time spent on a text (Tinker, 1939). In still another situation, one in which a subject reads a sentence and decides whether it is true or false of an accompanying picture, gaze duration appears to be an appropriate measure. The task difficulty is most closely related to total gaze duration on the sentence, irrespective of the durations of individual fixations within the gaze (Carpenter & Just, 1976; Just & Carpenter, 1976a). What is important in all these situations is the time spent processing a particular symbol, not the number of fixations nor the duration of individual fixations.

In the following experiments, the main dependent measure is gaze duration. The individual word is used as the unit of analysis, and consecutive fixations on that word are aggregated and treated as a single gaze. These gaze durations can be compared across different experimental conditions, defined by the semantic properties of the various sentences. Thus, we will examine the evidence for semantic influences on the temporal characteristics of the gaze.

FIXATION LOCUS AND SEMANTIC PROCESSING

While duration is one measure of reading performance, the issue of the semantic control of eye fixations traditionally has been defined primarily in terms of the *locus* of eye fixations. Does the computation of semantic information on the nth fixation determine the location of the $n + 1$st fixation? Although this question is still unresolved in the domain of forward fixations (cf. O'Regan, 1975), we have reported studies in which semantic processing directed the locus of regressive fixations (Carpenter & Just, 1977a). Regressive fixations are particularly susceptible to semantic control because the processor already has a record of the location of the relevant word or sentence.

Historically, regressive fixations have been associated with poor readers (Buswell, 1937) and were considered an unimportant component of the normal reading process. However, experimental artifacts and constraints reduced the number of recorded regressions, so that their frequency was underestimated. For example, some researchers instructed their subjects not to look back at previously-read lines of text. Others used eye trackers that detected only horizontal eye movements, so that upward regressions were not monitored. Finally, the reading tasks often did not require much integration across the various parts of the text, so there may not have been much reason to look back. With all these constraints, the type of regressive fixation that was most likely to show itself was the regression within a line of print, namely leftward eye movements. Many of these were semantically uninteresting, since they were corrections for undershoot of the return sweep from the right-hand extreme of one line to the left side of the next line. When some of these artificial constraints are removed (and perhaps new ones added), regressive fixations are often closely linked with comprehension processes.

Certain regressive fixations are indicative of comprehension processes and are correlated with the interpretation given the passage. For example, readers will tend to make regressive fixations to the referent of a pronoun (Carpenter & Just, 1977a). In that experiment, subjects read passages containing pronouns. The sentences preceding the pronoun contained two nouns that logically could have been the referent of the subsequent pronoun. The following is a typical example:

1. The guard mocked one of the prisoners in the machine shop.
2. The one who the guard mocked was the arsonist.
3. He had been at the prison for only one week.

The experiment focused on the interpretation of the pronoun *He* in Sentence 3. There are two possible antecedents for *He*; one is the arsonist/prisoner and the other is the guard. The linguistic structure of the second sentence focuses on the arsonist. Linguistic analysis suggests that this noun, in general, should be interpreted as the pronominal referent. (Other factors like serial position and agent—

object relations were taken into account.) When reading the pronoun sentence, subjects made regressive fixations to a potential referent about 50% of the time. Moreover, the regression was usually to the referent that was the focus of the preceding sentence and the pattern of eye fixations correlated with eventual recall. For example, subjects tended to recall the pronoun sentence in the example above as being about the arsonist. Thus, some regressive fixations are semantically driven and indicate what is being comprehended and what is being stored.

The following experiments examine the locus and duration of both regressive and forward fixations in more detail. The goal is twofold. On one hand, the results will be used to investigate the semantic influence on eye fixations. Here the issue is whether underlying semantic processes, such as inference-making, influence the duration and location of forward and regressive fixations. The second issue is the substantive question of inference-making. Fixation patterns will be used to examine inference-making and to determine when and how lexically-based inferences are made.

INFERENCES BASED ON VERBS

The primary interest of this research is how and when a reader infers the relation between a verb, like *murder*, and an entailed agent, like *killer*. (For convenience, we shall use the term *agent* to refer to all three kinds of entailments — agent, instrument, and manner.) Such an inference must take a certain amount of time to compute, and this time might be influenced by the lexical relationship between the verb and agent. In particular, the closer the semantic relation between the two lexical items, the less time it should take to compute the relation. For example, the relationship between the verb *murder* and the agent *killer* is direct. It is easy to integrate two sentences that refer to these concepts, for example:

1. The millionaire was murdered on a dark and stormy night.
   The killer left no clues for the police to trace.

By contrast, consider the relationship between *die* and *killer*. If someone dies, it does not necessarily mean that a killer is involved. Thus, if one sentence refers to someone dying and the next refers to a killer, it might take more time to infer the relation, for example:

2. The millionaire died on a dark and stormy night.
   The killer left no clues for the police to trace.

This study examined whether such indirect inferences take longer and how the additional time is distributed during reading.

At this point one might hypothesize that semantic distance would account for inference making. Perhaps the ease or difficulty of making an inference depends only on how far apart two concepts are in the reader's semantic space. If so, then the computation time should not be affected by the serial order of the two concepts to be related, since the distance between remains unaffected. To investigate this issue, we varied the serial order of the verb and agent sentences. The agent could either follow the verb sentence (as in Examples 1 and 2 above) or the agent could precede the verb, as in Example 3:

3. The killer left no clues for the police to trace.
   The millionaire died on a dark and stormy night.

If the time needed to make an inference linking two concepts was simply dependent on the interconcept distance, then the indirect inference condition (*e.g., killer–died*) should still be more difficult than the direct inference condition (e.g., *killer–murdered*). The additional time to make the indirect inference would be reflected in the extra time to read the indirect verb sentence. Alternatively, semantic distance may not be a sufficient explanation for inference making. For example, if the reader knows that there is a killer, then it may be equally easy to infer that someone else *died* or that someone was *murdered*. In other words, the "direct" and "indirect" inferences might be equally easy to make. In this case, the serial order of the agent and verb sentences would influence the relative ease of making an inference. The difference between the direct and indirect inferences might be eliminated when the agent sentence precedes the verb sentence.

Method

The main independent variable was the semantic relation between the verb in one sentence and the agent in another; the relation could be either direct or indirect. Examples of agents (in the sense described previously) and the directly and indirectly related verbs are: the killer, murder — die; the car, drove — went; the seller, bought — got; the will, inherited — received; the hill, climbed — walked. The second independent variable was the serial order of the verb and agent sentences.

Each paragraph had a total of five sentences: one containing the verb, one containing the agent, and three filler sentences. In half of the paragraphs, the filler sentence in the fourth or fifth position contradicted information in the earlier sentences, as illustrated below:

1. The millionaire was murdered on a dark and stormy night.
2. The killer left no clues for the police to trace.
3. The millionaire was found in his bed by the housekeeper.

4. There was no electricity in the house because of the storm.

5. It was the butler who discovered the body.

Each subject saw 32 paragraphs, half of which contained a directly related verb and half an indirectly related verb. In half of the paragraphs the verb sentence preceded the agent sentence and in the other half it followed. There were two versions of the design, differing only in whether the particular verb was directly or indirectly related to the agent sentence. Half of the subjects received one version and half received the other.

Procedure

The subjects' task was to read each sentence in a paragraph and determine whether or not it contradicted any information in a previous sentence. This task was used to ensure that the subject would integrate the sentences. The subjects' response latencies were recorded and their eye fixations were monitored as they read and responded to each sentence.

In this experiment and in the others that follow, eye fixations were monitored by a corneal-reflectance eyetracking system (see Just & Carpenter, 1976b, for more details). This system beams a small spot of light onto the subject's cornea and captures the reflection. As the eye moves, the angle of reflection changes approximately linearly with the amount of movement. The system is calibrated for each subject so that the locus of the reflection corresponds to the locus of fixation.

The subject's eye fixations were monitored while he read successive sentences of a paragraph on a video monitor and decided whether each was consistent with or contradictory to the previous sentences. Each sentence was started on a new line of the video display. Before a sentence was displayed, a fixation point was presented at the starting position of that sentence. The trial did not start unless the subject was fixating that point and pressed a "ready" button. Half a second later, the current sentence appeared, along with all of the preceding sentences. When the subject made a judgment about the current sentence, the entire display was blanked. Thus, only the first sentence was displayed during the first trial, the first and second sentences during the second trial, and so forth. Reading and judging the five sentences of the paragraph constituted five separate trials.

The average length of the agent word was 5.5 letters. The third and fourth words averaged 4.7 and 4.4 letters, respectively. The viewing distance was adjusted for each subject to equalize the excursion of the eye spot, but on the average it was 82 cm. The average visual angle subtended by the agent word was 2.5° and the angle subtended by the first four words of the agent sentence was 8°.

Twenty subjects participated, ten in each version of the experiment. The subjects were volunteers from an introductory psychology course.

Total Response Time

First, consider total reading time when the agent sentence followed the verb sentence. As predicted, subjects took longer to process the agent sentence in the indirect inference condition. The response time for the indirect inference condition (3277 msec) was 454 msec longer than the response time for the direct inference condition (2823 msec), $F'(1, 31) = 8.14, p < .01$. This supports the view that inferences are more difficult in the indirect condition. The greater response time in the indirect condition was found for 17 of the 20 subjects and for 14 of the 16 agent sentences. Some responses (less than 2%) were discarded because of an incorrect response or because the response time was over 10 sec. These trials were equally distributed between the direct and indirect inference conditions.

When the agent sentence was specified first and the verb sentence second, there was no significant difference between the indirect and direct inference conditions. Subjects took about the same amount of time to read the verb sentence in the indirect inference condition (3188 msec) and the direct inference condition (3220 msec). Thus, the order of the verb and agent sentences did influence the relative difficulty of making an inference, and semantic distance alone cannot account for the difficulty of inference making. Semantic distance is symmetrical; the distance between concepts A and B is the same as the distance between B and A. Distance considerations alone would predict that indirect inferences would take longer, regardless of whether the verb precedes or follows the agent. A more adequate explanation will consider the information entailed by sentences. For example, the existence of a *killer* entails someone's death by murdering. When a subsequent sentence refers to either of these concepts, they are equally available. The reader can construct a link back to the concept of killer. By contrast, when the verb is specified first, different information is entailed in the direct and indirect condition. Thus, the ease of subsequently relating the two sentences is different in the two conditions.

An alternative possibility is that there may be asymmetries in the comprehension of nouns and verbs that interact with their order in a paragraph. For example, many theories postulate that verbs play a central role in establishing the framework of the passage (cf. Norman & Rumelhart, 1975). Hence, a particular verb could influence the comprehension of subsequent sentences more than any particular noun. While several theories distinguish between noun-like structures and verb-like structures, such explanations require more investigation.

The agent sentence in the first position provides a control demonstrating that there was no a priori differences among the agent sentences. The reading time should be equivalent for the direct and indirect conditions, since the same sentences were used in both conditions. In fact, the two response times are similar, 3162 msec in the indirect condition and 3227 msec in the direct condition.

EYE FIXATION ANALYSIS

The distribution of eye fixations on the agent sentence might indicate when a reader makes the linking inference. The assumption underlying this analysis is that the reader will tend to make the inference at the same time in the direct and indirect inference conditions. However, the inference is more difficult in the indirect condition, so the reader spends more time gazing at the agent sentence. The locus of this additional time indicates where the inference was made. Thus, the fixation analysis compares the distribution of gazes on the agent sentence in the direct and indirect inference conditions.

Fixations within the agent sentence were classified as either forward or regressive fixations and aggregated into gazes. The easiest way to explain the classification is to consider a hypothetical sequence of fixations where the numbers 1 to 11 indicate the sequence of fixations:

    2 14 3 5 6   7 8 10 11   9
The killer left no clues for the police to trace.

Fixations 1 and 2 would be aggregated into the first gaze on *killer*. The total gaze duration would be the sum of the durations of Fixations 1 and 2. Fixation 3 would be a gaze on *left*. Fixation 4 would be classified as a regressive to *killer*. Fixations 5 to 9 are forward gazes on their respective words. Fixations 10 and 11 would be aggregated into a regressive gaze on *police*.

The distribution of gazes on the agent sentence was analyzed for 14 of the 20 subjects. Three subjects were not analyzed because their overall response times did not show the advantage for the direct inference condition. One subject could not be analyzed because of problems with the tracking apparatus and two others were dropped randomly to have an equal number of subjects from each version of the experiment. Eleven per cent of the agent sentences could not be included in the analysis because of loss of eye spot or head movement. These were equally distributed between the direct and indirect inference conditions. The total response time was 3340 msec for the indirect inference condition and 2688 msec for the direct inference condition, $F(1, 27) = 26.98, p < .01$.

Figure 1 shows the average duration of gaze on the first four words of the agent sentence for both the direct and indirect inference conditions for each subject. Twelve of the fourteen subjects spent more time on the agent word in the indirect inference condition. This effect was present for 12 of the 16 agent sentences.

Figure 2 shows the effect averaged over subjects. The gaze on the agent word itself was 65 msec longer in the indirect condition, $F'(1, 25) = 4.03, p < .06$. The gaze on the definite article preceding the agent word was 13 msec longer in the indirect condition. The gaze on the word following the agent was 24 msec longer in the indirect inference condition and on the fourth word, it was 44

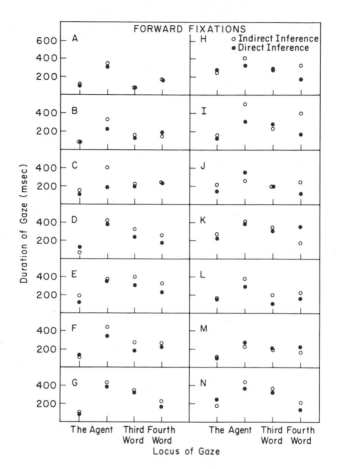

FIG. 1.   The gaze duration computed from forward fixations for each of 14 subjects (labeled A–N). The duration is shown for each of the first four words of the agent sentence for the indirect and direct inference conditions.

msec longer. On the average, subjects spent almost 145 msec extra in forward fixations on the agent sentence in the indirect inference condition. These data are interpreted to suggest that on some trials readers infer the relation between the agent and prior sentence immediately upon fixating the agent word itself.

Regressive fixations were of two kinds; there were regressions within the agent sentence and regressions to the preceding verb sentence. Within the agent sentence, subjects spent 84 msec more on regressive fixations to the agent word in the indirect inference condition, as shown in the bottom of Fig. 2. They also spent about 10 msec more on *The* and 61 msec more on the third word, the word following the agent word. Thus, regressions accounted for 155 msec of the difference between the indirect and direct inference conditions.

Subjects also made regressive fixations to the opening sentence that contained the verb. As in a previous experiment (cf. Carpenter & Just, 1977a), subjects spent more time on the verb sentence in the indirect inference condition (288 msec) than in the direct inference condition (131 msec). These regressions were generally made after reading the entire agent sentence. Thus, regressions within the agent sentence and regressions back to the verb sentence accounted for a total of 310 msec of the 652 msec difference between the two conditions.

The results indicate that readers sometimes make the inference relating an agent to a prior verb immediately upon encountering the word denoting the agent. This inference process takes longer in the indirect inference condition, and some of the additional time is reflected in the longer gaze duration on the agent word and the immediately adjacent words. The rest of the additional time is spent in regressive fixations to the sentence containing the verb. As the semantic path between the two concepts is constructed, the related words tend to be fixated.

The Effect of the Task

The next experiment examined the generality of these results in another task environment, one that did not involve consistency judgments. It examined the same inference-related variables in the context of a reading task. The subject read each sentence and pressed a button when he had understood the sentence. The subject made no consistency judgments and no inconsistent sentences were presented. At the end of a paragraph, the subject was asked to recall as much as he could, although memory performance was not stressed. Again, the primary question was the processing of indirect and direct inferences.

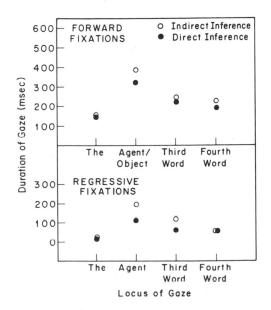

FIG. 2.   The gaze duration averaged across subjects. The top panel shows the gaze duration computed from forward fixations. The bottom panel shows the gaze duration computed from regressive fixations.

Method

The design was similar to that of the previous experiment. In this experiment, the particular verb used was the same in both versions of the experiment, but the serial order of the verb and agent sentences was varied. In one version, the verb sentence appeared first and the agent second. In a second version of the experiment, their order was reversed although the same verb was used. Half of the verbs were from the indirect inference condition and half from the direct inference condition.

Ten subjects were run in each version of the experiment. None of the subjects had participated in the previous experiment.

Results

The major results support those of the consistency judgment task. When the agent sentence followed the verb, reading times were 182 msec longer in the indirect condition (3124 msec) than in the direct condition (2942 msec). However, the difference was much more variable and not statistically reliable, $F'(1, 18) =$ 1.25, n.s. Again, when the verb sentence followed the agent sentence (e.g., *killer—died*), the indirect and direct inference conditions took about equally long. Reading times for the verb sentence were 3090 msec in the indirect condition and 3123 msec in the direct condition. Thus, the asymmetry found in the first experiment was also present here. When the reader already has information specified about a killer, it is no more difficult to make an inference relating that to a death than it is to make the inference relating it to a murder.

The condition in which the agent sentence followed the verb sentence produced results similar to those of the previous experiment. However, the difference between the direct and indirect inference conditions was smaller than that observed previously and was less consistent across subjects. One possibility that may account for the difference is that the consistency judgments of the preceding experiment forced subjects to integrate the sentences within a paragraph. In the current task, there was no way to insure integration.

EYE FIXATION ANALYSES

The analyses focused on six subjects, three from each version of the experiment, whose eye movement records had the least amount of noise and head-movement, and who had large differences between the direct and indirect inference condition. Their mean difference between the direct and indirect inference conditions was 430 msec.

Figure 3 shows the gaze durations on each of the first four words of the target sentence (when it appeared in the second position). All six subjects showed an increase in gaze duration on the target sentence in the indirect inference condi-

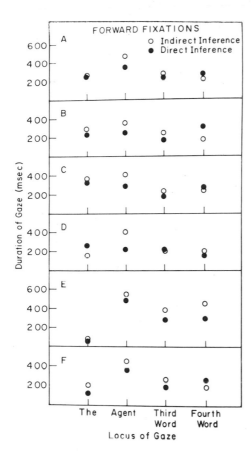

FIG. 3. The gaze duration computed from forward fixations for each of 6 subjects (labeled A–F). The duration is shown for each of the first four words of the agent sentence for the indirect and direct inference conditions.

tion. For most subjects there is also an increase on the third word, the verb or auxiliary following the agent word. However, by the fourth word, the difference between the direct and indirect conditions is less consistent. Figure 4 shows the results averaged over all six readers. The time spent on the agent word is 105 msec greater in the indirect inference word. There is also slightly more time spent on the following word (55 msec). The differences in time spent on the definite article (12 msec) and on the fourth word (−11 msec) are insignificantly small. Thus, the gaze duration does show a selective increase as found in the previous experiment.

The second panel in Fig. 4 shows the duration of regressive gazes on each of the first four words of the target sentence. These regressive gazes also demonstrated the effect of semantic processes on reading fixations. First, there were seldom any regressive fixations to the definite article. The regressive fixations occurred on the agent and the subsequent words. Second, the duration of regressive gazes was 71 msec longer on the agent word in the indirect inference condition. Thus, both the duration of forward and regressive gazes demonstrates the increased difficulty of the indirect inference condition.

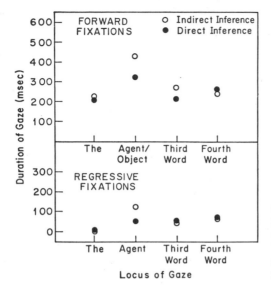

FIG. 4.   The gaze duration averaged across subjects. The top panel shows the gaze duration computed from forward fixations. The bottom panel shows the gaze duration computed from regressive fixations.

There was one final aspect of interest in the pattern of gazes on the target sentence. Very often, the final forward fixation on the sentence was extremely long. To quantify this effect, we measured the duration of the last forward fixation in the sentence plus any other consecutive fixations on the same word. The duration of this gaze averaged 462 msec in the direct condition and 538 msec in the indirect condition. These gazes are certainly longer than the last gaze observed in the previous experiment (352 msec for the indirect condition and 368 msec for the direct condition). One explanation is that the long gazes occurred during or at the end of the sentence because subjects were rehearsing the sentence, perhaps in preparation for recall. Rehearsing an entire sentence or even simply its major constituents required more time than encoding and comprehending a word or phrase.

DISCUSSION

Temporal Aspects of Inference-Making

In both experiments, there was an increase in gaze duration around the agent word. This result suggests that, at least in some paragraphs, the reader made an inference relating the agent word to the preceding information immediately upon encountering the agent word itself. Since this inference was more difficult in the indirect condition, it manifested itself as an increased gaze duration on the agent word. However, because the extra time spent on the agent was not equal to the total response difference between the indirect and direct inference conditions, the readers did not always make the linking inference immediately upon encountering the agent word.

The distribution of regressive fixations suggests that sometimes the inference-making process was accompanied by regressive fixations. The reader fixated more than the agent word, perhaps the entire subject—verb phrase or the sentence, before linking information in the previous sentence to the currently-read sentence. The linking inference is accompanied by a regression to the agent word or to the previous sentence. Regressions to the previous sentence generally occurred after the entire agent sentence was read. These data suggest that inferences relating two sentences may be made at various times. The two shortest times may be either when the related lexical item is first encountered or at the end of the clause or sentence.

The Mechanism of Inference-Making

The current experiments also suggest that semantic distance may not completely account for lexically-based inference making. Both experiments showed an asymmetry in the effects of the order of the agent and verb sentences. A verb that is related to a subsequent agent facilitated comprehension of that sentence. However, the converse did not occur. When the agent was read first, the direct and indirect verbs were equally easy to link. Thus, the information value of the second sentence was important. When the second sentence was deducible from the first, comprehension was not more difficult even if the two concepts were in some sense semantically more distant.

There are two main ways that the verb-based inference could be made. One possibility is that when a verb like *murder* is encountered in text, the verb and all of its associated cases (like a killer, a victim, an instrument, and a manner) are explicitly represented, even if the cases are not explicitly mentioned in the sentence (cf. Fillmore, 1968; Schank, 1973). This will be called a forward inference, because the cases are represented before they are required (Clark, 1975). If a later lexical item refers to a previously unspecified case, the item can be integrated easily because the case is already represented. Thus, after reading a sentence with *murder*, it would be easy to integrate *killer* because the representation of *murder* already contains the concept of a killer. By contrast, if the verb were *die*, then an additional inferential step would be necessary to integrate *killer*, consuming extra time, as the results showed. Consequently, *murder* (with its entailed extra cases) might be expected to take longer to represent than *die*, according to this formulation. However, the reading times were close for *die* and *murder* sentences in the opening position, and if anything, verbs like *murder* took less time.

An alternative possibility is that case relations are not represented until they are required (Clark, 1975). In the current experiment, no agent would be represented on encountering either *murder* or *die*, so reading time for the sentences with the verb in the opening sentence should be equal, as they were. When the agent sentence is read, only then would the agent (or other case) be represented and an inference made relating that representation to the representation of the sentence with the verb. This will be called a backward inference.

Presumably, the inference would be easier when the verb and agent were semantically more related, that is, in the direct inference condition. This model predicts the pattern of reading times in both the opening sentences and the agent sentences.

Semantic Control of Reading Fixations

The selectivity of the eye fixations demonstrates that gaze location and duration are sensitive to underlying semantic processes. When the individual word is adopted as the unit of analysis, there is no lag between the inference process and its manifestation in gaze duration. The reader spends longer on the agent word itself.

The duration of gaze on the words around the critical word also showed some selective increase in the indirect inference condition, particularly the word(s) following the agent word. There are at least two interpretations of this effect. One possibility is that sometimes the reader makes the inference after encoding more than just the agent word itself. For example, perhaps the inference is made after the verb is encoded. Thus, the increased duration on the verb would reflect the fact that the reader is making the inference somewhat later in the sentence. This is a reasonable interpretation of the effect, since the evidence from the regressive fixations indicate that sometimes the linking inference is not made until much or all of the sentence is read.

A second possibility is that the increased gaze duration reflects a "smearing" of duration of the main inference. The duration of the inference might be manifested over a number of fixations. With this interpretation, the longer gaze duration on the verb would reflect an inference process initiated when the agent was fixated, but which was longer than a single gaze. (See Russo, Chapter II.3, this volume, for a more detailed discussion of this hypothesis.) Of course, both interpretations could be correct also.

Regressive fixations are fairly prominent in the current experiments for both their frequency and regularity. Their prominence raises the question of the functional role of regressions during reading. Why do good readers tend to make regressions within and between sentences? The traditional interpretation was that regressions are "holding patterns" that allow the reader to maintain an optimal temporal relation between what is fixated and what is processed. If a reader has several processes to execute at one point, he might make a regression until the cognitive load is lightened. While this hypothesis might account for some regressions, it does not explain why the locus of the regressive fixation is so selective. Regressive fixations occurred on particular words that correlated with the inference that was being processed.

An alternative explanation is that the reader regresses to check some information. This explanation would account for the selectivity of the locus of a regressive fixation. However, the meaning and function of the "checking" process requires some clarification. Presumably, checking does not mean that the reader totally forgot some information. If he had, his regressions should be less selective since he would have to reread more than one element. A more likely interpretation is that the reader is confirming some interpretation of an element and regresses to check his interpretation.

A third possibility is that regressive fixations play a place-keeping role. The reader may fixate a particular word to keep track of the inference he is executing. For example, if he were making an inference about the killer, he would look at that word. Then, when the inference was complete, he would continue reading new textual elements. A closely related version of this hypothesis is that regressive fixations are correlated with certain semantic processes. In reading, as in many other cognitive domains, there may be a tendency to fixate the referent of the concept being processed. In this view, such regressions may not be functional. The reader may not be encoding information from the text. Rather, the fixation may occur because there is a spatial index to a particular concept that he is thinking about. (These hypotheses are outlined in the domain of spatial information processing in Chapter III.1 by Carpenter & Just in this volume.) Of course, there may be many kinds of regressions so that several of these alternative explanations may be necessary to account for regressions. In any case, the data suggest that regressions are an index of semantic processes such as inference making.

The results of these experiments show that reading eye fixations are sensitive to semantic processes during comprehension. This does not mean that semantic processes are the only factors that influence reading eye fixations. Visual processes certainly play a role as, perhaps, do oculomotor processes. For example, there might be a general scanning rule to fixate the next word or phrase that is out of the area of clear vision. However, this general scanning rule can receive interrupts from semantic and visual processes. These interrupts could increase the duration of a fixation, cause a refixation, or even a regression. The current data argue very strongly for at least some semantic control of reading fixations. For this reason, eye fixations may be a valuable tool for examining substantive issues about the nature of the underlying semantic processes.

DISCUSSION

FISHER: In the pronoun study, could readers be using their knowledge of the world, knowledge about landlords and electricians, to choose a referent for the ambiguous pronoun? Second, how do you know that subjects are looking back to what they want as a referent, rather than looking back to what they do *not* want as a referent.

CARPENTER: We have independent evidence to indicate that readers tend to look back at the referent, rather than looking back at the rejected alternative. We asked subjects to recall the paragraphs at the end of each presentation. When they recalled the sentence with the ambiguous pronoun, they would tend to disambiguate it. The disambiguation they provided in recall tended to match the word they made a regressive fixation to during comprehension.

You also asked whether the reader might choose a referent for the pronoun on the basis of their semantic knowledge about landlords and electricians, rather than on the basis of the linguistic cue provided by the cleft sentence. To control for this effect, there was a baseline condition in which the pronoun sentence immediately followed the opening sentence. In this case, semantic knowledge would play a primary role because there was no cleft device to influence the assignment of pronominal reference. Then, the other condition had the cleft sentence precede the ambiguous pronoun sentence, and the results for this condition were compared to the baseline.

FISHER: I thought it was refreshing to see someone working with, or at least having available, scanpath data. What is the angular extent of the regressive movements?

CARPENTER: We have classified regressive movements according to the word fixated in the previous sentence. Thus, the angular extent depends on which word is fixated. The vertical extent between one sentence and the preceding sentence was 3° of visual angle.

IV.3

Relation of Eye Fixations to Old—New Information of Texts

Leonard F. Scinto, Jr.[1]
Harvard University

THEME—RHEME STRUCTURE OF TEXTS AND EYE MOVEMENTS

Background

Within the human organism every level of what might be called the life process, from the strictly biological to the social, is interactive with some 'environment' outside itself. This interaction is critically dependent on the intake, processing, and exchange of information. The external environment as "information" source for man is constantly showering him with signals of various density, modality, and intensity. The capacity of an individual to absorb and process this flow of information is limited. As a consequence humans are endowed with a set of receptors that select consequential signals according to a set of laws, some of which are well-documented both on the physiological and psychological level. The perceptual system apart from the senses serves as a reduction device, in essence a shorthand, for the efficient construction of what is called subjective reality experience.

Two subsystems of the human 'system' are the focus of this paper, namely, visual sense and language. The visual system is concerned with the intake of information in the broadest sense of the word. Language, from a functional viewpoint, is concerned with communication, that is, the encoding and exchange of information. It is in the domain of print that these two systems come to interact. Our aim is to explicate the nature of the interaction of the visual and

[1]I wish to express my special thanks to Professor Gerald S. Lesser and Barbara Flagg for making available to me the laboratory facilities necessary to complete this study.

language systems where they interface in the intake, encoding, and exchange of information.

Information Structure and Language

Language when viewed from a functional perspective is analogous to the perceptual system in that it is a shorthand for the organization of information flow from the environment, both physical and cultural, in order to permit the coherent and efficient intake, processing, and exchange of information. A question arises as to the extent to which some common basic organizational or process algorithm underlies both the perceptual and language systems in the selection and organization of information. More precisely our goal is to determine empirically to what extent the semantic structure of language constrains and guides the intake of information in the visual processing of language texts.

Text as Basic Unit of Analysis

It is an intuitive observation that the natural unit of expression in natural language is not the "sentence" or "proposition," but the text or discourse whose units in turn are sentences, fragments of sentences, clauses, words, or propositions. We will not argue extensively here for the empirical validity of this observation but simply point out that there is increasing recognition of the limitations of sentence grammars for linguistic analysis. (For further documentation and argumentation of this assumption see especially Daneš, 1974; Sanders, 1969; Scinto, 1977; & Van Dijk, 1972.) It is sufficient for our purposes to point out that formal sentence grammars are incapable of handling certain basic language phenomena such as anaphora, pronominalization, and ellipsis as well, and more importantly for this study, basic facts of semantic interpretation, especially questions of presupposition and entailment and communicative function. We will therefore assume for the purposes of this study that the text is the empirically valid unit of analysis.

Level of Analysis

A number of investigators (Gibson, 1969; Gregory and Poulton, 1970; McConkie & Rayner, 1973; Mehler, Bever, & Cary, 1967), in order to articulate an account of the visual processing of printed textual material, have accomplished this by focusing on what we would term a micro-level of analysis. These studies and many like them have used as key variables such textual characteristics as word length. spacing between words, letter shape and delineation, and a number of syntactic characteristics such as constituent boundaries and transitional connectives.

While perhaps of value in elucidating certain basic aspects of stimulus discrimination, such a micro-analysis fails to address two crucial aspects of textual processing. It fails to take into account the semantic nature of the material (i.e., text), which has a holistic integrity and organization. Further, this attention to physical characteristics ignores the functional aspect that the text as a whole serves, namely, to act as a vehicle for the communication of information.

The present analysis focuses its attention on a macro-level of analysis in contradistinction to the studies cited above. Such an analysis addresses the two aspects of semantic integrity and the communicative function of texts. It is our contention that in the case of competent adult readers, information structure is a more powerful heuristic for the decoding or processing of text at the semantic level. It is our contention that attention to this variable will allow us more accurately to account for the processing of text on the semantic-language level.

We must emphasize that we do not wish to argue that the micro-analysis of shape, size, length, and spacing is not a valid form of analysis, but simply that in a perceptual sense it is a processing of text prior to language. It is prior to language in the sense that the kind of recognition it addresses itself to is a primary perceptual experience. We assert that the investigation of such variables as have been the concern of micro-analysis is an investigation of primary visual perception and not an investigation of language processing. The process of decoding "texts," whether they be language "texts" or static visual "texts" or dynamic visual "texts," consists of levels of processing matrix. Is is crucial in speaking of the visual processing of texts to distinguish the particular level of processing we are analyzing. The mistake is to assume that in explicating one level of processing we account for the entire process.

Redundancy and Visual Processing

As we have stated initially, the purpose of this analysis is to determine to what extent if any the underlying structuring of information within texts determines the visual processing of such texts. If in fact there is any empirical validity to the claim that such an underlying information structure as represented by Theme—Rheme plays a significant role in guiding the visual processing of textual material, then we would expect that the duration of fixations over areas of Theme—Rheme, representing old—new information, would vary significantly.

It is of some note that studies investigating the processing of static visual displays (cf. Mackworth & Morandi, 1967; Salapatek & Kessen, 1966; Zavalishin, 1964; Zusne & Michels, 1964) have noted that subjects tend to fixate most frequently areas high in information (i.e., unpredictable) or areas that are nonredundant. Many studies of fixation patterns on varying kinds of visual displays have made at least sketchy references to predictable versus nonpredictable and redundant versus nonredundant aspects of these displays and the role they might play in guiding fixation patterns. (For a comprehensive survey of a number of such studies, see especially Rayner, 1975). Yet no major or significant attempt has been made to document specifically the role that such a stimulus characteristic as predictable/nonpredictable, redundant/nonredundant, or old/new might have in guiding visual inspection or processing of static displays.

Within major studies of reading (Goodman, 1968; Hochberg, 1970b; Kolers, 1972; Levin & Kaplan, 1970; Wanat, 1971) the fact of the redundancy of language has been noted and some attempt has been made to incorporate this fact into models of the reading process. Yet these studies have not focused their attention on, nor exploited, the basic fact of redundancy. Where the concept of redundancy has been incorporated into processing models, it has usually been on the level of and in terms of the frequency distribution of letters, words, or the recurrence of certain syntactical patterns. The concept either on the semantic level or the level of information distribution within texts has been given little if any attention.

We would suggest that the concept of redundancy can and should be interpreted within the framework of Theme—Rheme structure of texts. Theme, encoding old or known information, represents recurring therefore redundant textual elements. Rheme, encoding new information, represents unpredictable and therefore nonredundant textual elements.

Theme—Rheme Structure

Our basic contention is that a text, insofar as it serves as a vehicle for communication, encodes its information inter alia by a dichotomy of old—new information represented in the structure of the text itself by the progression of Theme—Rheme.

Thought of in a simplified way, every constituent element of a given complete text consists of at least one element that serves as topic, i.e., given or known information, and at least one element that serves as comment, i.e., the critical new information crucial to pushing the communication forward. Consider the following fragment of a text:

1. My brother Leander bought a new car.
2. It was a green Audi.
3. It had a sun roof.
4. This could be opened from a control on the dashboard.
5. He gave me a drive in it the other day.
6. It rides very smoothly.

Presuming that you are familiar with the speaker's family, the element "My brother" serves as known information and in this case Theme. What is predicted of Leander is the "new" information. What is critical for pushing the communication forward in the first instance is to make known that a car was bought. In the second element "It" referring to the car now serves the function of "Known" information (hence the shorthand of pronoun) and the fact that the car was an Audi is the new information which again pushes the communication forward.

The process continues through the succeeding elements. If the point of the text was to tell us something about Leander's car, we can easily observe how this is done through the interplay of T–R.

We can represent this progression of old (i.e., known or recoverable from previous discourse) and new information in the following way:

$$
\begin{aligned}
&1.\ T_1 \rightarrow R_1 \\
&2.\ T_2(=R_1) \rightarrow R_2 \\
&3.\ T_2 \rightarrow R_3 \\
&4.\ T_3(=R_3) \rightarrow R_4 \\
&5.\ T_1 \rightarrow R_5(+R_1) \\
&6.\ T_4(=R_1 +R_5) \rightarrow R_6
\end{aligned}
$$

With this formal representation we can observe how the Theme–Rheme structure serves to build an interlacing pattern in order to push the communication forward. New information is linked on to known information and in turn becomes built on itself as it assumes the function of old information.

Theme–Rheme and Communicative Dynamism.   With one exception the example represents the simplest case of a Theme–Rheme structure. New information succeeds known information in a steady progression. There is a clean dichotomy between known and new information throughout. This holds until we reach element five in the text.

We can observe that element five has a Rheme that is partially recoverable from previous discourse, namely the reference to "in it." The Rheme then in element five is in some sense "less new" than other Rheme structures in the text. This variation in "newness" of given textual elements has been noted by Fribas (1964, 1975) who has termed the phenomena "communicative dynamism" (=CD). Fribas states (1975, p. 317):

> . . . the concept of CD is based on the fact that communication is not a static but a dynamic phenomenon. By CD I understand a quality displayed by communication in its development (unfolding) of the information to be conveyed and consisting in advancing this development.

Fribas concludes that while a discourse or text consists of a linear progression of information units, some old and some new, which in toto combine to form the "message" of the text, there is not always a clear delineation between the old and the new information. Text elements carry relative degrees of newness.

Those elements with a low degree of newness will be low in communicative dynamism (i.e., the degree to which they push the communication forward). Those elements with a high degree of newness will correspondingly exhibit a high degree of CD (i.e, they will be primarily responsible for pushing the communication forward). We will have occasion to return to this notion of CD at a later point.

Definition of Old—New Information Units

The Theme—Rheme or Topic—Comment articulation of a text or discourse then represents an efficient and underlying structure for encoding the information content of any communicative message. So far we have linked the term old or known information with Theme or Topic and new information with Rheme or Comment. We will here define these concepts of old—new, known—unknown and given—not given more precisely.

Information is essentially linear as is the text. Further, information can be thought of as varying in its probability of expectation or occurrence as can the elements in a text. In a significant work on information theory in psychology and education Walter (1971, p. 8) states:

> The more unexpected a sign the greater its information. Its information approaches zero when the receiver can expect the sign with near certainty. In the restricted sense of information theory, information is a measure of the novelty value of the sign for the receiver. One may also consider information as a measure of the uncertainty of a situation, which will be removed by the occurrence of an event from the field of possible events.

It is in this sense of "probability of expectation," derived from information theory, that we define the concepts of old—new, known—unknown, and given—not given textual elements. By new information we will understand any linguistic—semantic token that is textually or contextually not recoverable or nonderivable. By old information we will understand any linguistic—semantic token that is textually or contextually recoverable or derivable.

Every textual element, insofar as it occurs in a well formed text whose goal is communication, will exhibit an information focus. This information focus will be that portion of the element that represents new information in the sense we have defined new. We have observed above that it is those new information units that carry the most information and push the communication forward.

We can empirically observe that this information focus exhibits certain consistent structural characteristics within a text. We observe that the information focus, i.e. new information, is usually (a) noninitial, (b) nonanaphoric, and (c) occurs within the Rheme component of a textual element. On the other hand known information is usually (a) initial, (b) anaphoric, (c) often deleted by ellipsis (this is especially true in the case of spoken discourse), and (d) occurs in the Theme component of a textual element.

We can conclude that Theme can encode known information and will represent the starting point of a text or discourse. Rheme in turn will serve to encode new information and represent the information focus of a textual element. Rheme will be mapped onto Theme and serve the primary function of pushing forward the communication.

Theme—Rheme Hypothesis

We can formulate the hypothesis of the present study in the following way:

If Theme—Rheme structure of Texts represents an underlying processing algorithm of old—new information for such textual material we would expect that the duration of fixations over Theme—Rheme portions of textual material will vary significantly.

Using a notation developed by Daneš (1974) with modifications developed by Scinto (1977) we can characterize in a graphic fashion any particular text according to its information distribution of Theme—Rheme progression. Earlier I gave an example of simple text characterized according to its Theme—Rheme structure.

The notation essentially consists of two categories: T representing Theme, i.e., old information, and R representing Rheme, i.e., new information. Any element of text then can be characterized as consisting of a Theme and its corresponding Rheme. So then the sentence, "Leander is at least five feet tall" can be defined in the following way.

$$T_1 \qquad\qquad R_1$$
Leander is at least five feet tall.

that is, $T_1 \rightarrow R_1$

Given two sentences, between which there is a relationship, such that the Theme of the first is also the Theme of the second, they may be depicted as follows:

$$T_1 \rightarrow R_1$$
$$\downarrow$$
$$T_1 \rightarrow R_2$$

An example of such a pair would be the sentences:

$$T_1 \qquad\qquad R_1$$
The book was bought yesterday.

$$T_1 \qquad\quad R_2$$
It was published by Oxford.

A Rheme of one sentence may in turn become the Theme in the succeeding sentence. Such a relationship can be demonstrated by the following configuration:

$$T_1 \rightarrow R_1$$
$$\downarrow$$
$$T_2 \, (=R_1) \rightarrow R_2$$

An example of such a pair would be:

The paper was written for the conference.

The conference was held in Monterey.

The examples given illustrate the basic notation of Daneš. The examples are trivial in the sense that they illustrate only simplex sentences with a single Theme and Rheme. The notation is, however, adequate to handling more complex structures such as those involving coordination and subordination. In the case of such structures the expansion is as in the simplex cases but in a horizontal fashion. In the case of a coordinated structure the articulation might look like the following:

$$T_1 [T_1' + T_1''] \rightarrow R_1$$

An illustration of such a structure would be a sentence such as:

$$T_1 \qquad T_1$$
Leander and his brother left for Boston earlier.

The same would be true of a coordinated Rheme as in the following sentence:

Most of my time is spent writing papers trying to impress people.

R_1' = is spent writing papers

R_1'' = trying to impress people

The same notation is further capable of capturing the heuristic Theme—Rheme structure of other complex clauses which are the result of relativization and other concatenating processes.

However, to characterize adequately the semantic relationships between Theme and Rheme and succeeding textual elements, some further notation is necessary. In order to capture the nature of relationship of textual elements in their Theme—Rheme articulation, we propose to introduce the following additional vocabulary to the basic notation.

(a) = will represent an exact equivalence or paraphrase of T or R

So we may have: $T_1 \to R_1$
$$\downarrow$$
$$T_2 \, (=T_1) \to R_2$$

where $T_2 \, (=T_1)$ is an exact lexical copy, a synonym or a pronominalization of T_1.

(b) U will represent a subset or subelement of the set introduced by a previous T or R

So we may have: $T_1 \to R_1$
$$\downarrow$$
$$T_2 \, (UR_1) \to R_2$$

where T_2 the new Theme is a subset of the set defined by R_1. Often such elements will be introduced by a lexical marker such as: some . . ., few . . ., etc.

(c) ~ will represent the contrary or negative of the set defined by T or R.

So we may have: $T_1 \to R_1$
$$\downarrow$$
$$T_2 \, (\sim T_1) \to R_2$$

(d) $\not\to$ following T or R will represent an entailment, implication or consequence of T or R.

So we may have: $T_1 \to R_1$
$$\downarrow$$
$$T_2 \, (R_1 \not\to) \to R_2$$

where T_2 is an entailment, implication, or consequence of R_1.

The notation outlined above should be adequate in characterizing the information structure of texts in this study. For a further elaboration of this notation see Scinto (1977).

Experimental Paradigm

In order to test the empirical validity of the hypothesis, it was necessary first to select a text whose Theme—Rheme structure could be characterized fairly clearly in order to establish independently of observation of eye movement data its old—new information components. Next, once the selected text was characterized according to its old—new information structure, it was presented to subjects who were to read the text for information while their eye movements (especially fixations) over the text were recorded. The pattern of fixations and their duration, as they were distributed over identified old—new information portions of the text, were compared to ascertain whether there was a reliable difference between portions.

Experimental Text. It is unfortunate that there exists no standardized typology of texts that might characterize them in some systematic fashion as to their information structure, communicative function, or other characteristics. We only have at our disposal those textual classifications as they have come down to us from a classical tradition of rhetoric. These categories usually consist of the following classifications: fable, narrative, descriptive, expository, argumentative, discourses. Each of these categories can be and often are confounded with one another to form complex patterns.

As no index of well defined structural characteristics existed to allow us to choose between such types of discourses for experimental consideration, it was necessary to generate a set of criteria for selecting type of text for this study.

Criteria for Textual Choice. The following guidelines were established for the selection of an experimental text:

1. Its Theme—Rheme structure should be sufficiently direct so as to permit clear distinction between old—new information elements.
2. Its communicative function should be a single one and not an admixture of several to permit us to specify processing for a single purpose (e.g., information).
3. Contextual presuppositions for the text should be shared and accessible to as wide an audience as possible (a scientific text on quantum physics would hardly be appropriate).
4. The text should exhibit many phenomena of old or given information such as pronominalization, anaphora, and ellipses, to facilitate distinction between old—new information areas.
5. The CD structure of the text should be such as not to confound to a high degree the distinction between Theme—Rheme areas.
6. The text selected should be a communicative whole (i.e., form a complete message) and yet not exceed a reasonable length for presentation.

Given these criteria the text selected was a narrative fable by Aesop as retold by Anne Terry White. The text is reproduced below.

I

There once was a man who loved
money very much. He loved
money so much that he would
not spend a penny if he could
help it. All the miser wanted
to do was hold his money in
his hand and gloat over it.

II

At last he decided to sell
nearly everything he had and
change his money (into gold).
But then the miser was afraid
that someone would steal it.
So in the end he dug a hole
near the wall of his garden.

III

In this hole he buried his
treasure. Every morning he
would go to the garden and dig
up his treasure and look at
it. Then he would bury it
again. One morning he went
to his garden as usual.

IV

To his horror he saw that
someone had been there before
him. The ground was all dug
up. And the gold was gone.
"Thieves! Thieves!" he cried.
"I have been robbed!" He
began to cry and moan.

V

He cried so loudly that his
neighbor came running. When
he heard what had happened he
comforted the miser. "Nothing
so terrible has happened to
you. Just bury a stone there
and pretend that it is gold."

VI

"Since you never meant to spend
your treasure, a stone is as
good as a lump of gold."

Theme—Rheme Structure.   The experimental text may be characterized
in the following way using the notation established above:

$$n_1 \quad \text{To} \rightarrow R_1 \ [(\rightarrow \quad T_1 \ (=R_1) \rightarrow R_2)]$$

$$n_2 \qquad\qquad T_1 \rightarrow R_3 \ [(UR_2) \not\rightarrow T_1 \rightarrow R_4 \ (T_1 \rightarrow R_5 \ (UR_4)]$$

$$n_3 \qquad\qquad T_2 \ (=T_1) \rightarrow \quad R_6 \ (UR_2) + R_7$$

$$n_4 \qquad\qquad T_3 \ (=T_2) \rightarrow \quad R_7 \ [(UR_2) + R_8 \ (UR_2)]$$

$$n_5 \qquad\qquad T_4 \ (=T_2) \rightarrow \quad R_9 \ [\rightarrow (T_4 \rightarrow R_{10} \ (=R_8)]$$

$$n_6 \qquad\qquad T_5 \ (=T_3) \rightarrow \quad R_{11}$$

$$n_7 \qquad\qquad\qquad T_6 + \ T_7 \ (=T_2) \rightarrow R_{12} \ (UR_8)$$

$$n_8 \qquad\qquad\qquad T_8 \ (=T_2) \rightarrow R_{13} \ (\sim R_{12} + UR_8)$$

$$n_9 \qquad\qquad\qquad T_9 \ (=T_2) \rightarrow R_{14} \ (=R_{12})$$

n_{10} $\qquad$ $T_{10}\,(=T_2) \to R_{15}$ ———————

n_{11} $\qquad$ $T_{11}\,(=T_2) \to R_{16}$ $\quad [\to T_{12}\,(=T_4) \to R_{17}\,(UR_2 + UR_8)$

n_{12} $\qquad$ $T_{13}\,(UR_{15}) \to R_{18}$

$\qquad$ $+$

n_{13} $\qquad$ $T_{14}\,(=R_8) \to R_{19}$

n_{14} $\quad$ (Focus) $R_{20} \leftarrow T15\,(=T_2)$

n_{15} $\qquad$ $T_{16}\,(=T_2) \to R_{21}$

n_{16} $\qquad$ $T_{17}\,(=T_2) \to R_{21} + R_{22}$

n_{17} $\qquad$ $T_{18}\,(=T_2) \to R_{23}\,(=R_{21})\ [\to T_{19} \to R_{24}]$

n_{18} $\qquad\qquad\qquad$ $T_{20}\,(=T_{19}) \to R_{25}$

$\qquad\qquad\qquad$ $+$

$\qquad\qquad\qquad$ $T_{20}\,(=T_{19}) \to R_{26}\,(+T_2)$

n_{19} $\quad$ (Focus) $R_{27} \leftarrow T_{21}\,(=T_2)$

n_{20} $\qquad$ [ellipsis] $\to R_{28} + R_{29}$

$\qquad$ $T_{22}\,(=T_2) \to R_{30}$

n_{21} $\qquad$ $T_{23}\,(=R_{28}) \to R_{31}$

Delineation of Old—New Information. Having characterized the text as to its T—R structure, we can now clearly delineate those portions of the text which fall respectively under the classifications of old—new information. We will consider each sentence of the text in order of appearance. Elements that comprise old information will be enclosed in square brackets [ ] and elements comprising new information will be enclosed in parentheses ( ).

n_1 $\quad$ (There once was a man) [who] (loved money very much.)

n_2 $\quad$ [He loved money] (so much) (that) [he] (would not spend a penny) if [he] (could help) [it].

n_3 $\quad$ (All) [the miser] (wanted to do) (was hold) (his money) (in his hand) and [. . .] (gloat over) [it].

n_4 $\quad$ (At last) [he] (decided to sell) (nearly everything) [he] (had) and [. . .] (change) [his money] (into gold).

n_5 $\quad$ (But then) [the miser] (was afraid) that (someone would steal) [it.]

n_6 $\quad$ So in the end [he] (dug a hole near) (the wall of his garden.)

n_7 $\quad$ [In this hole] [he] (buried his treasure.)

n_8 $\quad$ (Every morning) [he] (would go to) [the garden] and (dig up) (his treasure.)

n_9 Then [he] (would bury) [it] (again.)

n_{10} (One morning) [he] (went to) (his garden) (as usual.)

n_{11} (To his horror) [he] (saw that someone had been) [there] (before) [him.]

n_{12} [The ground] (was all dug up.)

n_{13} And [the gold] (was gone.)

n_{14} ("Thieves! Thieves!") [he] (cried.)

n_{15} [I] (have been robbed!)

n_{16} [He] (began to cry and moan.)

n_{17} [He cried] (so loudly) (that) (his neighbor came running.)

n_{18} (When) [he] (heard) [what] (had happened) [he] (comforted) [the miser.]

n_{19} ("Nothing so terrible has happened to you.")

n_{20} [ellipsis] (Just bury a stone) [there] and [ellipsis] (pretend) (that) [it] (is) (gold.)

n_{21} "Since [you] (never meant to spend) (your treasure), [a stone] (is as good as) (a lump of gold.)

Subjects. Five subjects were solicited for the experiment. All subjects participating in the experiment were members of the Harvard University graduate and undergraduate community. Subjects were screened for the following two characteristics: (a) subjects' first language was English, and (b) subjects had not participated in a speed reading course or similar reading course.

Since it was strongly suspected that a developmental progression existed in the ability to produce and process textual material, only adults were chosen as subjects in this initial experiment.

Stimulus Presentation. The textual material was generated by a video character generator and recorded on video tape. Characters in the text were limited to upper case printed letters. Textual material was generated on the tape in six blocks or scenes of approximately the same length, with the exception of the final segment. Segments were broken at those points in the text which seemed to form natural divisions. As a consequence each of the six blocks had a semantic integrity of its own and formed natural subunits of the text as a whole.

Each of the segments was exposed for 9 sec. The exposure time was determined by taking the average time spent processing a similar amount of textual material in a pilot study. The textual segments were preceded by calibration material and faded in and faded out by means of a special effects generator during production of the stimulus material.

Spacing of characters and lines were subject to the constraints imposed by the video character generator and the manner of stimulus presentation (i.e., via television screen). Placing material too close to the edges of a television screen causes distortion of material and loss of data during eye-movement recording. In order not to project material too close to the edges of the screen, underscanning monitors were used during production of stimulus material. Lines were double-spaced in order to reduce ambiguity in scoring of fixations and to allow for later digitizing of the fixation data for off line computer analysis. Subsequent to production on videotape, textual material was transferred to cassette tape and frame coded for presentation in the laboratory.

Facility and Equipment

The experiment was carried out in the Eye Movement Laboratory of the Laboratory of Human Development, Harvard University. The Laboratory employs a Gulf & Western Eye-View Monitor system (Model 1994) employing a pupil-center corneal-reflection technique. All stimulus presentations in the Laboratory are through a video cassette deck. Subjects view the stimulus presentation while seated three feet in front of a seventeen-inch television monitor. Output data are recorded on half-inch video tape which records the stimulus presentation with crosshairs superimposed over the scene, the intersection of which marks the subject's point of fixation. Data are also recorded in digital form with frame code on nine track computer tape for off line analysis. Data samples are taken thirty times every second.

The Gulf & Western camera is situated one- and one-half feet in front and to the left of the subject. This positioning has not proved obtrusive to subjects. The system tolerates gross head movement within a one-cubic inch space. Subject's head movement is restricted by the use of a padded head rest which surrounds the temples and back of the head.

Experimental Task

Subjects in the experiment were fully cognizant of the purpose of the experiment. Subjects were told, before viewing the texts, that they would be asked to write a short summary of the story subsequent to reading it on the screen.

Subjects were seated before the screen and the necessary adjustments were made to the equipment. They were then informed of the calibration task and that following calibration they were to read silently the text as it appeared on the screen. Subjects were also instructed to read through the text only once, and having read through it, to fixate a small asterisk in the lower right corner of the screen.

After viewing the text subjects were asked to write a summary of the text. It was hoped that by requiring them to write a summary of the text material subsequent to viewing we might exercise some measure of control over the purpose for reading.

Method of Analysis

Data were collected on tape as outlined above. All video output was hand scored to yield locus of fixation and duration of fixation.

A tape deck with a stop-frame and slow motion feature was used in the scoring of all data tapes. We controlled the advance speed of the video tape so that one field dropped on the monitor screen at a rate which permitted the determination of the duration and the locus of fixation.

Locus of fixation was determined by observing the position of the intersection of the cross hairs in relation to the textual material. Duration of fixations was determined by counting the number of frames that dropped during the fixations. As every frame has a duration of one-thirtieth of a second and is composed of two fields, counting the number of fields that drop and dividing by sixty yielded a measure of duration.

Operational Definitions. The video data tapes yield thirty samples per second. In order to determine individual fixations, it was necessary to establish criteria for defining fixations. The following criteria were used:

1. Fixation — Any stabilization of the cross-hairs which has a duration of at least two frames will count as a fixation.
2. Duration of Fixation — Duration of fixation will be determined by counting frames of stabilization beginning after the initial two frames of stabilization.
3. Termination of Fixation — A fixation will be considered terminated at the last frame prior to dissolution of cross-hair stability (often observed as a collapse of the cross-hairs backward).

Results

Results given in Tables 1 and 2 represent the data output on five subjects, four males and one female. Here the total numbers of fixations, the distribution of these totals over old and new information areas, and the mean duration of fixations over old and new information areas are shown. Mean durations were determined by dividing total duration of fixations over areas of old and new information by the number of fixations over the respective areas. New information areas of text occurred more frequently than did old. The mean fixation durations on old and new information areas were found to be significantly different ($t_{(4)} = -6.67$, $p < .01$) and might be attributed to the artifact that new information units are on the average longer (i.e., in terms of character length) than old information units.

It is yet to be demonstrated empirically that stimulus length is directly correlated with fixation duration. However, it appears that the analysis indicates that

TABLE 1
Number and distribution of fixations

Subject	TF[a]	FO[b]	FN[c]
01	189	38	151
02	178	39	139
03	121	24	97
04	132	31	101
05	120	25	95

[a]TF = total number of fixations over all areas;
[b]FO = fixations on old information areas;
[c]FN = fixations on new information areas.

TABLE 2
Mean duration of fixation (msec.)

Subject	MFO[a]	MFN[b]	TFDO[c]	TFDN[d]
01	.14	.17	5.45	25.55
02	.15	.18	5.66	24.72
03	.10	.15	2.46	14.58
04	.11	.13	3.53	13.47
05	.11	.15	2.70	14.30

[a]MFO = mean duration of fixations on old information areas;
[b]MFN = mean duration of fixations on new information areas;
[c]TFDO = total duration of fixations on old information areas;
[d]TFDN = total duration of fixations on new information areas.

duration is correlated with the information value of stimulus events. Intuitively, it might be expected that the greater the length of stimulus units, the greater the number of fixations over those units. This question of the relation of length to fixation duration remains an empirically unanswered question, for it was decided to control for stimulus length in the comparison of fixation durations on old and new areas.

The following formula and procedure was devised to account for varying stimulus length. When the mean character length per word was calculated for old and new information portions of text the following values were obtained: old = 3.09 CL/W; new = 4.03 CL/W. In order to enter this value into the calculation of fixation duration units for comparison the following formula was used:

$$\text{TFD} \div (\text{TNF} \div [\text{MCL/W}]) = \text{Units of comparison}$$

Total fixation durations (TFD) on given areas of old and new areas of text were divided by a value obtained by dividing the total number of fixations (TNF) on the given area of text by the mean character length per word as determined for that area of text.

In this way it is possible to control for the fact that there is a greater probability of fixations occurring on new areas of text.

Rather than enter the total number of fixations on a given area of text in determining a mean fixation duration, we enter a total number of fixations value corrected for the differing length of units for that area of text. Now we are able to weight the units of comparison for the difference in both the number of old–new information units and the difference in length of those units. We obtain a fixation duration per fixation per character length per word.

Given in Table 3 are the total numbers of fixations corrected for character length per word. When total fixation durations are divided by the corrected value for number of fixations we obtain the values shown in Table 4. The comparison of these weighted means yielded a significant difference between the old and new information ($t_{(4)} = -14.07, p < .001$).

TABLE 3

| Subject | TNFO[a] | TNFN[b] |
	(as corrected for CL/W)	
01	12.30	37.47
02	12.62	34.49
03	7.77	24.07
04	10.03	25.06
05	8.09	23.57

[a]TNFO = total number of fixations on old information areas;

[b]TNFN = total number of fixations on new information areas.

TABLE 4

Subject	Old	New
01	.44	.68
02	.45	.72
03	.32	.61
04	.35	.54
05	.33	.61

Discussion and Implications

Results from the analyses reported here suggest a relation between the underlying information structure of texts and the visual processing of such texts. Based on these results we can formulate a suggestion for a processing rule for textual material. Such a rule might read as follows:

$$\epsilon \quad n \quad [(n + x) \rightarrow (t - x)] \quad V \quad [(n - x) \rightarrow (t + x)]$$

Given a set of textual elements whose probability of occurrence is some factor n: spend less time processing those elements with n + x probability of occurrence and more time processing those with n − x probability of occurrence.

While such a rule specifies an adequate description of what textual processing might look like on a macro-level there still remains the task of explicating how the process comes to recognize, distinguish and compute those elements with (n + x) or (n − x) probability of occurrence.

Such a task is clearly beyond the scope of this paper. In fact, it is probably beyond the state of the art in either psychology or psycholinguistics today. For a first attempt at delineating what might be involved in the specification of how the process alluded to above takes place, see especially Katz (1975) and Miller and Johnson-Laird (1976).

However, if we assume that the process involves some sort of internal computation (as my own biases and intuition lead me to believe), we would suggest the following sort of mechanism. Given that the linguistic—semantic tokens are assigned internal representations (for purposes of processing) one of which is an index of their "information value," these representations are in turn computed in a hierarchical order. Once a given level of a token's representation has been computed, the subject must then make a decision as to whether to continue processing beyond this point. At any level of processing a decision point is reached as to whether to continue or terminate, based on the information available about the stimulus input at that point. This process we assume occurs in real time — within the time that the token is being fed to the representational system through the visual sense, and is available in short-term store. With tokens whose information index assigns a high probability of occurrence we would expect processing to be terminated as an earlier stage than would the processing of tokens with a lower probability of occurrence. This should be reflected in length of fixation on the stimulus. Given that a token has been encountered in previous discourse, more information about the token would be available at a much earlier stage of computation than would be true for newer tokens.

The kind of process suggested above agrees in part with models of information processing suggested by Broadbent (1958) and by Triesman (1964). A full explication must await the results of more empirical observation and manipulation.

Emphasis is on a macro-level of textual processing. The analysis does not challenge the validity of explanations of primary visual perception in the processing of texts but instead clearly delineates a necessary distinction: that in decoding text there is a "levels of processing matrix." If we seek to discover what is distinctively involved in the visual processing of language *qua* language, fully satisfying answers will not be found on the level of primary perceptual processing but by consideration of whatever is distinctive to the stimulus under consideration. In the case of language, success in elucidating the production and decoding process lies in a consideration of the functions that language serves and of how those functions are realized within the unit text.

DISCUSSION

ROTHKOPF: First of all, I think it's very nice that you stressed the analysis of the functional aspect of text. I'm somewhat less optimistic about analyzing the semantic content of text itself. Before I go to that, though, I want to say that the tradition of estimating semantic content of text in information terms is pretty old, dating back at least to Taylor's (1957) analysis.

SCINTO: I have not tried to determine any kind of quantitative measure of information within textual material. What I have done was to take a distinction first proposed by Mathias (in Vachek, 1966) and the Prague School of Linguistics that states that texts embody two basic fields or types of information, namely, old or previously known information and new information. I have attempted to determine whether this basic distinction in type or kind of information is reflected in actual textual processing.

ROTHKOPF: There are many quantitative data around in some sense more reliable than the essentially subjective analysis that's involved here, and the kind of morphological analysis of text that you do. There have been experimental manipulations of information content. Some have had rather contradictory findings. For example, the Morton (1964) Successive Approximation to English studies showed no effect on duration of fixation.

SCINTO: I am aware of the kind of studies you refer to. What I wish to point out is that if in fact weak correlations between duration and information processing have been found in the past, this may in large measure be due to the way in which the stimulus texts have been characterized. Alternatively, such weak correlations may be the consequence of looking at the stimulus text at too fine a level of analysis.

What I have suggested in the paper is a different way of characterizing the textual material along a nonquantitative dimension that was developed independently of eye-movement recording. Upon testing out this characterization with eye-movement recording, we found strong correlations between duration of fixation and theme—rheme structure.

WISHER: It seems from the example that you've given, the old information is often signalled by reference and relative pronouns and the new information tends to be introduced by grammatically more complex structure. I wonder if the increase in duration reflects not that it's old or new, but is the result of the inherent processing difficulties of these syntactic structures.

SCINTO: As a broad generalization that is true. I should point out that the old—new information distinction can cut across syntactic and constituent boundaries. It is not always the case that the relation you point out exists. Theme—rheme form a hyper-syntax of their own which is independent of lexical content and syntactic categories.

IV.4

Ocular-Motor System Control of Position Anticipation and Expectation: Implications for the Reading Process[1]

Gerald Leisman
Brooklyn College of the City University of New York
and *East Orange, New Jersey VA Hospital*

Reading is one of the most complex of human activities involving the extraction of meaning from language, an intricate interaction between visual information processing and ocular-motor function. Yet little is known about how visual information is received, processed, stored, and retrieved (Gibbon, 1975).

Vision is the dominant sense in humans. More brain area is devoted to the acquisition and processing of visual information than to any other sense. It is interesting to note that, despite the amount of information it provides, the eye is actually a limited receptor of visual information. The fovea, which constitutes a small region of the retina, corresponding to 0.6 to 1° of visual angle, is capable of resolving images with a high degree of acuity. However, acuity decreases sharply with increasing distance from the fovea (Alpern, 1962). Therefore, in order for information to be effectively received, the fovea must be aligned with the intended target. Saccades and fixations are required to perform this process, and they have been described elsewhere in relation to reading (cf. Leisman & Schwartz, 1976; Monty & Senders, 1976; Yarbus, 1967). It is important to note that visual sensitivity is reduced by a factor of between 2 and 3 during the period just prior to and during a saccadic eye movement (Haber & Hershenson, 1973; Volkmann, Schick, & Riggs, 1968). Thus, one must question whether any useful information enters the visual–perceptual system during such movement.

Somehow, from successive small samplings of information, the brain is able to construct and maintain a meaningful representation of presented text, thus making reading possible. Since the receptive powers of the eye are limited, the

---

[1]This work is supported by the Medical Research Service of the Veterans Administration.

ocular-motor system must perform efficiently to allow the brain to analyze and integrate limited input.

Another reason for moving the eye during reading is to change fixation by traveling from the end of one line to the beginning of the following line. This large saccade is called a return sweep. In order for this aspect of the reading process to be most efficient, the eye must accurately move to the beginning of a line, neither stopping before the target area (undershoot) nor stopping past the target area (overshoot).

The smaller the degree of error, the greater the efficiency, since any error forces the reader to refixate, that is, to determine where to move next and to make a small saccade to get there (Abrams & Zuber, 1972). These extra movements require as much time as "normal" saccades; therefore, reading speed decreases when these movements are made.

Leisman and Schwartz (1976; 1977) have formulated a model of the reading process based on a discrete edge transmission model of vision that is summarized in Fig. 1.

Implicit in this theoretical formulation is the notion that two types of processes occur during the fixation pause. First, text material is transmitted and processed (text processing) (cf. Gaarder, 1975; Leisman, 1976a). Second, position information is processed through the ocular-motor system to determine where the eye will move next (position processing) (Abrams & Zuber, 1972). The analysis of information necessary to direct the return sweep to the beginning of the following line occurs during position processing.

Inspection of eye movement patterns recorded during reading indicates that there are two distinct processes that determine position of the return sweep. The first process appears to be *position anticipation*, where all of the necessary information regarding the beginning position of the following line enters the

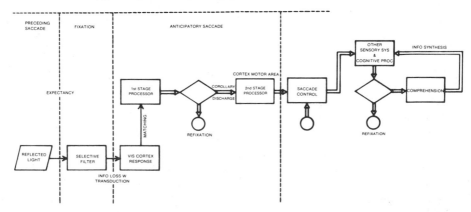

FIG. 1.   Model of visual information transmission in the reading process. (From Leisman & Schwartz, 1976a. In R.M. Knights and D.K. Bakker (Eds.) *The neuropsychology of learning disorders: Theoretical approaches.* Copyright 1976, University Park Press, Baltimore.)

visual system during one of the fixations on a preceding line, and is utilized during the first few lines of the text. After anticipation has been in operation for several lines, and if all lines start in the same horizontal position (i.e., left justified), the second process, *position expectation,* utilizes previous position information to determine where each of the following lines begin.

Abrams and Zuber (1972) make the assumption that the last fixation on a line involves less text processing than other fixation pauses, primarily because the position information necessary to direct the return sweep is being processed. Although their data seems to support this assumption, the work of several researchers (McConkie, 1976; Poulton,1962; Rayner, 1975; Taylor, 1976) leaves open the possibility that when a reader fixates the end of a line, the beginning of the next line would be too far into the periphery for sufficient position information to enter the visual system.

The importance of anticipation and expectancy mechanisms should not be minimized. For example, Leisman and Schwartz (1976) have noted that a difficulty frequently associated with reading disability in childhood is the inability of the child to attend to and select from various sensory stimuli impinging on him at any given moment. Attentional handicaps, especially those associated with reading disorders, have a marked visual component. We have reported data indicating that many individuals with such disorders demonstrate variable patterns of scanning and fixation and do not demonstrate anticipatory saccades (Leisman, 1973; 1974; 1975; 1976b). By further analogy, some children may be unable to expect forthcoming stimuli as demonstrated by reduction or absence of the *contingent negative variation* (CNV) or *expectancy wave* and the P_{300} wave in the computer averaged evoked response (cf. Sutton, Tueting, Zubin, & John, 1967; Walter, 1964). When paired flashes of light are presented over many trials, the interstimulus interval defines the CNV potential. These potentials are frequently absent or reduced in children with reading disorders (Mackworth, 1973).

The sequential nature of the reading process, the ability to recognize small differences between visually similar items, the necessity of remembering and recognizing orientational differences, and the importance of an adequate ocular-motor and visual processing apparatus all become important considerations in the development of any model of the reading process.

EYE MOVEMENT PRECISION PROGRAMMING IN READING

Dallos and Jones (1963) show that an observer who makes a series of successive saccades in a regular sequence will anticipate the target to some degree after the fourth or fifth jump. Monkeys fail to make such predictive saccades (Fuchs, 1967), as do significant numbers of reading retarded children (Leisman, in press; Leisman, Sprung, Ashkenazi, & Schwartz, in press). The ability to anticipate correctly a target in a sequence depends on the precision of eye position encoding. Without precision, a correct anticipatory set cannot be efficiently formed.

The duration of the return sweep requires that these movements be pro-grammed to anticipate future events, allowing ocular-motor performance to keep in phase with developing cognitive situations. The minimum length of time over which such programs operate depends on factors related to ocular-motor reaction time (Leisman, 1975, 1976b, 1977a); age (Gatev, 1968; Leisman, 1975, 1976b); practice on task; and sequencing regularity.

Each saccade is a controlled event upon which the clear reception of visual information depends. In reading, prediction is necessary, because if the eye movement is to occur when it should, it must have been planned in advance. Further, prediction is essential because saccades are essentially ballistic, unmodi-fiable once they have begun.

Prediction, therefore, means that eye movement cannot depend on a simple connection between stimulus and response, but involves multilevel distribution of control. Ballistic means that the fixations and saccades are phased-and time-sequences of muscular contractions and relaxations that are initiated as wholes (cf. Leisman & Schwartz, 1976). Therefore, in reading one usually does not fixate a letter or word, but larger units (Rayner & McConkie, 1976; Gaarder, 1975). In the case of reading, there is a complex interaction based not only on the immediate stimulus, but also upon the future goals, past experiences, and concurrent factors such as head position changes. Therefore, while progressive saccades are in a sense similar from one scan to the next, in another sense they are never the same. Eye movement in reading, therefore, should require active updating and reading efficiency should be related to anticipation.

THE RELATIONSHIP BETWEEN INTERMITTENCY IN VISION AND CONTROL OF POSITION INFORMATION

Studies of eye movements may be broadly classed into two categories. The first is how the nervous system converts the retinal pattern into a fovea-target error marker. The second category deals with the conversion of the error marker into motor commands. The assumption implicit in our studies is that the presence of nonfoveal retinal stimulation leads to the generation of error markers.

Fleming, Vossius, Bouman, and Johnson (1969) have presented evidence in support of the contention that the saccadic eye movement system is independent from retina to extraocular muscles and operates on displacement error signals. While the visual system may intermittently take information because the saccadic system does not provide a continuous input, the perceptual system must con-tinually process information (Gaarder, 1975; Latour, 1962). This is in addition to the well-known elevation in visual threshold accompanying a saccade that begins prior to the movement (Volkmann et al., 1968).

Considering the available knowledge of the return sweep process, one can only speculate the course of events between retinal stimulation and actual saccadic return sweep movements. MacKay (1973) developed what appears to be a reasonable explanation of the perception of change in the visual environment. By placing the events related to the return sweep into MacKay's format, an explanation can be developed for the return sweep process. He points out that the perceptable world can be regarded as a source of constraints on both internal and external action, and on the organization of such action. Thus, sensory perception has two basic functions: (a) to update the evaluation and selection of onging effector action, and (b) to update the conditional readiness of the organism to take account of the contents of its environment when organizing action.

MacKay discusses the ideal situation in which the perceptable environment does not change. Here changes in sensory input could only be caused by movements of the retina relative to the environment. Since objects are stable, the eyes function as ongoing supplier of feedback about where the organism was positioned in relationship to the objects in its environment, thus enabling the organism to move effectively among these objects. Since the contents are fixed, their location could be represented in some form within the brain. This would impose conditional constraints on the planning of locomotion in a way similar to the effect of a map on the driver of a car. As long as the environment is fixed, once the map is produced, there would be no further need for any coupling to it from sensory input, since only 100% redundant information would be produced. Sensory input would still be important, however, in relation to locomotor feedback. Thus, in a stable world, sensory signals would have a high selective-information rate, with respect to locomotor guidance, but a negligible selective-information rate, with respect to internal map-making.

If we now look at a page of text, we find that, for analytic purposes, it can be equated with MacKay's stable world, since words do not move in relation to the page. Visual information, concerning the position of points of interest, impinge upon the retina, allowing for the ongoing reestablishment of an internal map. With such a map, the eyes can be guided within and between lines of text. Although the specific sensory input affecting eye movement across a line changes from line to line, those affecting margins, and therefore return sweeps, are usually constant. When a page of text is both right and left justified (all lines begin in one vertical column and end in another vertical column), the only place where position deviations will appear is at the beginning and ending of paragraphs. One of the principles of MacKay's system is acceptance of the null hypothesis that the map is correct until sufficient evidence is received to the contrary. If such a parsimonious approach is followed in the reading of text, then once the map coordinates for the beginning of lines have been established, and a program to execute the necessary eye movement from the right justified position to the left justified position has been generated, no updating need be necessary until an error (deviation) is detected. What is necessary, however, is an ongoing informational evaluation, where an expected event, represented on an internal map and instituted as a corollary discharge, is compared to a current event, represented by an incoming signal. It is this process, whereby the establishment of a map can be utilized repetitively to guide eye movements, that we refer to as *position expectation*. Since one need only detect a difference between two signals, it is expected that less processing and, therefore, less processing time should be utilized than in the situation where coordinates must be calculated and a new saccade program generated.

Thus, there appears to be evidence supporting two processes related to saccadic movement of the eyes during reading. One process, position anticipation, deals with the utilization of the sequential input of visual information for the generation of a new program to direct each saccade. The other process, position expectation, deals with the establishment, in storage, of spatial location values related to a particular reoccurring saccadic movement for the generation of a program utilized whenever the need for that particular saccadic movement is encountered.

If we now look at these two processes in relation to the return sweep, we can begin to formulate hypotheses with regard to the nature of the motor encoding of the return sweep in reading. Our primary concern is with the nature of the encoding of position information related to saccades in general and the return sweep in particular. Further, control mechanisms underlying anticipatory saccades and the prevention of undershooting and overshooting of return sweeps are of interest. Opening a servo loop to analyze eye control systems has been accomplished by both optical and electronic techniques (Dichburn & Ginsborg, 1952; Ford, White, & Lichtenstein, 1959; Leisman, 1973, 1974, 1976c; Riggs, Ratliff, Cornsweet, & Cornsweet, 1953). Both methods add eye position to target position in a fashion that cancels any effect of eye movement on reducing fovea target error.

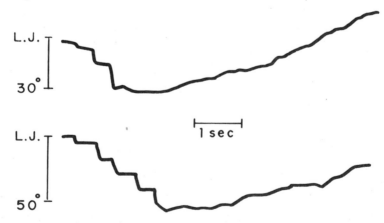

FIG. 2.   Electro-olulographic record of subjects' left eye movements while viewing right and left justified text generated on CRT subtending. (A) 30° and (B) 50°, with paralysis or right eye and occlusion of left. Deflections are from fixation at left justified (L.J.) position.

TABLE 1

Saccades Recorded From Occluded by Mobile Left Eye of Subject[a]

	Average Width of Text (in deg)	Average Saccade Displacement (in deg)	Total Saccades
Noncomplex Text	10	3.7	28
(RGL = 8.3)	20	2.6	29
	30	2.4	62
	40	2.0	74
	50	2.0	82
Complex Text	10	4.6	31
(RGL = 12.8)	20	3.8	43
	30	2.9	68
	40	2.5	79
	50	2.1	87

[a]Indicated under complex text presentations to paralyzed right eye and subtending between 10 and 50°.

Using a method previously reported by Fleming et al. (1969) and Kulikowski and Leisman (1973), we attempted to demonstrate the effects of a pharmacological open loop situation on the directional coding of saccadic eye movements in reading. Retrobulbar *lignocaine* anesthetic was administered to a subject's right eye with bilateral pupil dilation and restriction of accomodation achieved by the topical instillation of *cyclopentolate*. The details of these procedures are reported elsewhere (Leisman, 1977b). EOG was recorded from the mobile eye, which was occluded so that only the paralyzed eye was exposed to a computer graphics terminal screen. In other words, the eye that could see could not move, and the eye that could move, could not see. Unfamiliar text, right and left justified, which subtended either 10, 20, 30, 40, or 50° at a distance of 1 m was generated on the CRT. The subject was required to read the text presented on the screen under each condition.

Figure 2 demonstrates that an increase in the angular subtense of the text on the screen results in an increase in the number of saccades made by the occluded eye. The mobile eye continues to make saccadic movements as the reading of the line progresses. However, when it reaches the end of the line, as Fig. 2 illustrates, the occluded eye, displaced anywhere between 10–50° from the left justified position, does *not* perform a return sweep, but instead drifts gradually towards the left text margin. These drifts require times ranging from 10 sec for a 10° deviation to 55 sec for a 50° deviation. When the occluded eye does return, it consistently overshoots the left justified text position. Also *no* regressions were noted in any of the records. Even when text is erased, the occluded eye makes a slow return drift, similar to that which takes place when the paralyzed eye is occluded and the moving eye views the text on the screen.

This example is consistent with the notion that an uncorrectable error signal drives the saccades in the mobile eye until it reaches a maximum displacement. This effect might be related to relative retrieval position cues from both eyes, rather than to inappropriate disparities in the position of the eyes.

Nodine and Simmons (1974) and Rayner and McConkie (1976), among others, have indicated a relationship between the level of text complexity and the number of saccades per line. In Table 1, it can be seen that for two 150 word passages of text of varying complexity, that is, *Reading Grade Level,* the indications are that the number of forward saccades vary primarily as a function of the angular subtense of the line, with wider text greatly limiting the extent of the total displacement of the moving eye. Although textual complexity plays a relatively minor role here, both parameters influence the number of saccades made.

It is not likely that the observations were due to inconsistent position information from the eyeball, for no proprioceptors exist in the extra-ocular muscles (Brindley & Merton, 1960). The slow drift "return sweep" may have been the result of a release of a tonic holding mechansim and an example of movement without proprioception described by Bossom (1974).

INNERVATION OF THE RETURN SWEEP IN READING

Eye muscles can be innervated in two ways. First, the bilateral and symmetrical nerve supply can create tonus in extra-ocular muscle and, second, tonus may be created by means of a reflex position innervation dependent on fixation, luminance, and attention. The preceding example showed that even though binocular innervation had been supplanted in part by monocular controlling centers, the voluntary nerve supply still exhibited some inhibitory control over the "intact" eye.

To illustrate the relative effects of eye position and the role of the locus of retinal stimulation on the latency of the return sweep under the anaesthetized condition previously described (Leisman, 1977b), text was again presented left and right justified, subtending, in steps of 10°, between 10–50° of visual angle. The subject viewed the screen binocularly with base-out prisms of .5, 1, 1.5, 2.5 △ placed over the left unanaesthetized eye (Fig. 3). Eye movements were recorded electrooculographically while the subject viewed the screen at a distance of 1m.

With base-out prism in excess of + .5△ inducing deviation of the "intact" eye, the normal characteristics of the return saccadic sweep are restored. Increase in the amount of prism has no observed effect on the duration of the return sweep independent of the width of the text on the screen. Figure 4 gives

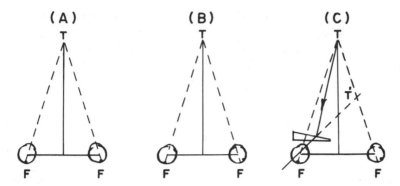

FIG. 3.   (A) indicates the normal vergence of the eyes without paralysis while fixating on marker superimposed on text on CRT; F represents fovea. (B) indicates the position of the eyes with lateral movements of right eye paralyzed on retinal stimulation of the right paralyzed eye displaced from the foveal area. (C) indicates the presentation of base-out prism over the mobile left eye that displaces the retinal image on the left moving eye temporally, resulting in the reinstitution of the return sweep and backward saccades.

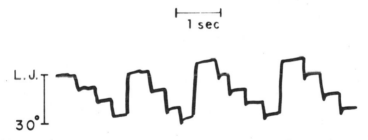

FIG. 4.   Eye movement record of subject while viewing right and left justified text subtending 30°, presented on CRT screen with paralyzed right and .5 base-out prism over moving left eye.

an example of an eye movement record obtained while viewing text subtending 30° with .5△ base-out prism over "intact" left eye with binocular viewing.

Basically, two neural systems signal movement: the *image/retina* and the *eye/head* systems (cf. Gregory, 1958, 1966). Each cancels the other out during an eye movement, to give stability to the visual world. Sherrington (1906) had proposed an *inflow theory* in which signals from the extra-ocular muscles are fed back to the brain when the eye moves to cancel the movement signals from the retina. Helmholtz (1896) on the other hand, thought that central signals from the eye fields programmed eye movements. This has been referred to as an *outflow theory*.

Hochberg (1976) and Fisher (1976) in a discussion of the question of the programming of eye movement in reading, suggested a number of possible control mechanisms. One of these was that information acquired in the visual periphery directs eye movement. This might explain the observed phenomenon when coupled with Yasui and Young's (1976) comment that cancellation is associated with an outflow mechanism that is less than complete — on the order of 60 to 70%.

Additional questions need to be answered in order to understand the nature of the control of the return saccades in reading. Examples are: Why is it that saccades can be performed by the nonparalyzed eye? Why is it possible to have the return sweep, and all movement away from the paralyzed eye, drift or stop?

In answer to the first question, it would appear that the return sweep saccade is a yoked movement. Even with the paralysis of one eyeball, the innervation should be equal and reciprocal. The ability to perform progressive saccades and the inability to perform adequate regressive movements, however, indicate the existence of multiple control functions consistent with Stark's notions on saccadic control.

Stark (1971) has indicated that when plotting phase plane trajectories, the trajectories were found to be suboptimal for a controller that supposedly minimizes the time necessary to make an eye movement such as a return sweep. He had calculated that the actual movements take two to four times as long for completion as could be obtained if the system operated with the maximum tension and attempted a minimal time policy. Such suboptimal trajectories, reported by Stark, were hypothesized to be a consequence of a system being computationally bound on one level and requiring multilevel distribution of control.

One possible explanation of the phenomenon is that the retina of the paralyzed eye has created a large error marker in relation to the saccadic movements of the occluded left eye, which does not get past the now "opened" saccadic control path. This then might cause an inhibitory process to occur that would cancel the anticipated return sweep. In Stark's (1971) terms, the "first level" error path has been open-circuited and the higher level cancellation paths remain in operation.

A second possibility is that the return "sweep" drift may be reflective of an instability in the ocular-motor system. Under normal circumstances, eye movements serve an adjustive function for getting information from the periphery to the fovea, that is, bringing text to that portion of the retina with the greatest visual clarity. With minimum clarity in the periphery and paralysis of the seeing eye, the return sweep may have been cancelled.

A third possibility to explain the return sweep drift involves Ludvigh's (1952a) notion of *parametric feedback* as related to the muscle spindle discharge. This discharge, according to Ludvigh, provides information regarding discrepancies in eye position and tonus. This mechanism is a good fit for the normal return sweep, in that it allows the eye to make a low error—high velocity shift after a latency of approximately 180 msec corresponding to the long last fixation on a line. According to Ludvigh, even a small difference in extra-ocular muscle tone or metabolism would make a movement such as a return sweep difficult to execute.

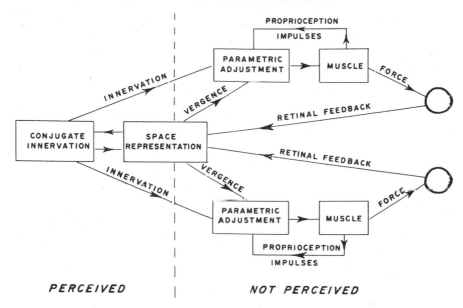

FIG. 5.   Schematic representation of Ludvigh's model of parametric feedback. (From Ludvigh, 1952b. *A.M.A. Archives of Opthalmology, 48,* 442–448. Copyright 1952, American Medical Association.)

Figure 5 is a schematic representation of Ludvigh's (1952b) model of parametric feedback. The system is based on retinal feedback to conjugate eye fields. It is possible, then, that our observations may have resulted from a lack of adequate retinal feedback.

IMPLICATIONS FOR THE READING PROCESS

Most saccades are goal-directed eye movements and are to a large extent preprogrammed to meet the intended visual target (Brooks & Jung, 1973). Brooks and Jung conclude that attentive expectancy and preprogramming play an essential role in the preparation and timing of goal-directed saccades in visuo-spatial location. Both interfixation and return sweep saccades are of a goal-directed nature. It is, therefore, expected that as reading proceeds, and as the eyes move from one fixation to the next, each fixation will be prepared by saccades directed toward an anticipated target to allow for a sequence of visual information input. It is this process that has been referred to as position anticipation.

In order for the return sweep to be most efficient, the eye must move accurately from the end of one line to the beginning of the next, neither undershooting nor overshooting the target area. The duration of a saccade is related to its amplitude; if a positioning error is made, the duration of a saccade needed to correct for that error will depend on the amplitude of that error. Therefore, the greater the error, the longer the latency of the correction, and the slower the reading speed. Thus, reading speed should be affected by the accuracy of saccadic eye movement and, hence, the correctness of anticipatory programs.

In eye movement studies of skilled reading, it is difficult to examine the effects of text processing in isolation from position processing. This is especially true in light of Abrams and Zuber's (1972) succinct observation that the major portion of the fixation pause is not spent in the acquisition of textual information. In the same vein, anticipatory saccadic mechanisms related to reading cannot be studied in isolation, as reading dynamics confound concepts of a preprogrammed eye movement.

DISCUSSION

VAUGHAN: I will briefly restate your findings in my own terms and then make a suggestion. When the seeing eye is paralyzed and the moving eye is occluded, saccades in the direction of reading occur in the occluded eye, but return sweeps do not. The stimulus presented to the paralyzed eye is directly in front of it, so that this eye is presented with textual material in either hemiretina and, therefore, there is text to the right of the point of fixation. There is a stimulus for making eye movements to the right. Since the paralyzed eye does not move and, therefore, the point of fixation is never located at the right end of the line, the effective stimulus for the return sweep is never presented to that eye.

LEISMAN: The point is that this effect is found independent of the length of the line. At 30° perhaps one does not see the end of the line and the stimuli are certainly blurred. At 10° there would at least be parafoveal vision of the end of the line, but the return sweep is still cancelled.

VAUGHAN: But the direction of gaze is never *directed* at the end of the line. Even in the 10° case the end of the line would always be 5° to the right.

LEISMAN: Yes. But the latency of the return saccade decreases with increasing time after initial paralysis. If what you suggest was correct, one would expect an all-or-nothing situation, which was not found.

GOLDBERG: Although I'm an amateur in the reading business, I am somewhat disturbed by the concept that there might be some fundamental difference between progressive and return saccades. The data on the open loop experiment are somewhat reminiscent of the Flemming, Vossius, Bouman and Johnson (1969) open loop experiments, in which the eye, when it gets to the end of the orbit, gives up and returns to central fixation. As the fixed eye has no way of knowing that the first progressive saccade has occurred, might it not be that the saccade system is just generating the same first saccade over and over again? Perhaps it is that the occluded eye reaches the end of the orbit and then gives up, rather than a case of the eye being able to make a series of progressive saccades and being unable to make a return sweep.

LEISMAN: In other words, what you're saying is that we are dealing with the repeated programming of a single movement.

GOLDBERG: Yes, and that you are not looking at the natural progression of saccades that one would ordinarily see.

SKAVENSKI: I think Goldberg's comments are exactly right. What the subject is trying to do in this situation is to make small saccades from the beginning of a line of text to the next word. Since the seeing eye cannot move, when he makes the saccade, it looks like the whole sheet of text has stepped in the direction of that first saccade because the eye really cannot get to the second word, so after another saccadic latency you do it again. With this chain of saccades, the whole page of text should now appear when the eye reaches the end of its mechanical limits. What then happens is that the nonparalyzed occluded eye simply stops making saccades and the eye simply goes back as it does because it has no stimulus.

LEISMAN: I do not think that we are dealing with the programming of single rather than successive saccades for a number of reasons. First, the return sweep latency varies with the time subsequent to anesthetic administration. One might expect an all-or-nothing situation if the effects observed in the demonstration were due simply to the incomplete programming of a single movement. Secondly, base-out prism over the intact nonparalyzed eye, on the one hand, returns the regressive saccades to the msec time frame, but on the other, still manifests significant latency differences between normal and paralyzed/prism conditions, as we have reported elsewhere (Leisman, 1977b). Also, it is not as if the nonparalyzed eye was required to perform a maximum displacement in the orbit on each trial. Progressive saccades of less than 40° still resulted in regressive drift when redirection was required. The most compelling reason that I do not think that we are dealing with the repeated programming of a single uncompleted saccade is that the displacement of the intact, occluded eye corresponds with the angular subtense of the line presented to the paralyzed eye.

IV.5

Analyzing Eye Movements to Infer Processing Styles During Learning from Text

Ernst Z. Rothkopf[1]
Bell Laboratories

The primary aim of this research is to understand how people learn from written material. My associates and I have concentrated on examining the control of processes by which readers extract information from text when they are reading for specific purposes. In this connection we have developed techniques for recording and analyzing eye movements during prolonged reading in realistic settings. I will describe these techniques and illustrate their usefulness with results from experiments on goal-guided learning and on text readability.

GENERAL NATURE OF RESEARCH

We have sought a better understanding of basic psychological processes during purposeful reading in the hope that it will help in writing clearly and in fostering effective study of written teaching materials. Much of our work has been focused on factors that influence effective, purposeful reading in realistic settings. We have attempted to identify attributes of the instructional environment that shape and maintain effective processing activities, and to use this information in designing aids for learning from text.

Typically, in our experiments with adjunct aids, we have used instructional passages that ranged in length from 2000—9000 words. The subjects read through these passages at their own pace under systematically controlled conditions.

---

[1]P. Staum and M. J. Billington made important contributions to the work reported in this paper. Staum wrote several of the computer programs used in the eye movement analysis. Billington extended these programs and developed practical techniques for their use in experiments.

Most commonly, the nature of the written material is held constant while instructional contingencies or task demands are systematically manipulated. We then measure what students learn under various conditions. The experimental manipulations may involve, among others, the use of text-embedded questions, interactions with teachers or teacher surrogates, and the use of directions that specify instructional goals to students.

We assume in our research that the students' processing activities are at least as practically important as text characteristics; that processing activities determine the nature of the effective stimulus; and that the effective stimulus, in turn, determines what is learned.

WHY RECORD EYE MOVEMENTS?

Concern with the role of the learner has led us to postulate a class of activities, called mathemagenic activities (e.g., Rothkopf, 1971, 1972, 1976). *Mathemagenic* is a coined word derived from Greek roots that mean *giving birth to learning.* Mathemagenic activities are those activities that are relevant to the translation of the written stimuli into internal representation. Included here are not only the primary translations of written symbols into usable internal codes, but also the concatenation of dispersed information, inferences, and other constructive or mnemotechnic activities during reading.

The mathemagenic activities that are most interesting from a psychological point of view are largely invisible. In our research, inferences about these mathemagenic activities have been made indirectly, usually through measurements of what was learned. It has long been hoped that some other ways of indexing processing activities by readers may become feasible in realistic instructional settings. Two kinds of measurements offered some promise as additional indices of mathemagenic activities. These were the measurement of inspection time and eye movements during reading. Our work on inspection time has produced some interesting results (Rothkopf & Billington 1975a, 1975b, submitted for publication [a]). Two years ago we began to investigate eye movements during the study of written materials in order to obtain a descriptive model of the subjects' activities during purposeful reading.

METHODS FOR OBSERVING EYE MOVEMENTS

We chose a method that would meet the following requirements. First, we needed a technique that would allow observations of eye movements during 5—60 min of reading under conditions that resembled reading assignments in realistic instructional settings. We did not want to alter reading conditions in such a way as to interfere with the student's persistence during study or to change the student's usual approach to the study of written material. For example, we judged it unacceptable to unduly restrict the student's head movements or to burden the student with devices that might alter his usual reading style. Second, we needed a technique that would allow study without significant interruptions or other interferences not directly related to the reading demands being made on the student. Third, we needed a method that was clearly within existing technology of eye movement measurements and was both reliable and technically simple. Direct mapping of eye movements on the experimental text was not considered necessary, although we would have been pleased to have that capability if it had been practicable. As it is, we found that an indirect mapping technique, nystagmography, suited our purpose well.

The procedure was as follows: The experimental text was prepared on negative 35 mm slides and presented by rear projection. Slides were presented in sequence and controlled by the subjects with a switch. A blank slide appeared between text slides. The subject's head was supported by a chin rest 80 cm from the rear projection screen. A line of text on the screen subtended a visual angle of approximately 25°.

A 16 mm silver chloride skin electrode (Beckman) was placed approximately 2 cm laterally from the external canthus of each eye. These electrodes were used to record the corneo-retinal potential relative to an 11 mm reference electrode which was fastened to the dorsal surface of the left ear lobe. Only horizontal eye movements were recorded.

Prior to placing the electrodes, the skin surface was cleansed with isopropyl alcohol. The electrodes were filled with *Synapse* electrode cream (Med-Tek Corp.) and fastened to the skin with Beckman plastic adhesive collars of appropriate size.

The signal from the electrodes was amplified by AC techniques with a 3-sec time constant using an input coupler (Beckman, Type 9859) connected to a Beckman RM Dynograph. The amplified position potential and its derivative (obtained by use of a Beckman, Type 9841, nystagmus velocity coupler) which corresponds to the velocity of the eye motion, was recorded on FM magnetic tape. An Ampex Model 500 Recorder/Reproducer operating at a speed of 7.5 in per sec was used for that purpose. The operation of the slide changing mechanism was also recorded on tape. The eye movement potentials as well as the slide change record was visualized by a rectilinear pen linkage on paper tape and also on a large-screen (39 x 28 cm), multiple trace oscilloscope.

The principle analysis was performed on the velocity signal (first derivitive of EOG output). The recorded output of the velocity channel, sampled 100 times per second, was fed into a PDP–11/40 computer for analysis after the completion of the experimental session.

Several analysis programs have been developed. The major relevant programs were based on the principle that within 10–12° of ocular movement, angular excursion is approximately linear with velocity of eye movement (Fuchs, 1971,

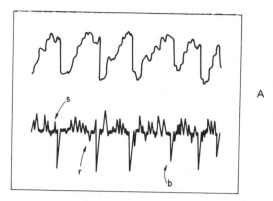

A

ELECTRO-OCULO-GRAM RECORD   SUBJECT 1302   PAGE 2

PARAMETERS: 2050   401   400   -400   -401   -1700   -1701   -2050

10 F	-608 R	14 F	862 S	18 F	1622 S	46 F
1442 S	14 F	875 S	17 F	-742 R	10 F	-406 R
5 F	799 S	21 F	-2048 B	210	38 F	-547 R
33 F	-1064 S	21 F	1331 S	22 F	989 S	18 F
723 F	10 S	-449 R	5 F	460 S	26 F	-1120 R
28 F	1056 S	8 F	-2048 B	263	37 F	2047 S
12 F	-514 R	55 F	-1066 S	17 F	1101 S	16 F
745 S	40 F	-421 R	9 F	-2048 B	227	9 F
-1469 R	31 F	1553 S	13 F	565 S	18 F	-945 R
16 F	929 S	15 F	833 S	17 F	-561 R	14 F
1656 S	16 F	-446 R	15 F	1190 S	52 F	-2048 B
278	9 F	-914 R	18 F	655 S	14 F	1267 S
21 F	1312 S	20 F	650 S	17 F	-1084 R	20 F
609 S	21 F	-2048 B	189	8 F	-899 R	35 F
1314 S	15 F	1155 S	16 F	1174 S	14 F	-2048 B

B

ELECTRO-OCULO-GRAM RECORD   SUBJECT 1302   PAGE 2

PARAMETERS   2050   401   400   -400   -401   -1700   -1701   -2050

BACK SWEEP LINE AMPL	TOT ELAPSE SEC	TOT FIXATN SEC	NO OF FIX	NO OF SAC	NO OF REG	AVG FIXATN SEC	AVG FRWRD FIX	AVG BKWRD FIX
4 -2048	2.100	1.550	9	5	3	0.172	0.210	0.097
5 -2048	2.630	2.090	10	6	3	0.209	0.204	0.220
6 -2048	2.270	1.860	7	4	2	0.266	0.244	0.320
7 -2048	2.780	2.160	11	6	4	0.196	0.200	0.190
8 -2048	1.890	1.400	8	5	2	0.175	0.170	0.190
9 -2048	1.250	0.880	5	3	1	0.176	0.132	0.350

C

FIG. 1.   Electronystagmogram and two of the printouts produced by the computer analysis of the velocity signal. The top record in Panel A is the primary positional trace. The bottom of the trace corresponds to the left edge of the text. The bottom record of Panel A is the first derivative of the top record and corresponds to velocity of the eye movement. The features marked s, r, and b are examples of a saccade, regression, and backsweep respectively. Panel B shows the features of velocity records from Panel A. The parameters specify from left to right the upper and lower limits for labeling features, as saccades (S), fixations (F), regressions (R), and backsweeps (B), respectively. Records in the printout provide a numerical code corresponding to the maximum velocity occurring within features S, R, and B. For fixations, (F), the numbers correspond to temporal duration (.01 secs.). Panel C shows the summary of eye movements for approximately the lines shown in Panel A.

p. 346). The computer analysis uses prespecified magnitudes and directions of the eye velocity signal to define: (a) left to right saccades, (b) regressions, (c) the duration of fixations that follow these two types of movements, and (d) return sweeps (movements of the eye from the right margin of the page to the left).

The statistical rationale for specifying the upper and lower velocity boundaries that identify the eye movement characteristics listed above has not yet been established in rigorous detail. However, empirical techniques for approximating these boundaries have been developed and provide reliable results. This is achieved by using a sample page, specifying boundary estimates, and then comparing the results against tracings of the positional signal. Marked discrepancies between the results of the velocity analysis and positional data are corrected by revising the velocity boundary parameters. The estimation procedure is repeated until uniformly satisfactory results are obtained for the entire trial page.

Once satisfactory velocity boundaries have been established for the several eye movement characteristics of interest, suitable computer programs provide line-by-line analysis of horizontal eye movements for each text slide or for any prespecified set of text slides. A sample nystagmogram and two sample print-outs resulting from its computer analysis are shown in Fig. 1.

RESULTS

Results obtained by our method for analyzing eye movements will be illustrated using data from experiments on the effects of descriptions of learning goals on learning achievements, and from experiments on text readability. The use of computer storage and subsequent analysis of large numbers of horizontal eye movements that occur during a substantial period of reading has made it possible to investigate phenomena that were difficult to examine in detail in the past. These include, among other things, the determination of eye movement patterns for selected text segments and the nature of individual readers' reactions to task demands.

LEARNING PRESPECIFIED INFORMATION FROM TEXT

Providing readers with explicitly described learning goals has a very marked effect on what the readers remember about a text. The number of goal-relevant questions correctly answered on a postreading test has been observed to be two to three times greater than questions about incidental (not goal-relevant) text information (e.g., Gagné & Rothkopf, 1975; Rothkopf & Billington, 1975b; Rothkopf & Kaplan, 1972). Several studies showed that the amount of incidental information remembered by goal-guided students was somewhat lower than that remembered by a control group who was directed to learn as much about the text as possible and not provided with explicit learning goals (Gagné & Rothkopf, 1975; Roth-kopf & Billington, 1975b), although reversals of this effect have also been reported (Kaplan & Rothkopf, 1974; Rothkopf & Kaplan, 1972). The literature on learn-ing prespecified information from text has been reviewed in detail elsewhere (Rothkopf, 1976).

In attempting to examine the effects of prespecified learning goals on reading, eye movements were observed under various experimental conditions. Subjects memorized six learning goals and then studied a 1498-word passage on ocean-ography presented on 35 mm slides, each containing 150–200 syllables of text (Rothkopf & Billington (b), submitted for publication, (b)). Six of the slides in the experimental series contained *no* information relevant to learning goals. These will be called *incidental* slides. Each of the other six slides included exactly one goal-relevant sentence as well as two or more incidental sentences. These will be call *goal-relevant* or *mixed* slides.

Our recording method avoids technical problems that arise in mapping eye movements on the text by direct observation. The following procedure was developed to infer eye movements in goal-relevant text neighborhoods of mixed text slides. The procedure was based on the assumption that subjects inspecting text slides used *one* of two inspection styles. These were (1) the incidental mode, which included the text for goal-relevant information; and (2) processing aimed at learning goal-relevant information.

Eye movements during processing of a goal-relevant sentence, in slides con-taining a mixture of incidental and goal-relevant material, can be reconstructed in the following way. The total observed quantity of each of the various classes of eye movements for mixed slides was divided into two components: those eye movements generated during background reading, and those produced during goal-processing. The basis for the division was the number of *objective text* lines that were expected to be read in the background, incidental mode (I). In the Rothkopf and Billington (submitted for publication (b)) experiment, there were on the average 12.3 lines of incidental text and 2.2 lines of goal-relevant material on each mixed slide. The number of text lines in a mixed slide that were read in the incidental style (I) was therefore 12.3, plus the portion of the 2.2 goal-relevant lines that was read in the incidental style. The latter quan-tity was 2.2 k, where k is the proportion of the goal-relevant sentence read in the background mode, that is, an estimate of how much of the goal-relevant sen-tence was read in the incidental style before goal-relevance was detected and the subject switched to the goal-processing mode. According to this conception, the number of objective text lines on a mixed slide that were read in the incidental style (I) was:

$$I = 12.3 + 2.2 \, k$$

We then calculated, on the basis of data from purely incidental slides, how much of any eye movement characteristic should have been produced by (I) lines of incidental text. This quantity was subtracted from the observed quantity of that eye movement characteristic for mixed slides and the remainder was attributed to goal-processing activities.

The general procedure can be summarized as follows. All quantities, unless otherwise indicated, were those appropriate for mixed slides (i.e., those which included a goal-relevant sentence).

(1) Number of text lines read in background mode (I) = Number of incidental text lines $+ k \times$ Number of goal-relevant text lines

(2) Eye movement characteristics generated by background mode = Number of text lines read in background mode (I) $\times$ $\dfrac{\text{Eye movement characteristics observed on incidental slides}}{\text{Number of text lines on incidental slides}}$

(3) Eye movement characteristics generated by goal-processing = Total eye movement characteristics observed on mixed slides $-$ Eye movement characteristics generated by background mode

The only quantity used in this procedure, not directly or indirectly based on observation, was the constant of proportionality k. It seemed reasonable to assume $0 < k \leq 1$. We determined a plausible value for k by asking observers to judge at what word in a goal-relevant sentence they felt certain that the sentence was relevant to a particular goal. The average value of k obtained by this method in the Rothkopf and Billington (submitted for publication (b)) experiment was .64.

Using this technique we found that an average sentence composed of 20.7 words and covering 2.2 text lines resulted in the model inspection pattern summarized in Table 1.

TABLE 1

Modal Inspection Patterns for a 20.7 Word Sentence
(2.2 Text Lines) when it Contained Goal-Relevant Information
and when it Included only Incidental Matter

	Goal-Relevant[a]	Incidental
Line Scans	3.76	2.24
Saccades	19.52	10.10
Regressions	15.71	6.01
Duration of Fixation after Saccades (in secs)	.233	.216
Duration of Fixation after Regressions (in secs)	.212	.184

[a]Includes inspection in the incidental mode prior to detection of goal-relevance (k = .64) for all except the duration of fixation entries.

As can be seen, the inspection of goal-relevant material involved 1.52 more line scans, 9.42 more saccades, and 9.7 more regressions than incidental material. Duration of fixation was 17 msec longer after saccades and 28 msec longer after regressions with goal-relevant material than with incidental sentences.

Similar results were obtained in two experiments. They suggest a simple descriptive model of subjects' responses to task demands. When a sentence is goal-relevant, the density of fixations is increased, and the durations of fixations are lengthened. It would be but a small leap of the imagination, though one still consistent with the current Zeitgeist, to translate density of fixation into the likelihood of appropriate internal representation of text components, and to equate the small increases in the average duration of fixations with greater depth of processing. Both the likelihood of appropriate internal representation (e.g., Rothkopf, 1976) and increased depth of processing (e.g., Craik & Lockhart, 1972) have been reported to increase instructional achievement.

Because our method allows us to collect very substantial amounts of eye movement data from each reader, it becomes possible to analyze style differences among individual subjects in their response to reading demands. The results of this kind of stylistic analysis suggest that the kind of modeling described above is inappropriate in certain details. There are two kinds of problems. First of all, the averaged group responses to the demands of learning goals are poor descriptions of the inspection patterns of individual readers. Second, comparison of the eye movement patterns of individual subjects in goal-relevant and incidental text neighborhoods does not predict relative achievement on goal-relevant and incidental materials well.

INDIVIDUAL RESPONSES TO TASK DEMANDS

Readers respond to the demands posed by learning goals in several distinctive individual styles. Some readers change the manner in which lines are scanned. Others reread lines or vary both rereading and line scans. Certain subjects have the same inspection patterns for both goal-relevant and incidental portions of the text. These style characteristics are not related in any simple way to differential learning of goal-relevant and incidental information. We analyzed individual responses to task demands in the following way. A measure of each of three eye movement characteristics on goal-relevant slides was compared with the corresponding measure on incidental pages for each subject. The eye movement characteristics were: (a) number of lines scanned, (b) number of fixations per scanned line, and (c) the average duration of fixations that followed saccades. Table 2 was obtained by determining, for each of 32 subjects, whether goal-

TABLE 2
Number of Subjects Showing Consistently
Greater Measures on Goal-Relevant
than on Incidental Text Portions
in Each of Three Eye Movement Characteristics

Number of Subjects	Lines Scanned	Fixations per Scanned Line	$\bar{X}$ Duration, Forward Fixations
7	R > I	—	—
2	—	R > I	—
5	—	—	R > I
5	R > I	R > I	—
2	R > I	—	R > I
3	—	R > I	R > I
1	R > I	R > I	R > I
7	—	—	—
Total for Each Eye Movement Characteristic	15	11	11
Chance Expectation	4.0	4.0	4.0

relevant slides consistently exceeded incidental slides on measures of these eye movement characteristics throughout the experimental reading sequence.[2]

The data in Table 2 indicate that the majority of subjects displayed different eye movement patterns in goal-relevant text neighborhoods than in incidental text portions. But there appears to be very substantial diversity in the style in which inspection patterns are altered by task demands. Some subjects vary one or more aspects of the way each line is scanned. For others, the scanning style for each line does not differ between goal-relevant and incidental text segments, whereas the number of lines scanned is altered between conditions. Other subjects do not differentiate between goal-relevant and incidental slides at all. The data in Table 2 suggest individual styles in response to task demands. Averaged group data may be useful in indexing passage difficulty or the influence of a particular task demand on inspection activity. But averaged group data are not good descriptions of the reactions of individual readers.

---

[2]Goal-relevant and incidental slides were compared for each third of the experimental text. Differences between the treatments for any given eye movement measure were judged *consistent* if all three comparisons showed a larger measure for the goal-relevant condition. This procedure is equivalent to a criterion of $P \leqslant .125$.

INDIVIDUAL INSPECTION STYLE AND LEARNING

Differences in eye movement characteristics between goal-relevant and incidental text are not simple predictors of differences in learning between goal-relevant and incidental information. Rothkopf and Billington (submitted for publication (b)) have found that differentiation in eye movement patterns between goal-relevant and incidental text and differentiation in the relative amount of learning on the two types of material were weakly correlated.

Results for eye movement patterns in the Rothkopf and Billington study (submitted for publication (b)) are summarized in Table 3. It is reasonably clear from an inspection of this table that subjects who showed no differences in inspection patterns between goal-relevant and incidental text neighborhoods remembered more goal-relevant than incidental information. Learning achievements on goal-relevant text material were not simply related to inspection activities as indexed by eye movements. Similar results have also been obtained for differences in inspection time between goal-relevant and incidental text slides. The correlation between differential inspection rate in syllables per minute and differential learning on goal-relevant and incidental text was significantly different from chance but small ($r = -.296$).

Preliminary analysis of two additional experiments suggests that the individual style differences observed in goal-guided learning also occur to a somewhat lesser degree in subjects' inspection of text of various difficulty (readability).

TABLE 3
Differences in Eye Movement Characteristics
Between Goal-Relevant and Incidental Text
and the Recall of Goal-Relevant and
Incidental Information

Eye Movement characteristic in which goal-relevant text exceeds incidental	Proportion correct responses on recall test			
	Goal-relevant information		Incidental information	
	$\bar{X}$	σ	$\bar{X}$	σ
Scanned Lines	.73	.28	.34	.15
Fixations per Line	.83	.14	.34	.14
Fixation Duration	.76	.23	.30	.15
No Differences	.83	.29	.26	.04

TABLE 4
Eye Movements on Eight High and
Eight Low Readability Passages[a]

Eye Movement measure	Readability		
	Low	High	P
Lines Scanned per Passage	20.80	18.00	$<.02$
Number Saccades per Scanned Line	5.70	5.83	$>.05$
Number of Regressions per Scanned Line	2.42	2.30	$>.05$
$\overline{X}$ Duration, Forward Fixation	.243	.227	$<.001$
$\overline{X}$ Duration, Backward Fixation	.215	.201	$<.05$

[a]Average Flesch Reading Ease Index was: High = 87.53
(σ = 7.28), Low = 29.10 (σ = 15.32).

Eye Movements and Readability

The effect of readability on eye inspection patterns was studied using techniques similar to those described above (Rothkopf & Billington, unpublished manuscript). Subjects read 16 passages that varied widely in the Flesch Reading Ease Index. The passages were 93–159 words in length. Each passage was photographed on a separate negative slide. The subjects were requested to learn as much about each passage as possible. This request was reinforced by money incentives for high recall test performance. Order of presentation of the passages was randomly varied among subjects.

Averages for various eye movement characteristics were obtained for each of the 16 passages. Means of representative measures for the eight high and the eight low readability passages are shown in Table 4. This table shows significantly more lines scanned with difficult than with easy text. Duration of fixation, both after saccades and after regressions, were longer with less readable material.

The results of another recent study also support the finding shown in Table 4. Rothkopf and Krudys (unpublished manuscript) using the same 16 passages found that number of fixations per scanned line was relatively unaffected by readability. The correlation between number of fixations per scanned line and the Flesch Reading Ease Index was not significantly above zero (r = $-.16$). The total number of fixations per unit text, on the other hand, decreased with reading ease (r = −.45). This implies that if group trends are considered, the number of fixations per scanned line remains constant regardless of readability, but that the average reader increases the number of scanned lines when the text becomes more difficult. This interpretation is consistent with the results in Table 4. Rothkopf and Krudys (unpublished manuscript) also confirmed that duration of fixation increases with text difficulty. The correlation between reading ease and average duration of fixation was −.69.

Both the data in Table 4 and the results of the Rothkopf and Krudys study reported above were based on group averages. Just as in the studies of goal-guided learning, individual style analysis of the readability experiments indicated that averaged group results provided a somewhat misleading picture of what individual subjects were doing to cope with text difficulty. These aspects of the eye movement pattern, number of lines scanned, number of fixations per scanned line, and duration of fixations, observed for eight highly readable passages, were compared with those of the eight difficult slides for each individual reader. One-tailed t-tests (p < .1) were used for each measure. Among the 27 subjects used in the Rothkopf and Billington (unpublished manuscript) and the Rothkopf & Krudys (unpublished manuscript) subjects, six of these showed no reliable differences between the eye movement patterns observed for difficult and easy text. Fifteen subjects had longer fixations, and six scanned more lines on difficult than on more readable text. The number of subjects who had more fixations per scanned lines on difficult than on easy text were about what might be expected by chance.

Our method for analyzing nystagmograms by computer appears to be a useful tool for studies of reading. The estimation procedures allow inferences about how particular text neighborhoods are inspected. The estimation procedure makes it possible to avoid presenting the text one sentence or other small unit at a time. Fragmenting text in this way is one option for investigating inspection of individual sentences when means for mapping eye movements directly on print are not available. Such fragmentation appears to be a suspect research strategy when it is used to investigate persistence in reading, or when selective attention is of interest. The method allows the capture of very substantial eye movement records per subject. This makes it possible to undertake serious investigations of individual reading styles. Such investigations appear to have been somewhat neglected in previous research on eye movements in reading. The findings of Rothkopf and Billington (submitted for publication (b)), Rothkopf & Billington (unpublished manuscript), and Rothkopf & Krudys (unpublished manuscript) indicate that individual readers respond to task demands in markedly different styles. These results raise a number of empirical and theoretical questions that deserve investigation.

There are strong hints in our results that eye movements are not a super highway to the discovery of fundamental psychological processes during reading. The eyes may be the windows to the soul, but they may also provide views of unoccupied rooms. The weak and complex relationship between differential eye movement patterns and differential learning from various text segments suggests that visible inspection patterns include many ineffective and superstitious components. The discriminations necessary for the discovery of goal-relevant information in the text may be sufficient for the marked advantage in the retention of goal-relevant information over the retention of background material. The discovery of goal-relevant information could, in addition, result in a variety of additional inspection activities that add little or nothing to the learned performance of the reader. Substantial portions of the systematic eye movements observed during reading may reflect superstitious inspection activities of that character. Our results indicate the need for caution in interpreting eye movement data as indicators of underlying processing activities during learning from written material.

DISCUSSION

JUST: In 1930 Judd reported some experiments in which he varied the difficulty of the text to see how this would affect eye fixations. He wanted to see whether there were more or longer fixations, or both. He found that some subjects produced longer fixations and some did both. Essentially, those results are very similar to yours. Different subjects adapt differently to more difficult text. This did not make Judd think that eye fixations aren't the royal road to the study of reading, he simply thought that he hadn't quite gotten the right way to analyze the behavior, and I wonder if this doesn't apply to your results as well.

ROTHKOPF: It is possible. I certainly am not prepared to rule out the possibility that a change in procedure could alter the observed relationship between learning results and eye movement data. However, I can't see right now what procedures are likely to produce these changes.

JUST: Let me suggest that you're throwing away the most important data by not looking at the fixations of those sentences that contain the answers to your questions. That's what the subjects are reading for. You measure whether they acquire certain information from those test sentences and you have the data to show how they read, how they scan those test sentences. Now, if those two measures don't correlate very highly I would be very, very surprised.

ROTHKOPF: You may be right. We could get more insight into what is happening if we could map eye movements directly on the text. However, this would require us to break the text into small segments. This has some undesirable consequences because we alter the inspection activity of the subject in unknown ways. It would confront the subject with a reading situation that is substantially different from that in which people read ordinarily.

The complex relationship between eye movement and learning surprises you. We find similar variations among subjects with gross inspection time measurements. In several experiments we have found that the times readers allocate to intentional and incidental text portions, respectively, were weakly but significatly correlated with relative retention of intentional and incidental information. But in these experiments, there are subjects who spend no extra time in the goal-relevant text portions and yet remember all goal-relevant material while recalling very little incidental information. They have responded to the treatment perfectly as far as learning is concerned, but inspection time data do no reflect this.

I would like to draw your attention to a hypothesis that makes good sense with our data and to which I have alluded in my paper. It is that the act of discriminating goal-relevant text portions from background is sufficient for the better retention of goal-relevant material. This act may not take very much time. Finding goal-relevant material may, in addition, elicit time-consuming superstitious activities on the part of the reader. This conception leads to predictions of weak correlations between time spent on goal-relevant material and intentional learning. This is because the time-consuming superstitious activities would take place only when goal-relevant information is found. Naturally, heightened recall of goal-relevant information can also be expected only if it is found.

JUST: One of your points was that you should not average over strategies, and I think nobody would disagree with that. At the same time you said something about box models — I'm not exactly sure what you mean by box models. I'm not sure what you're proposing as an alternative, and I'm not sure what this has to do with averaging over strategies.

ROTHKOPF: You detected a bias on my part. Box models are quasi-theoretical models where internal events occupy small rectangles and are connected to other internal events by arrows. Box models are popular now, but they don't appeal to me. One problem with box models is that they are frequently more complicated than the data they are trying to explain.

Many box models are proposed as models of how all human beings behave in a given experimental situation. Averaged data are therefore commonly used to test such models. Models that can handle style differences among subjects are uncommon.

JUST: I suggest that the weak correlation between time spent or duration measurements and relevance versus incidental information might be a function of how you define relevance and incidental information. I would also suggest that the stimulus material itself has a way of structuring information, so that if you can capture that independently, you would be more successful in showing that the recall of information and time spent on different portions of the text are in fact more strongly correlated than your data suggests. And to this point I'd like to ask how you define relevant vs. irrelevant or incidental portions of textual materials.

ROTHKOPF: For any experiment we will take the set of goal statements, that is those statements that subjects in the experiments memorize and ask another group of subjects to map these statements on the text. We give subjects the text and a goal and say, "Will you underline those portions of the text that are relevant to this goal." We get very high consensus among subjects about what text elements are relevant to each goal. The consensus is of the order of anywhere from 99 to 100%. We get high agreement because we repeat the mapping procedures 3 or 4 times with different subjects. When we observe disagreement, we modify the text until consensus is obtained. That's the definition for goal relevance that we use. Furthermore, in some of these experiments we counterbalance. Incidental slides in one treatment are goal-relevant slides in another because the subjects have been asked to memorize a different set of goals.

IV.6

Eye Movements in
Reading Disabled Children[1]

Lester A. Lefton
University of South Carolina

Perceptual and cognitive psychologists are becoming increasingly involved in the investigation of reading disability. They have taken up the challenge by examining the potential perceptual and cognitive variables that might enter into the inability of subjects to read. This is clearly not a new field. Educators and psychologists have been examining the abilities of readers for many decades, yet their success has been moderate at best.

One of the principal explanations that has been used to explain reading disability has been the notion of a "perceptual deficit." This notion suggests that disabled readers suffer from an inability to perceive the world, and particularly alphabetic material, the way normal readers do. A perceptual deficit is often considered to be a relatively low-level problem compared with cognition and comprehension. Typically, studies in support of a perceptual deficit explanation show that poor readers do not perform as well as good readers on discrimination tasks. A large experimental and clinical literature developed to support this notion. Yet, as Larsen and Hammill (1975) indicate, "the educational usefulness of this important theoretical construct has never been fully substantiated, (p. 282)." Indeed, recent work has suggested that neither good nor poor readers have trouble with discriminating letters (Lahey & McNees, 1975). This, of course,

---

[1]This research was supported by grants from the National Institute of Education (NE-G-00-3-0017) and from the U.S. Army Human Engineering Laboratory and Army Research Offices (DAAG 29-77-G-0035). No official endorsement of NIE, HEL, or ARO should be inferred. This paper may be reproduced in full or in part for any purpose of the United States Government. Gratefully acknowledged is the help and co-operation of the parents, teachers, and administrators of Sandhill Academy, and the Richland and Lexington County School districts. I thank Benjamin Lahey and David Stagg for their important help and ideas.

raises the possibility that although reading disability and visual discrimination indeed may be correlated, there is no causal relationship. This becomes particularly important when we realize that many children are diagnosed as reading disabled based on tests of visual perception, for example, the Bender Visual Motor Gestalt Test (Bender, 1957). Zach and Kaufman (1972) examined childrens' scores on the Bender and compared these with their ability to perform discrimination tasks using the same forms. They found it was possible for a child to discriminate forms well and still obtain a score on the Bender that indicated a "perceptual difficulty." In examining the relationship of visual perceptual skills and academic achievement, Larsen and Hammill concluded that visual perception skills are not essential to academic achievement and that children who fail in school do so for reasons other than visual perceptual deficits.

This brief review of some of the controversy on the notion of perceptual deficits is not meant to be exhaustive, but rather to point out the diversity of approaches to reading disability. The controversy over perceptual deficits and visual abilities will likely continue. The present study examines eye movements of normal and reading disabled children when they are engaged in a task involving visual discrimination. Its goal is to assess the potential contribution of eye movements to the etiology of reading disability.

There have been many investigations of the letter discrimination abilities of good and poor readers and many of these used tachistoscopic tasks that showed a "perceptual deficit" (e.g., Bender, 1957; Coleman, 1959; and Lyle, 1969). However, Lahey and McNees (1975) have recently found that neither good nor poor readers had trouble discriminating single letters when provided with an *untimed* match-to-sample task.

Most studies on the discrimination of letters deal only with single letters. One recent study, however, used multiletter discriminations (Lahey & Lefton, 1976) in a match-to-sample task. Children in the second, third, and fifth grades who were in either the upper or the lower portion of their class served as subjects. They were presented either single letter items or items that were 2, 3, 4, 5, 6, or 7 letters in length. There were seven alternatives from which they had to choose to match to the sample. The results of this study were straightforward: children made more errors on match-to-sample problems composed of several letters than those composed of single ones and, more importantly, poor readers made relatively more errors than good readers on the longer items. In a second part of the study, spacing between the letters was varied, so that the letters within the item were as normally spaced (i.e., one-half space between letters), or three or six character spaces apart. The major reason for this manipulation was to force the subjects to fixate several times on each item in hope of reducing errors. Results were as predicted: earlier findings were replicated, and when the items were spaced apart, to force more fixations, subjects made significantly fewer errors.

This study has subsequently been replicated with normal children and children diagnosed as reading disabled (Lahey, Sperduto, Beggs, & Lefton, unpublished

TABLE 1
Sample Stimulus Array

BPRDT	BPRTD	PBTRD	BPTDR	BPRDT

manuscript) with the same results. Reading disabled children make more errors than normal readers in this *untimed* match-to-sample task, and this is particularly true with increasing numbers of letters in the stimulus array.

The critical question is why reading disabled children make more errors. Clearly, the introduction of more letters into the items has elicited more errors because it made a harder task. But when the letters were spread apart and subjects were forced to look at them longer, they made fewer errors. The possibility exists that the reading disabled had not been examining the items. The errors of the reading disabled may have had nothing to do with visual discrimination, but instead may have been an attentional phenomenon. (The reading disabled are known to be impulsive and have short attention spans [Ross, 1976].) Perhaps the reading disabled children do not look at the stimuli and therefore make more errors. An alternative to the "not looking" hypothesis is that disabled readers may be doing just the opposite. They may look more often but not examine closely the letters each time they look.

The present study was primarily an attempt to replicate our previous results with reading disabled children. A second purpose was to examine the frequency of fixations of disabled children compared with normals. A third purpose was to assess the possibility of using eye movements to validate a theoretical position and to evaluate the possibility of using eye movements in a match-to-sample task as a diagnostic tool.

The subject pool consisted of 24 subjects at each of 4 grade levels: third graders, fifth graders, adults, and reading disabled children who were matched for age with the fifth graders. A reading disabled child was defined as a child who scored normally on intelligence tests, had no sensory defects, but who was performing at least one and one-half grade levels behind their age-matched counterparts. The average age of these fifth graders and the disabled group was 10 years, 8 months.

All the subjects were presented with the same match-to-sample stimuli. As is shown in Table 1, these were typed upper case letters in which a sample was typed on the left-hand side of a card and four alternatives typed horizontally across the card. Each item on a card consisted of five typed upper case characters separated by six blank character spaces. Each five-letter item subtended 1.6° of visual angle. The items were combinations of five different visually confusable consonants. The same five consonants were used to make up all five groups of any one stimulus card. The entire array subtended 15-½° horizontally. The sample was always presented to the left and the four alternatives to the right. The subject's task was to choose from the alternatives the one which precisely matched the sample.

Counterbalancing was used so that each of the four correct possible positions was sampled three times in a randomized order. To control for possible specific item difficulty, four decks of stimuli were used to counterbalance the alternatives as well.

The subjects were seated in front of a Biometric Eye-Trac machine which uses a photoelectric principle to measure eye movements. They were told the nature of the task and asked to locate the alternative that looked exactly the same as the sample on the far left. It was made clear that this was not a timed task and that they could look as often and as long as they wished. Subjects were given practice trials and calibration trials at the beginning of the testing period. Calibration preceeded each new trial. When subjects throught they had found the correct alternative, they closed their eyes as a signal to the experimenter and then indicated as quickly as possible the alternative they had selected.

Scoring the data consisted of counting the number of fixations made per trial and measuring fixation duration. On any given trial, 5.7, 7.4, and 8.2 fixations were made by adults, fifth, and third graders, respectively, providing support

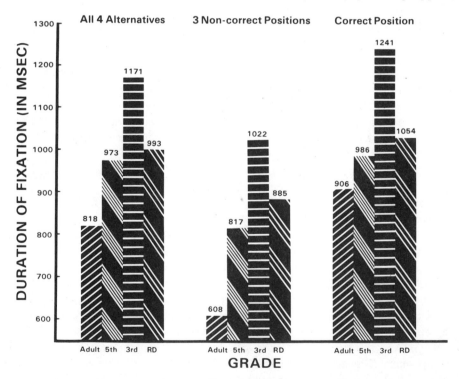

FIG. 1.   The mean duration of a fixation is presented in milliseconds as a function of grade level. (RD stands for reading disabled. The left panel represents the data collapsed for all four positions, the middle panel presents the data collapsed across the three non-correct alternatives; whereas the right panel has the data just for the correct position.)

for a distinct developmental progression. The reading disabled group required 9.3 fixations, more than any other group. The analysis of variance showed a strong effect of grade level. In addition, there was also a strong effect of position; when the correct position was on the right-hand side of the display, subjects used more fixations than when it was on the left-hand side. This finding was true for all grade levels.

The mean fixation duration decreased as grade level increased. Overall, the adults spent 818 msec per fixation compared to 973 and 1171 msec for fifth and third grade subjects, respectively. However, a different pattern of results emerges for the reading disabled subjects. As can be seen from the left-hand panel of Fig. 1, reading disabled children only spend 20 msec more per fixation than their fifth grade counterparts. The times per fixation for the three noncorrect positions are also shown in Fig. 1.

The reading disabled group spent about the same amount of time per fixation as other children of their age, yet made more fixations. Intuitively, it might have been expected that they would be different − spending either more time per fixation (because of task difficulty) or less time per fixation (because of in-attention). Neither was the case.

Predictably, the reading disabled children made significantly more errors (13.2%) than any other group. Third graders made 4.8% errors, fifth graders made 6.5% errors, and the adults made 9.7% errors. The older subjects who were spending less time and looking less often, made more errors. The reading disabled group, who were age-matched with the normal reading fifth graders, made twice as many errors as their counterparts. Because this was an untimed task and the subject could look as often and for as long as he wished before making a choice, the error rate should have been very low. More errors were made when the item was in a correct position further to the right. For example, there were 2% errors when the correct answer was in Position 1 compared to 15% errors when the correct position was in Position 4.

To measure the efficiency by which the subjects were examining the stimulus arrays, eye movement sequences were analyzed. Of concern was where the subject was looking: at the Sample, or at the first, second, third, or fourth alternative. When the correct answer was in Position 1, virtually all of the subjects (97%) would look at the Sample. On the second fixation virtually all of the subjects (93%) would move their eyes to the first alternative. On the third fixation, however, variance was introduced because some of the subjects would typically look back to the Sample (78%) while other subjects might move their eyes to Position 2 (20%).

The aim of this analysis was to find the most likely fixation sequence and to see if this fixation sequence correlated to any extent with the subject's ability to correctly respond in a match-to-sample task. Table 2 summarizes these data by showing the *most likely* fixation strategies for each of the different groups. Not every subject followed the fixation strategy presented, although many did.

When the correct position was Position 1, we see that third graders started at the Sample (97%), then moved to the first alternative (93%). The next most likely fixation was back to the Sample (80%), back to the first alternative (72%), back to the Sample (70%), back to the first alternative, and then they terminated their search. As can be seen from Table 2, fifth graders and adults used a similar strategy but stopped examining the alternatives after fewer fixations. The reading disabled group used the same strategy as all the other groups, except that they went back to the Sample and the first alternative more frequently. Further, the percentage of other fixations was slightly higher for this group. The reading disabled subjects were more likely to adopt an alternative set of fixations, perhaps looking at Position 2 or 3. Also, in Table 2 we see the most likely fixation strategy when the correct position was Position 2. Again, all the groups used a

TABLE 2
Most Frequent Fixation Positions

					Fixation Number					
Grade	1	2	3	4	5	6	7	8	9	10
					Correct Position = 1					
Third	S	1	S	1	S	1				
Fifth	S	1	S	1	S					
Adult	S	1	S	1						
RD	S	1	S	1	S	1	S			
					Correct Position = 2					
Third	S	1	S	2	S	2	S			
Fifth	S	1	S	2	S	2				
Adult	S	1	2	S	2					
RD	S	1	S	1	S	2	S			
					Correct Position = 3					
Third	S	1	S	2	S	3	S	3		
Fifth	S	1	S	2	S	3	S	3	S	
Adult	S	1	2	3	S	3				
RD	S	1	S	1	2	3	S	3		
					Correct Position = 4					
Third	S	1	S	2	S	3	4	S	4	S
Fifth	S	1	S	2	S	3	S	4	S	
Adult	S	1	2	3	4	S				
RD	S	1	S	1	S	4	S	4	S	3

relatively systematic strategy going from the Sample to Position 1, back to the Sample, and so on. The older subjects checked less frequently, and the reading disabled checked more often.

When the correct alternative was at Position 3, the third graders adopted a slightly different strategy than the adults. The third graders went Sample, 1, Sample, 2, Sample, 3, and then checked again by going back to the Sample and then to Position 3. The fifth graders used a similar strategy. The adults, however, instead of going back to the Sample after each alternative, seemed to be using memory. They looked at the Sample and then at Positions 1, 2, 3, returned to the Sample, and checked one more time at Position 3. This is most likely due to their greater memory span and their ability to remember that an alternative was correct or not correct. What is most interesting about these data is the pattern of the reading disabled. These children seemed to try to behave the way adults did. Rather than adopting the relatively conservative strategy of a third grader who returned to the Sample after each alternative, they apparently tried to hold the sample in memory as they looked at the alternatives. This strategy did not fare them well, because when the item was in Position 3 they were making many errors.

When the correct item was in Position 4, third graders again adopted the same strategy as did fifth graders. Adults, using memory again, looked at the Sample and then all four correct alternatives, then back to the Sample. The reading disabled subjects provided an interesting pattern of results. Their strategy resembled neither that of the third graders who were adopting a conservative checking approach, nor that of the adults. Rather, the fixation sequence seems somewhat random. Indeed, a close analysis of the positions at which the reading disabled children looked showed a semirandom pattern. The data are presented in Table 3.

TABLE 3
Distribution of Fixations (In Percent)
Reading Disabled: Correct Position 4

Fixation Number	N	Sample	1	2	3	4
1	57	98.2	1.8	0	0	0
2	57	1.8	80.7	3.5	5.2	8.8
3	57	73.7	0	22.8	1.8	1.8
4	56	7.1	35.7	26.8	16.1	14.2
5	54	42.6	1.8	29.6	14.8	11.1
6	52	30.8	9.6	21.1	13.4	25.0
7	50	30.0	10.0	22.0	28.0	10.0
8	45	35.5	4.4	4.4	22.2	33.3
9	39	33.3	7.7	10.2	17.9	30.8
10	34	38.2	5.9	8.8	26.4	20.6

NOTE: N is the number of subjects still making fixations.

Younger children looked more often, for more time, and were relatively conservative in their strategy. While adults looked less often and spent less time per fixation, they too adopted a systematic approach. The reading disabled group is the most interesting, for they looked more frequently than anyone else, although they did not spend more time than their age-matched group. Yet, the sequence of fixations that they made was neither conservative nor systematic.

The lack of a systematic search by the reading disabled subjects most likely brought about the higher error rate. The reading disabled children were not obtaining an error rate of 50%; indeed, it was only 13%. Thus, they were able to discriminate letters. Remember, the adults were obtaining a 10% error rate. The higher error rate for the reading disabled children was most likely due to their unsystematic search and lack of a conservative approach. The adults were less conservative than the children, but they remained systematic and used memory.

Unlike the adults, the normal children were being conservative. They went back to the sample after each trial to see if the sample matched the alternative. This is consistent with our knowledge of the visual memories of young children. A large research body has shown us that children have poor memory spans compared with adults and would, therefore, need to check more often. Furthermore, children's sequential memory is worse than than of adults. Piaget and Inhelder (1967) suggest that young children do not readily perceive order and attach little importance to the spatial orientation of visual stimuli. Since the letters in a match-to-sample task are scrambled, it is not surprising that a reading disabled child who does not systematically check back to the sample will have trouble making a decision which requires strict match.

The reading disabled and normals all adopt a similar approach in the first eye movements. Most started at the Sample and then moved to Position 1 and then often went back to the Sample again. The breakdown in systematic eye movements seemed to happen after these first three eye movements. Part of this breakdown may be due to the secondary development of impulsiveness on the part of reading disabled children. It has been reported repeatedly in the literature thar reading disabled children have not only a short memory span but a short span of attention, and tend to be impulsive (Ross, 1976). After two or three fixations and no success in finding the correct alternative, the reading disabled child may make the impulsive decision to move his eyes not in a systematic conservative manner such as do his fifth grade counterparts, but by impulsive jumps to any of the other positions. Of course, his lack of systematic eye movements creates a more difficult task and he winds up making more fixations than necessary.

What is the role of visual discriminations in the etiology of reading disability? The reading disabled subjects made 13% errors, twice as many as their age-matched counterparts. Clearly, they were doing something wrong even though they made 87% correct judgments. They were able to discriminate the letters and most of the time to be correct in their match-to-sample. The notion of perceptual deficit, if it is at all valid, should not refer to the ability of a child to be able to make fine visual discriminations. At best, a perceptual deficit should probably be renamed a cognitive deficit. Any problems that the child has do not come from his inability to discriminate the letters but probably from his unsystematic strategy in examining the letters and his failure to use a positive systematic sequential examination. This is more a cognitive style and should at best be called a cognitive deficit. Interestingly, 20 years ago Vernon argued ". . . the child is unlikely to be greatly handicapped in learning to read by any deficiency in the visual perception of word shapes . . ." (Vernon, 1957, p. 30).

I'm not fond of any kind of label, but the notion of perceptual deficits has been shown to be minimal, at best. Further, attempts to train fifth graders to make better perceptual discriminations have often been shown to be a waste of time. Children who are in the fifth grade do not benefit from perceptual training (Allington, 1976; Hammill, 1972). They may benefit from training in more systematic searches, or in being less impulsive; but clearly, reading disabled children who are having trouble with match-to-sample problems are not having trouble because of their inability to make a proper discrimination.

What can we conclude from the present study?

1. We should discard the concept of perceptual deficits in favor of a cognitive deficit (Allington, 1976; Fisher, in press). Reading disabled children make errors, but not because they cannot discriminate letters. Whatever their problem, reading disabled children can discriminate letters. While Vernon (1957) made this point 20 years ago, it cannot be stressed enough. Reading teachers tenaciously hold on to the idea, practitioners still train in visual perception, and educators still advocate it.

2. The eye movement patterns of normals are systematic and predictable. Young children who have less experience and have shorter memory spans make more fixations and spend more time per fixation than adults. Their sequence of eye movements is systematic and cautious; after examining each alternative, they go back to the sample to check. The older subject is also systematic and relies to a great extent on memory.

3. In contrast with the normals, the reading disabled subjects are unsystematic and make more errors. They are not cautious, not conservative, and do not have an adult memory span. Thus, they adopt a hit-or-miss approach. Their problem is that they miss too often and have to make more fixations to achieve a modicum of success. They achieve 87% accuracy in this relatively simple task; but they do it at the expense of more fixations per trial. Part of the reason they make more errors might be that they are impulsive and lack the patience to be systematic and cautious.

4. Can the reading disabled be helped? I am of the firm belief that a majority of the reading disabled children have a neurological impairment that is not susceptible to correction by surgery or medication. As Fisher has argued ". . . dys-

lexia can't be cured — the brain will not stand for that, but the brain *is* susceptable to compensatory training which will allow the dyslexic to process visual verbal information" (Fisher, in press).

We can teach cognitive control. We can teach impulse control. We can teach more systematic strategies. Further, reinforcement techniques have been shown to be effective. Lahey has been able to increase the comprehension levels of reading disabled children two grades through reinforcement techniques (Lahey, McNees, & Brown, 1973).

5. Eye movements can be used to assess reading disability. Eye movements can be used to assess progress in teaching the disabled to be more systematic. Perceptual deficits should not be a major concern, rather researchers should focus on cognitive control. The automaticity of LaBerge and Samuels (1974) and the peripheral-to-cognitive search guidance systems of Hochberg (1970b), can become operative only when we teach systematic cognitive control. Since eye movements are a relatively important information-gathering mechanism, their measurement is a logical way to assess, evaluate, and remediate cognitive control.

6. Eye movements are only one aspect of reading disability. Indeed, they are probably only a peripheral cognitive component to reading. Further attempts at models of reading, reading disability, and remediation may be futile. It is time to collect data and investigate reading with existing models. Since eye movements are largely under voluntary control, they may be natural components of cognitive behavior to modify in the reading disabled. Eye movement training may not enable us to fix the reading disabled, but the teaching of systematic information gathering would be a start.

DISCUSSION

LEISMAN: I congratulate you for making a stand on the fact that the perceptual disorders which manifest themselves in reading problems are far too global to be studied. "Reading disabilities" is a rather gross, badly defined area and there are many associated problems with it. I'd like to propose an alternative explanation for your data. In a recent paper, Bouma and Legein (1977) have summarized some thoughts on the problem of dyslexia. They had explained deficiency in terms of one of a number of possible interactive factors, one of which was "inadequate eye control"; a second point that they brought up was of maturational lag; and a third was a problem in foveal as opposed to parafoveal detection. I'd like very briefly to go through these. The first factor was eye control. We set up a situation in which dyslexic and normal children and adults were required to change fixation rapidly between two circular red lamps at various distances and recorded their saccadic eye movements which ranged from 2° to 30°. The time, amplitude, and angular velocity were measured. We found significant differences between normal children and normal adults, but no significant differences between dyslexic and normal children. The differences can be explained on the basis of certain biophysical parameters like differences in the radius of the eyeball, the spring stiffness of the eye, and the moments of inertia. The conclusion is that as long as there are no significant differences between dyslexic and normal children, then the differences that are found between dyslexics and normal adults can be explained in terms of development criteria rather than any kind of basic deficit.

A second possibility lies in terms of the process of maturational lag or the developmental components of reading disability. We recorded EEGs in response to a number of tasks. We recorded EEG with electrode locations and made a number of analyses including cross-spectral densities and coherence values. We have found that independent of age, the particular characteristic indicative or predictive of reading disorders was a greater abundance of activity over the left-right occipital regions. This is true from ages 6–19. The conclusion seems to be that we're not dealing with a maturational lag, but rather with some specific deficit, or better, a difference between dyslexics or reading disabled children, as we call them, and those children not so affected. It seems to be essentially a word-finding difficulty. To the extent to which this exists, differences that we find in eye movement patterns are a reflection of a visual verbal matching problem and not a primary deficit. In other words, we're dealing with something that is reflective of a problem and not actually etiologically related to the problem. Therefore, eye movement training would be difficult to justify.

LEFTON: I don't believe in maturational lag either. The data do not support such a contention. What the reading disabled do if they are two or three years behind in ability is not the same as a child would do who is two or three years behind chronologically.

Second, you cannot examine the way children look at pictures or bouncing lights and talk about reading disability. I call these children reading disabled because they don't have other problems – they just can't read. You have to put subjects into *real* reading tasks not into other tasks which *might be* involved in reading. This is a mistake that many researchers have been making for a long time. A tachistoscopic task where words are briefly flashed is not reading. Similarly, if children bounce their eyes back and forth between lights, that is not reading either.

I'm not convinced that training eye movements is a way to help the reading disabled. However, the behavior modification psychologists take these children and train them to do all types of tasks and get significantly better performance out of them. If you can train eye movements and get better performance, why not do it? I don't think you'll ever teach them to read the way normals read. However, if you can get them to comprehend those words that are on the page better because they are moving their eyes more systematically, then do it!

PERLMUTER: I was wondering why your adults were making more errors than your younger children, and whether this has any bearing on your interpretation?

LEFTON: At first I couldn't believe that the adults were making more errors than the children. However, when you actually watch the testing, it's very simple. The adults (college sophmores) sit down at the machine, and *very* rapidly proceed with the task. By contrast, the third graders are so systematic and cautious, that they don't make errors. They go back and they check, whereas the adults use memory and are a little cocky about the whole thing.

LOFTUS: I've got a question about the theory you have postulated having to do with the sequence of fixations when the correct item was in the third and fourth position. It seemed that when it was in the third position, the disableds were acting like adults in the sense that they were going Sample, 1, 2, 3 — bingo. However, when it was in the fourth position they were doing something weird. They were going Sample, 1, 4. That doesn't seem to jibe.

LEFTON: There is some reaction time data in the literature to suggest that after about 4 or 5 seconds children get impulsive. For the first few fixations they move: Sample, 1, Sample, 2? however, after about 4 or 5 seconds they start bouncing around, exhibiting random appearing behavior.

RUSSO: If you were to ask your subjects what they were doing, especially your third or fifth graders, they would tell you "well, I go back and forth and I check them in order" and if you asked your adults they'd say they did the same thing, except they don't have to go back because they remembered the standards.

LEFTON: Correct.

RUSSO: If you ask your learning disabled children what they're doing, what do they say?

LEFTON: They might say "I looked at it, and then I looked at the others and I knew that was the one."

RUSSO: You mean they express confidence in their answer even though they have many more errors?

LEFTON: Yes, but remember that it was still a low error rate.

ROSEN: It is not quite clear to me why it takes adults 800 msec for each fixation and almost 6 fixations to do that task. That is an exceedingly trivial task. Subjects can add a series of four numbers in less than 2.5 seconds, why does it take your subjects so long?

LEFTON: If you get a set of angular letters — s, y, m, and z, and you start mixing those letters up, it takes a while to sort them out to get the correct ones. They are confusable. When you have o's and c's and s's all together, it also takes a while. Remember, the adults are using memory and taking 750 msec for a comparison. This doesn't seem to be an extraordinary amount of time.

ROSEN: I can't believe the adults make 10% errors on this relatively easy task. Can you comment on the patterns of fixations they make on error trials?

LEFTON: There weren't really enough data — only 10% of all the data were error data. Casual examination showed no systematic strategy because there were so few data across each of the positions.

Part **V**

LOOKING AT STATIC AND DYNAMIC DISPLAYS

V.1

Searching for Nina[1]

Calvin F. Nodine
Dennis.P. Carmody
Harold L. Kundel
Temple University

For over 30 years Al Hirschfeld has been testing the search performance of *New York Times* readers by hiding NINAs in wisps of hair, folds of clothing, or other unlikely features of his drawings of scenes from the theater and movies. Actually, artist Hirschfeld has been drawing for the *New York Times* for over 50 years, but it wasn't until the blessed event of the birth of his daughter that he began playing hide-and-seek with NINA.

The game he devised has all the properties that characterize a true visual search task. The target, NINA, is cleverly interwoven into the composition of a picture. In most cases, Hirschfeld camouflages his target by carefully embedding it in a scenic feature, so that the picture becomes *background* in the task of search for NINA. This is done by employing the same long flowing lines for the letters of the target, NINA, that are used to create the picture itself.

In addition to embedding the target so as to make it less conspicuous, Hirschfeld hides the target in a variety of background contexts. Sometimes, the target is embedded in a feature which characterizes the main theme. Other times, it is embedded in an obscure background detail. Even the most dedicated NINA-MANIAC will confess that Hirschfeld's choice of contexts is varied enough to keep them on their toes and this is, of course, an indispensable characteristic of visual search tasks.

---

[1] This research was supported, in part, by Grant GM 21474, National Institutes of Health, U. S. Public Health Service, and by Grant DAAG29–76–G–0313, U. S. Army Research Office. Portions of this paper were presented at the meetings of the Psychonomic Society, Denver, Colorado, 1975. The authors wish to thank Al Hirschfeld for giving us permission to use his pictures in this study.

Finally, Hirschfeld sometimes includes more than one target in the scene. When multiple targets were first introduced, they created such a stir that he was forced to devise a means of indicating how many targets each picture held. His solution was to punctuate his name with a number that represents the number of targets in the picture. You can imagine what happens when he occasionally makes an error.

Figure 1 shows one of the pictures used in this study, "The Apartment." The target in this case is embedded in a scenery detail in the background, the lamp.

From our viewpoint, Hirschfeld's pictures make ideal stimuli for the study of visual search, as they combine all the ingredients found in a task which involves searching for embedded targets in pictures. Our task is not dissimilar to that which faces the photointerpreter searching for a camouflaged tank in an aerial photograph, or the radiologist searching for a lung nodule in a chest x-ray. Both of these tasks require that the observer both sample and disembed the target from the surround. It is an interesting question to speculate which comes first, the sampling or the disembedding of the target. Most commonly it is assumed that the eye has to sample the area containing the target before disembedding it.

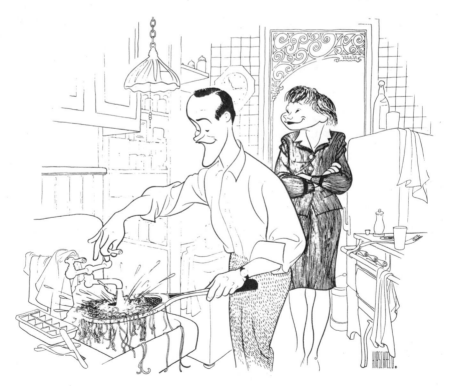

FIG. 1.   Scene from "The Apartment" with Jack Lemmon and Shirley MacLaine. (Reproduced from Hirschfeld, 1970, p. 104).

Thus, some kind of global survey is presumed to proceed detailed pattern analysis.

Most models that deal with the way people look at pictures distinguish between eye movements designed to survey general areas of the picture, and those designed to examine specific details within these areas. Two eye movement parameters, fixation duration and saccade extent, have been used to differentiate these two functional aspects of the eye movement pattern.

Fixations of short duration resulting from long saccades are usually interpreted as performing a survey function, whereas fixations of longer duration resulting from short saccades are interpreted as performing detailed examination of features (e.g., Buswell, 1935; Antes, 1974; Mackworth, 1976).

Behind this functional distinction in the eye movement pattern there is, of course, a cognitive plan. Hochberg (1970) has stressed this point by talking about schematic maps, and in a similar way Neisser (1976) has talked about the importance of anticipatory schemata that serve to direct percpetual exploration. Gould (1976) cited the importance of expectancy in "... constructing or synthesizing a stable, meaningful representation of the environment that he is successively sampling with his eyes. This representation *is* heavily influenced by expectancies . . . (p. 332)." Expectancies are not only important in organizing the way people look at pictures, but we believe they are also important in organizing an effective search for hidden targets in pictures.

With these points in mind, we began to study the ways people search for NINA targets by determining how visual search differs from a simple examination. Specifically, do subjects look at a picture differently when searching for a target than when simply examining it so that they might describe it to someone who has never seen it? This question defines a specific task for the subject, requiring that he extract and encode the key features of the scene that give meaning, at least in a descriptive sense. Or, more generally, specifying agent—action—object relationships.

We chose to use eye movements to measure task differences. A number of studies have been concerned with how people look at pictures (e.g., Antes, 1974; Brandt, 1945; Buswell, 1935), but there have been few comparisons of the same subjects performing under both examination and search modes.

Probably the closest study to the present one was performed by Yarbus (1967). He compared the fixation patterns or scanpaths of the same subject looking at the painting "The Unexpected Visitor" by Repin (p. 147) under a variety of tasks ranging from free examination, to estimating the ages of the people in the painting, to remembering the clothes worn by the people in the painting. Figure 2 shows the subject's eye movement record under a variety of task conditions.

Yarbus found that the scanpaths varied with the subject's task. When compared to the scanpath obtained under free examination, the different scanpaths "showed clearly that the importance of the elements giving information is de-

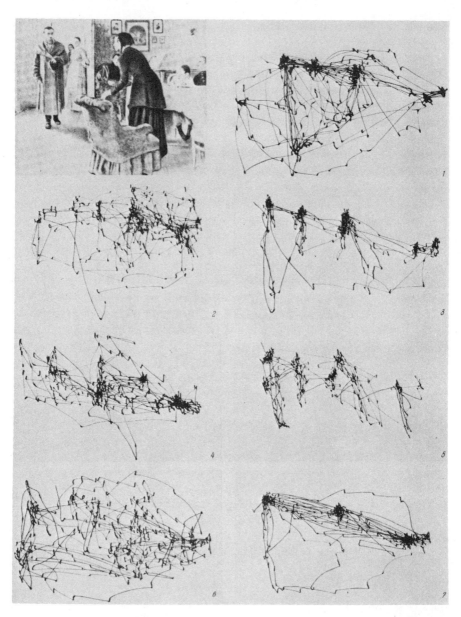

FIG. 2.   Scanpaths produced over a 3 min period as the same subject looked at Repin's painting "The Unexpected Visitor," under different task conditions. Scanpath in upper right panel (#1) was the result of free examination. Scanpaths in subsequent panels resulted from asking the subject to: estimate material circumstances of family (#2); give ages of people (#3); surmise activity of family prior to visitor (#4); remember clothing of people (#5); remember positions of people and objects (#6); and, estimate how long visitor had been away from family (#7). (Taken from Yarbus, 1967, Fig. 109, p. 174.)

termined by the problem facing the observer, and that this importance may vary within extremely wide limits (p. 193)."

Although Yarbus describes the focal points of the scanpaths resulting from different questions asked of the observer, there are no quantitative analyses of the eye movement records on which to make comparisons. We believe such quantitative comparisons would be useful in understanding how people look at pictures and how this looking is changed when the subject is searching for a hidden target.

PROCEDURE

We were interested in three questions: (1) Where does the observer think he should look for information when his task is one of simple examination vs. one of search? (2) Where does the observer look for information under these two conditions? (3) What aspects of looking distinguish a successful from an unsuccessful search when looking for a target?

Ratings of Informativeness and Hiding Potential

To answer the first question, each picture was divided into 64 cells, using an 8 x 8 superimposed matrix. These gridded pictures were then presented to two separate groups of subjects who were asked to rate each of the cells in each picture. One group of subjects was asked to rate the cells for informativeness, which we defined as the relative importance of each cell in describing the picture to someone who had never seen it before. A second group of subjects rated the cells for the potential of hiding a NINA target. Ratings obtained from those few subjects who were familiar with Hirschfeld's work were not included in the final ratings.

A five-level rating scale was used for both tasks, with one level reserved for those cells that were blank. The mean ratings for each cell were used to categorize areas of each picture in terms of either informativeness or hiding potential. A comparison of the ratings indicated that some cells were rated high on both informativeness and hiding potential. Typically, these areas contained the faces of the characters. Other cells were rated low in importance for each condition. These areas contained a minimum of picture detail. Figure 3 illustrates those cells rated high in informativeness, those rated high in hiding potential, and those rated high in both conditions for the picture "The Misfits."

Of interest were those cells that were rated high for one task but not the other. Figure 3 illustrates those cells, designated by E and S, that shift in importance between tasks, as well as those cells that were rated important for both tasks. We interpret these ratings as reflecting the expectancies of observers performing under Examination and Search tasks. These expectancies are presumably used in generating a cognitive scanning plan designed to seek informa-

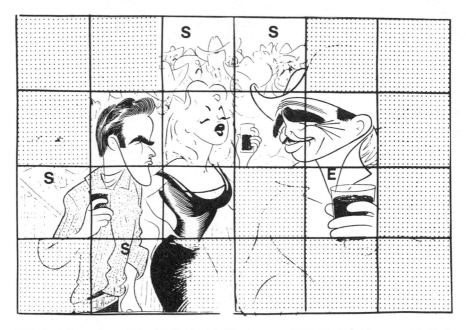

FIG. 3. Scene from "The Misfits" with Montgomery Clift, Marilyn Monroe, and Clark Gable. An 8 x 8 matrix has been superimposed over the picture. Different groups of subjects then rated the cells for either informativeness or hiding potential for NINA. Cells designated by E were rated important for Examination purposes. Cells designated by S were rated important for Search purposes. Clear cells were rated important in both conditions. Textured cells were rated unimportant in both conditions. See text for further explanation. (Reproduced from Hirschfeld 1970, p. 108.)

tion that would be useful in describing the pictures to someone else, or that would hide a potential NINA target. Thus, the sampling distribution of eye movements over the picture should fit the demands of the task, whether it be examination or searching for targets.

Areas rated important for a specific task should be sampled early and frequently throughout scanning, according to Mackworth and Morandi (1967), Antes (1974), and Loftus (1976).

Visual Sampling

Where does an observer look for information under these two conditions? To answer this question, we asked four subjects who were unfamiliar with Hirschfeld's pictures to serve in an eye movement study. The subjects were not aware that they would be tested under two task conditions. The eight pictures previously rated were used as stimuli. In the first task, the subjects were told to examine each picture so they would be able to describe the pictures to someone who had never seen them before. Each picture was individually presented for ten seconds, after which the subject described the picture to the experimenter. The NINA targets were not present in the pictures during this Examination task.

Following the Examination task, the subjects were asked to look at the pictures again to find the NINA target. The same eight pictures were presented in the same sequence for 10 sec each. Before each trial, the subjects were told how many NINA targets were hidden in each picture and were instructed to signal, using a hand held button, when a target was found. This signal terminated the trial. The subjects then described the target location(s). Viewing was terminated at the end of 10 sec if the subject did not signal a target detection.

Eye movements were recorded during both Examination and Search tasks using a Mackworth Wide-Angle camera running at eight frames per sec. The cine records were scored by projecting each frame onto the surface of an X, Y plotting table which was interfaced with a LINC-8 computer. This procedure yielded a series of X, Y loci that served as the basis for defining a fixation. Details of this procedure can be found in Kundel and Nodine (1973). Using this procedure, the accuracy of specifying fixation location was 1.4°. This error is less than one-half of the grid system superimposed over each picture in the rating task.

For analysis purposes, the information in each cell of each picture was defined in two ways. One was based on the ratings of informativeness, and the second was based on ratings of the hiding potential for NINA targets. Separate analyses of the eye movement data were performed by matching the appropriate ratings to the eye movement parameters during both the Examination and the Search tasks.

Two parameters of the eye movement data were considered for both tasks: the frequency of sampling each value of the rated cells (Values 1–4) and the duration of samples within each value of the rated cells.

Sampling Rate

A measure of the sampling rate was obtained by determining the number of fixations in each rated area over the 10 sec of viewing for each trial. An area was defined as a group of cells having the same rating value. The resulting frequencies were then adjusted for the size of the areas. This adjustment was performed for the Examination task and for the Search task using the missed target trials that contained a full 10 sec of viewing.

Table 1 compares the sampling rates, in terms of adjusted percentages, for both Examination and Search tasks. These data indicate that areas rated high in importance (1 and 2 ratings) were selected 3:1 over areas rated low in importance (3 and 4 ratings) for both tasks. However, the separation between areas 1 and 2 was greater in Examination than in Search. This could be attributed to the naiveté of the raters in differentiating between high (1 rating) and moderate (2 rating) ratings of potential hiding sites for NINA in Search.

TABLE 1
Sampling Rate (Percent Fixations/Adjusted Area)
over Pictures Broken Down by Areas Rated
For Importance for Examination and Search Tasks

Task	Rated Importance of Area[a] (1 = High, 4 = Low)			
	1	2	3	4
Examination	55	25	15	4
Search	41	34	20	5

[a]Ratings of informativeness for the Examination task were: 1 = Necessary for description; 2 = Supportive, 3 = Incidental; and 4 = Irrelevant. Ratings of hiding potential of NINA targets for the Search task were: 1 = High; 2 = Moderate, 3 = Low; and 4 = None.

Sampling Duration

Sampling rate is one measure of the distribution of the observer's attention over the pictures. Another measure is sampling duration, that is, how long each sample lasted as measured by the duration of each fixation. We were interested in whether sampling duration varied over ratings between tasks.

Table 2 compares the mean sampling duration as a function of the rating level for Examination and Search. Sampling durations were proportional to the importance of the rated area to the task except between ratings 3 and 4 in Examination. When areas rated high in importance (1 and 2 ratings) were combined and compared with areas rated low (3 and 4 ratings), the difference was significant during Examination (High = 576 msec vs. Low = 358 msec, $t(1) = 4.26$, $p < .01$), but not during Search. Thus, although areas low in importance were sampled less

TABLE 2
Mean Sampling Duration (Msec/Adjusted Area)
Over Pictures Broken Down by Areas Rated
For Importance for Examination and Search Tasks

Task	Rated Importance of Area			
	1	2	3	4
Examination	619[a]	516	360	437
Search	609	521	487	466

[a]Durations were obtained by converting frames to msec by multiplying them by .125 (8 fps).

frequently than areas rated high in Search, the durations per sample were not different. There was, presumably, a detailed examination of features in low rated areas (3 and 4) when they were sampled. But during examination subjects were highly selective in where they looked, focused on information that was relevant to the task of description, and sampled areas rated high in importance longer than areas rated less important to fulfill task demands.

Selective Looking Over the Course of Viewing

Was looking selective over the time course of viewing? Was this selectivity related to the rated importance of the sampled areas? The answer is yes to both questions, but there are some qualifications, as shown in Fig. 4. Here tasks are compared on the sampling rates for each rating level as a function of the course of viewing. Sampling was selective over the course of viewing in both tasks. Areas rated important received more attention as early as the first 2 sec interval of viewing. Areas rated least important were practically ignored throughout viewing.

The patterns of sampling differ over the course of viewing between Examination and Search. In Examination, sampling of areas rated highest for description decreased over time relative to areas rated of lesser importance. Areas rated 1, though, held a 2:1 sampling rate over the areas rated 2. In Search, sampling of

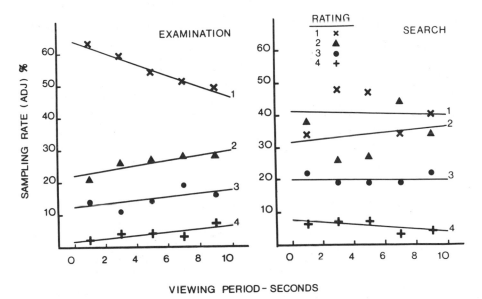

FIG. 4.   Sampling rates as a function of the rated importance of areas within the pictures, (1 = High, 4 = Low), over the course of viewing based on the means of 2 sec periods for Examination and Search tasks. Rates were adjusted by equating the sizes (number of cells) of the four areas.

areas rated high in hiding potential was stable over the course of viewing. This stability of sampling was evident for all rating levels in Search. However, the relative superiority of areas rated 1 to areas rated 2 was less (1.3:1) than that found in Examination. These data suggest that 1 and 2 areas competed for attention throughout viewing during Search.

Antes (1974) reports a tendency for the mean fixation duration to increase over the viewing period across subjects and pictures. He relates this tendency to a change of emphasis in the function of the scanpath from an initial survey phase to detailed examination later in viewing. To determine if similar changes in the function of the scanpath occurred in our viewing situations, the rates of sampling areas were compared with sample duration over the course of viewing.

Figure 5 shows how we differentiated samples on the basis of duration into short samples, durations of 125 msec (one frame), that are presumably designed to survey global areas of the picture, and long samples, durations of 500 msec or greater (four frames) that are presumably designed to examine detailed features within an area. Short samples comprised about 25% of the sampling distribution in Examination and 19% in Search, in contrast to the long samples, which comprised 48% in both tasks. The median fixation durations for Examination and Search were similar (2.7 vs. 2.8 frames respectively, or about 350 msec).

SHORT SAMPLES → 125 MSEC → SURVEY SAMPLING
LONG SAMPLES → ⩾ 500 MSEC → EXAMINATION SAMPLING

FIG. 5.   Diagram showing the relationship between sampling duration and sampling function.

Figure 6 presents the distribution of short and long samples as a function of the course of viewing for each area in each task.

In the first 2 sec interval of Examination, areas rated most informative, (1 rating), received over twice as many short *and* long samples when compared to areas rated 2. Over the course of viewing, the percentage of short samples decreased for areas rated 1 and increased for areas rated 2. The percentage of long samples to all areas remained relatively constant over time; areas rated most informative (1 ratings) and next most informative (2 ratings) received 63 and 25% respectively of these long samples.

These sampling patterns suggest that the time course of surveying pictures during Examination was dependent on those factors that lead to the rated importance of the areas. Areas important to the task received initial priority that later shifted to areas of lesser importance, but were still relevant to the task. Despite this shift in sampling location, areas rated high on informativeness receive 88% of the long samples, indicative of a detailed examination of features within these areas. Such features, consistent with Buswell's (1935) findings, were details of the faces, hands, and objects that comprised the most informative cells of each picture. Treated as a composite, these cells expressed the main ideas

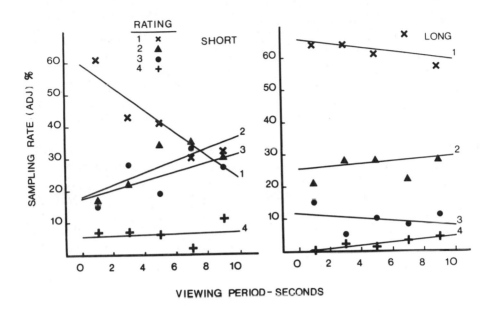

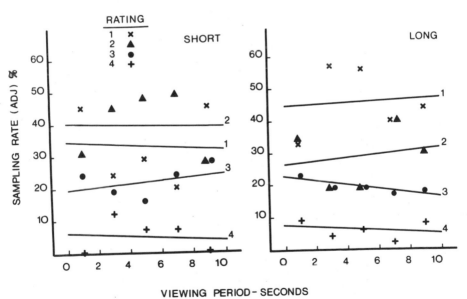

FIG. 6.   Sampling rates as a function of rated importance of areas within the pictures, (1 – High, 4 = Low), over the course of viewing (2 sec periods) for samples of short duration (.125 sec) and long duration ($\geqslant$ .500 msec.) in Examination (top) and Search (bottom). Rates were adjusted by equating the size (number of cells) of the four areas. Short durations presumably reflect survey-type scanning; long durations, examination-type scanning. See text for further explanation.

of the picture, by depicting the agent—action—object relationship. These features are the focal points of a detailed examination designed to encode the theme of the picture for the purpose of describing the picture to someone who has never seen it.

In Search, the sampling patterns over time for short and long samples were different. Short sample surveying of all areas tended to be relatively constant over time, although there was considerable noise about the best-fit linear functions. Also surveying tended to favor areas rated 2 in hiding potential rather than those rated 1. Interestingly, nine of the 13 NINA targets were located in areas rated highest in hiding potential, whereas only three were located in areas rated second highest. Thus, areas that received the most attention by survey-type sampling (one frame), were less likely to contain either an expected target (indicated by the ratings) or an actual target (NINA). However, areas that were highest in hiding potential, and that contained more targets, received more attention by examination-type sampling throughout Search. These long samples were presumably necessary to disembed the NINA target from the picture-context.

To determine if there were changes in sample duration over the course of viewing, the mean durations were calculated for four 20 frame intervals over subjects and pictures in Examination. Table 3 provides these data. There is a small though nonsignificant tendency for the mean sample duration to increase over the course of viewing, confirming what Antes found.

Antes (1974) reports a tendency for the mean interfixation distance to decrease over the viewing period. This is indicative of a shift in emphasis of the scanpath from an initial survey phase to a later detailed examination phase. To determine if similar changes occurred in our situations, the mean interfixation distance was calculated for four 20 frame intervals over the course of viewing in Examination. Table 3 provides these data. There is no tendency for the mean interfixation distance to change over the course of viewing in Examination.

Successful versus Unsuccessful Search

To this point, we have compared sampling strategies between Examination and unsuccessful Search, that is, sampling patterns that failed to detect a target. The

TABLE 3
Mean Interfixation Distance and Mean Sampling
Duration Over Quarters of Viewing Period
for the Examination Task

Variable	Quarters of the Viewing Period (2.5 sec Intervals)			
	1st	2nd	3rd	4th
Interfixation Distance (deg)	4.5	4.4	4.9	4.7
Sampling Duration (msec)	515	583	542	555

final question of concern is: *what aspects of looking distinguish a successful from an unsuccessful sampling pattern when looking for a target?*

A total of 13 NINA targets were hidden in the eight pictures. Half of the pictures contained single targets, three pictures contained two targets and the remaining picture contained three. All four subjects found the single targets in two pictures (DZ, FK) and three subjects found one of two targets (in the hair, CH) in a third picture. The remaining six targets that were found were distributed across pictures and subjects. Thus, about one-third of the targets (17/52) were detected within the 10 sec limit.

Relationship of Hits to Ratings

Table 4 provides an assessment of search performance on each picture. These data are interpreted as indicating that the probability of finding a NINA target was inversely related to the hiding potential rating of the cell containing the target. The hit rate per area was lower (7/36 = .19) for NINA targets located in areas rated highest (1) than the hit rate (9/12 = .75) for targets located in areas rated 2.

TABLE 4

A Listing of Pictures Indicating the Target Surround,
Target Cell Rating, and Median Duration of
Hits and Misses During Search

Picture Title	Target Surround	Target Cell Rating	Median duration of First Sample on Target Cell (Sec)	
			Hits (No.)	Misses (No.)
Never on Sunday (NS)	Hair	1	— (0)	.25 (4)
Odd Couple (OC)	Hassock (L)	2	1.0 (1)	—^{a}
	Hassock (R)	1	.88 (1)	.88 (1)^b
Doctor Zhivago (DZ)	Pants	2	1.25 (4)	—
Cherry Orchard (CH)	Cravat	1	.75 (1)	.12 (3)
	Hair	1	1.38 (3)	.50 (1)^c
Fugitive Kind (FK)	Box	2	.75 (4)	—
Rhapsody in Blue (RB)	Sleeve	1	— (0)	.12 (1)^d
	Tutu (L)	1	— (0)	.88 (4)
	Tutu (R)	1	— (0)	.38 (4)
The Apartment (AP)	Lamp	1	— (0)	.25 (4)
Misfits (MF)	Collar	1	1.75 (2)	.25 (2)
	Sleeve	3	2.0 (1)	.38 (3)
			Mdn =1.0 (17)	Mdn =.25 (27)

[a]Three subjects did not fixate target cell.
[b]Two subjects did not fixate target cell.
[c]One subject fixated target cell on start.
[d]Three subjects fixated target cells on start for mdn dwell of .2 sec.

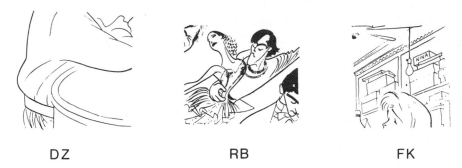

DZ   RB   FK

FIG. 7.   Close-up views of the NINA targets in three scenes "Doctor Zhivago," "Fugitive Kind," and "Rhapsody in Blue." All subjects detected the NINA targets correctly in DZ and FK pictures. All subjects failed to detect the three NINA targets in the RB picture. (Reproduced from Hirschfeld, 1970, and The New York Times.)

The suggestion of an inverse relationship between the probability of a hit and the ratings could be attributed to the greater amount of feature detail found in areas rated 1. These areas provide a noisier surround in which to embed the NINA target than other areas, and noisy surrounds have been shown to adversely influence search performance (Kundel & Nodine, Chapter VI.1, this volume).

Of the 17 hits, 15 (88%) occurred in target cells that shifted to a higher rating in hiding potential from a lower rating in descriptive value. None of the three NINA targets embedded in the folds of clothing in picture RB, and also located in cells rated 1 in both tasks, were detected. Figure 7 shows the way the targets were embedded in pictures DZ, RB, and FK.

All subjects found the single NINA in pictures DZ and FK, which were embedded in cells that shifted to higher ratings in hiding potential than descriptive value. It should be noted, however, that the NINA target in FK was the least embedded target that was presented.

Relationship of Hits to Sample Duration

How is sampling duration related to target detection? Table 4 provides the data indicating a positive relationship between duration and detection. The data were obtained by recording the duration of the first fixation that fell on the target cell and noting whether it resulted in a hit or a miss. Analysis of the data in Table 4 indicated that sampling durations were significantly longer for hits (Mdn = 1.0 sec) than misses (Mdn = .25 sec) by a median test, χ^2 (1) = 11.34, p < .001. In only two of the 17 hits was the duration of the first sample on target less than .88 sec (seven frames). Only five of the 37 missed records (14%) contained samples which equalled or exceeded .88 sec on a target cell. Thus, duration of the first sample on target was a good predictor of a hit. Also, a sample duration of at least .88 sec was necessary to resolve these NINA targets.

These data also suggest that examination-type sampling (long samples ⩾ .50 sec) preceded a hit, while misses were preceded by survey-type sampling (.12—

.38 sec). In support of this interpretation, a majority of the hits (65%) were followed by several additional samples within 3° of the target cell. The median duration of these follow-up samples was .88 sec. These follow-up samples were also
the result of short saccades (median distance = 2.9°) indicative of detailed examination-type sampling. Interestingly, the five false-positive responses were also
characterized by long sample durations (Mdn = .88 sec) on the false target.

Relationship of Hits to Interfixation Distance

The saccadic displacement, called excursion, prior to fixation on target was related to the success of the sampling pattern. Excursions to the target were significantly longer when the target was detected (Mdn = 5.2°) than when it was missed
(Mdn = 4.0°), χ^2 (1) 4.73, $p < .05$. Figure 8 illustrates the scanpath of one of the

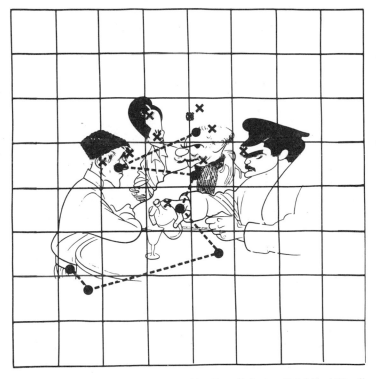

FIG. 8.   Scene from "Doctor Zhivago" with Alex Guinnes, Geraldine Chaplin, Ralph
Richardson, and Omar Sharif. The x's indicate the points sampled by subject M.L. during
the description phase. The scanpath during search for the same subject is indicated by
the dot pattern connected by lines. The grid squares were not present during viewing.
Overlap between sampling patterns for Examination and Search are minimal. The search
pattern is used to illustrate the large excursion to the target displayed by this subject.
Each grid square represents 3° visual angle. The distance traversed by the eye movement
was 9.1°. The median excursion to the target for this picture was 7° (N = 4). (Reproduced
from Hirschfeld, 1970, p. 121.)

TABLE 5
Transitional Probabilities of Long Excursions ($\geqslant 6°$)
Landing on Important Areas for Examination and Search Tasks

Importance of Launch Cell[b]	Importance of Landing Cell[a]				
	Examination			Search	
	To: High	Low		To: High	Low
From: High	.60[c]	.18		.39[d]	.26
Low	.18	.04		.31	.04

[a]Fixation location after excursion $\geqslant 6°$.
[b]Fixation location before excursion $\geqslant 6°$.
[c]χ^2 (1) = 80.8, $P < .001$
[d]χ^2 (1) = 18.8, $P < .001$

four subjects who detected the NINA target in picture DZ during Search. The median excursion to the target cell for subjects in this picture was 7.0°. In this case, the subject jumped 9.1° to the target. The location of the areas sampled by the same subject during Examination are shown in Fig. 7. Sampling during Examination concentrated on the faces of the characters and the hand holding the bottle. Of the eight cells sampled in Examination, six were rated 1 in informative- and two were rated 2.

Both Mackworth and Morandi (1967) and Antes (1974) have emphasized the role of peripheral vision as a component of selective attention, which edits sampling choices. However, Antes questions whether peripheral vision can be effective in guiding long excursions (e.g., those in excess of 5°) to informative areas in the picture. Our data indicate that even longer excursions landed more frequently on informative than non-informative areas, χ^2 (1) = 80.8, $p < .001$. Table 5 provides the transitional probabilities of landing on areas rated high in importance for excursions of 6° or better in both Examination and Search. Comparisons were made between areas rated high in importance (1 and 2 ratings) and low in importance (3 and 4 ratings).

Long excursions were generally preceded by short samples, which imply survey-type sampling of areas. The excursions of 6° and greater were preceded by a median duration of 240 msec in Examination and 370 msec in Search. Survey-type sampling may be guided by contextual cues derived from the picture as a whole. This view is consistent with the notion of a cognitive scanning plan. Such a plan presumably determines sampling choices on the basis of a holistic representation or schematic map that provides the viewer with a set of expectancies about the location of potential hiding places for NINA in the Search task. These expectancies may reflect rules for embedding imaginary NINAs within scenery details.

GENERAL DISCUSSION

Our subjects were unfamiliar with Hirschfeld's work and therefore had to rely on expectancies generated from looking at pictures in the past to guide search. These expectancies were different for the tasks of Examination and Search. In Examination, expectancies were used to locate informative areas in terms of descriptive value. In Search, expectancies were used to isolate areas likely to hide a NINA target. Agreement between the ratings of descriptive value and visual sampling of these areas during Examination indicates a high relationship between expectancy and looking. Information of descriptive value centered on agent—action—object relationships that helped to characterize the main theme of each picture. This same information was contained in the verbal protocols of the subjects after each picture viewing.

The relationship between expectancy and looking was not as high in Search. Subjects did not know what kind of picture surround would best hide a NINA target because they did not know what the target would look like in the picture surround. These expectancies could not take shape until after the observers had experienced finding NINA. Gregory (1973) talks about this problem as one of object recognition, that is, separating object from background. He emphasizes the importance of an object hypothesis to generate predictions (or expectancies) about the way the object will look in a given context.

Our data suggest that survey-type sampling is responsible for identifying potential target areas. Once identified, these areas are subjected to a pattern-recognition analysis which employs examination-type sampling. This detailed sampling might, for example, focus on a distinctive feature of the target. The "A" in NINA could be used as a distinctive feature in disembedding target from the background.

The major reason for search failure in our experiment was not inadequate sampling of target areas. Of the 35 targets that were missed, 31 were sampled. Thus, getting the eye on the target did not guarantee detection. The problem was one of recognition, which required disembedding of the target from the surround. Our naive subjects were simply unable to unravel NINA from the picture context. We believe this was primarily due, elaborating on Gregory's (1973) idea, to an inappropriate target hypothesis. The subjects did not know how the targets fit into the surround. These expectations come from knowing (a) what features of the target become distinctive when placed in the picture surround (e.g., the "A" in NINA), and (b) what features of the surround provide the focal points in a cognitive search plan. That plan is undoubtedly modified by what the subject sees as he searches the picture and by his past experiences in finding NINA targets, but that's another story.

DISCUSSION

STARK: Your subjects were naive at first, presumably became skilled as they performed the task, and maybe became NINAmaniacs eventually. Did you notice changes in their hit rate or search strategy or anything like that?

NODINE: No, I think this task provided them with a minimum amount of feedback. The targets that they hit were the targets that were in the pictures in the middle of the group of eight pictures, so there didn't seem to be any experience playing a role there. And, they only saw these pictures twice: once during examination when they didn't really think about finding targets, and then the second time when they were searching for a target. I think the role of experience in this task is minimized, although it's certainly a consideration.

SNYDER: Two questions come to mind. I'm not surprised that the background information is somewhat critical. In 1963 or 1964, using actual aerial photos, the Port Calhoun Study showed that the background cues rather than the target cues were used by about 60% of their subjects. More recently, it was found that microphotometric scans produced better information for finding objects from the background information than from the target. Perhaps you'd like to comment as to whether you're intending to generalize this type of information to scenes which are of use to someone like photo interpreters. I can see why you wouldn't use such scenes and photo interpreters, because you really wanted naive subjects; on the other hand, you did use naive subjects, so would you comment upon why you chose this task in order to get there.

NODINE: Well, this is the first of a series of projects that we have ongoing, and the next task is with experienced viewers. One of the problems is finding experienced viewers. We're in Philadelphia, and it is not as easy to find NINAmaniacs in Philadelphia, as it is in New York. I'm interested in the relationship of the surround information, in this case picture information, to the target information. That is, I'm interested in the fact that these surrounds do have meaning for the viewer, and that's why I'm using the pictures.

HANSELL: You mentioned two stages in your experiment, Examination and then Search. Can you describe the frequency of fixation duration of the two different stages?

NODINE: Examination and Search? I think I said that roughly 20% of the fixations were one frame or 125 msec, and about half, 48%, were five frames or greater in duration. The distribution tended to shift toward longer durations in Search than in Examination, so the peak of the distribution was greater at the short end for Examination and shifted toward the longer duration for Search.

V.2

Eye Movements During Inspection and Recall[1]

Warren H. Teichner,
Dean LeMaster,[2]
Patricia A. Kinney[3]
New Mexico State University

There are two persistent hypotheses that view eye movements as the mirror of memory. One, the *construction hypothesis,* is that eye movements play a role in the construction of memory images. The other, usually implicit, the *scanner hypothesis,* is that eye movements reflect the behavior of an internal memory image scanner. The implications of these hypotheses, if true, are enormous because they suggest that eye movements that are easily available can be used to study memory and thought processes and, in certain spheres of application, that eye movements may reveal private thought. For both reasons resolution of these hypotheses is of major importance.

The construction hypothesis has an historical background in the motor theory of thought and the concept of redintegrative stimuli discussed in the Titchener era. Hebb (1968) stated it by suggesting that an original visual impression is reinstated in the form of a visual image by sequential eye movements. He hypothesized that ocular movement is not only essential to visual memory images, but that it also serves to reconstruct them by mediating the separate visual impressions

[1]Experiment 1 was based upon the Master's thesis of the second author in 1971; Experiment 2 was based on the Master's thesis of the third author in 1973. The senior author prepared this paper and directed both theses. Experiment II was supported by the Air Force Office of Scientific Research, Contract AFOSR No. F44620-71-C-0072. We are grateful to Ms. Julie Goodrich for secretarial assistance and to Ms. Nancy E. Hutchcroft for preparation of figures.

[2]Now at Air Force Human Resources Laboratory, Williams Air Force Base, Phoenix, Arizona.

[3]Now at New Mexico Department of Transportation, Santa Fe, New Mexico.

that form the image. Hochberg (1968) and Neisser (1970) have made similar proposals.

The scanner hypothesis necessarily differs from the construction hypothesis in that, for it to operate, the memory image must already be present; whereas the construction hypothesis concerns the actual development of the image. Unfortunately, although the distinction is clear in principle, it is not clear in practice. A series of well-ordered eye movements consistent with the ordering of segments of a visual display, e.g., as in textual material, could be the same if an image were being constructed, or if an existent image were being scanned. This problem could be resolved if there were an independent nonsubjective criterion (Bugelski, 1970) for the presence of an image, so that the temporal order of eye movements and images could be determined. So far, however, all that has been suggested as criterion is eye movement!

A frequent experimental paradigm is one which presents a subject with a briefly exposed row of alphanumeric symbols and then requires a verbal report of the items in the row. Eye movements are analyzed to determine whether or not the subject either moved his gaze in the direction being reported or, if in doing so, his eye movements followed the positional sequence of his report of the items. Studies such as those of Crovitz and Daves (1962) and Winnick and Dornbush (1965) have found a congruence between eye movements and order of report; Bryden (1961) and Weitzenhoffer (1971) found a relationship only between the general direction of eye movement and the subject's report.

In contrast to the method of reporting all of the items, Hall (1974) used a Sperling (1960) post-stimulus cued, partial report design. The subject was presented with a 3 x 3 matrix of letters for 250 msec followed 300 msec later by a frequency-coded tone which designated the row to be reported. Hall found that the aiming point of the eyes during recall was to the row to be reported and concluded that eye movements are a correlate of an internal image scanner, and that intended tests of the construction hypothesis such as those just cited were probably contaminated by scanning.

A possible problem with the partial report method, as used by Hall (1974), is that the post-stimulus cue not only tells the subject what to report, it may also suggest or direct the subject to where he should look. Thus, the eye movement may depend on the cue and not on an internal scanner. The same problem appears in the whole report situation because the direction of reading is predetermined. In both cases, the direction of gaze may be an independent orienting response cued by stimuli in the task. This problem was avoided in the two experiments to be reported by post-cueing the subject with selected items and requiring that he report where those items were in the display.

Thus, there are two major confounding problems in this literature. One concerns the problem of distinguishing a constructional pattern from a scanning pattern of eye movements. The other concerns the use of external cues and configurations that may induce or suggest the direction or position of the gaze. The present study attempted to circumvent both problems.

A variety of other kinds of studies have been performed in an attempt to relate eye movements to visual memory images. Many of those studies were also concerned with a possible similarity between eye movements during the inspection of a scene and those made during recall or imagining of some sort. Interestingly, none of the studies available compared the two patterns or any of the parameters of each, but instead assumed an inspection pattern and generally accepted any kind of eye movement during recall as being related to an inspection pattern. Reviewing the literature, both Bower (1972) and Paivio (1973) concluded that the data are not yet convincing of a correlation between eye movements and memory images. We note, however, that a relationship need not be evident as a gross coincidence of images and eye movements. The relationship, if any, could be more subtle and could involve quantitative aspects of eye movements rather than their mere occurrence.

Both of the experiments to be reported provided the subjects with a row of alphanumeric symbols for inspection. After removal of the display the subjects were asked to report the location of a specific item. To accomplish that using an image would seem to require that an image of the entire array be available, and that it be searched for the target item. For the image to be available by the construction hypothesis, there should be a systematic pattern of eye movements some time after offset of the display, or after the post-stimulus cue. Then, if the information load in the display is sufficiently large and the positional arrangement sufficiently complex, a second pattern of eye movements should be observed if scanning is going on and eye movements are related to it.

Unfortunately, the construction hypothesis need not require that the pattern during recall closely resemble the inspection pattern. Instead, a recall pattern that is, in some sense, a fractional representation might suffice. In that case, unless the recall pattern is in some sense proportional to the inspection pattern, there is no way to interpret it. However, if the recall pattern were in opposition to the inspection pattern, some interference might be expected. Furthermore, if during recall no eye movements were present, neither construction nor image-scanning would be reasonable to infer if their presence were necessarily reflected by eye movements. Experiment 2 manipulated ocular activity during both inspection and recall; Experiment 1 was based on a logic that avoided eye movement patterns as such.

A very important concern is whether the image may persist as either a retinal or iconic storage long enough for it not to need to be constructed prior to scanning. Hall (1974) concluded that his subjects, as well as those of other studies using briefly-exposed displays, were scanning an iconic image, a brief, uncoded, large capacity storage, which has been proposed to be a post-retinal phenomenon. That they were really scanning an icon is unlikely, since iconic images move with eye movements (see Sakitt, 1976 for a review). Furthermore, even if it is post-retinal storage, an eye movement need not necessarily reflect the scanning of a visual-like image. Other questions about the validity of the icon concept as derived from the partial report technique have also been raised (e.g., Gardner,

1973). In general, these questions suggest that the partial report technique provides data that reflect a selective attentional process rather than an icon.

Of course, that the image is not an icon does not preclude the establishment of a coded post-retinal storage in the subjective form of an image or with the availability of an image. If so, eye movements might not have to precede the image. That is, there may be no need for a construction hypothesis. In fact, since none of the studies reported attempted to determine the temporal relationship between the eye movements observed and the subject's response, they can not be used to support either a construction hypothesis or a scanning hypothesis. However, if eye movements were found to precede the response, these hypotheses become plausible although such results do not yet rule out an independence between eye movements and image phenomena.

EXPERIMENT 1

A pilot study indicated clearly that after subjects scan an array and the array remains available, when asked for the position of a particular item, their gaze is directed instantly to the position at which they believe the item to be. Furthermore, if we do accept Hall's (1974) finding of a similar eye movement during recall, we can use this behavior as a model of what eye-aiming behavior should be when the array is not present but some form of visual image is. Accordingly, it might be expected that a coincidence of gaze and recall response should be found if a memory image of the array is available. However, if an image must be constructed before it can be scanned, the tendency of the eyes to be aimed at the position reported should be delayed compared to the first case, and the latency of the recall response should be longer. This experiment attempted to test these expectations.

Subjects who deliberately attempt to use memory images may have an advantage in being able to produce a better image than those who do not make such an attempt. Thus, if imagery could be maximized in one group, that group should have shorter response latencies and faster eye aiming to the position of recall than a group not so maximized. An attempt was made to develop such a distinction, although we acknowledge that such attempts do not ensure the use of images and that discouraging imagery does not preclude its use.

General Procedures

Horizontal eye movements were recorded by EOG during and following the viewing of a horizontal rectangular array of projected alphanumeric symbols. An illustration of the array is shown in Fig. 1.

As the figure shows, the display consisted of five cells, each containing three different characters, either capital letters or single digits. The characters, selected

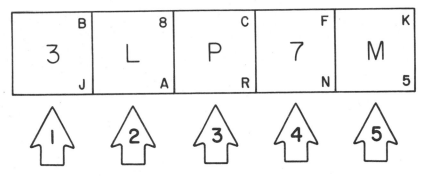

FIG. 1.   Illustration of stimulus display.

randomly without replacement, were always arranged so that a large character was in the center of the block and two smaller characters were in the upper right and lower right corners. The large symbol subtended a visual angle of 2.25° vertically and 1.75° horizontally; the small symbols were 1.50° vertically and 1.0° horizontally. The array itself was 50.0° wide and 10° high, with each cell being 10.0° square.

The slides were projected at eye level on a blank white wall by a projector with a lens-mounted electronic shutter. Arrows with digits (1–5, as shown in Fig. 1) were affixed to the wall for identifying the cells. The subject was seated at a table 2.44 m from the display. The only illumination was a ceiling-mounted fluorescent light 2.44 m behind the subject.

Following instruction and practice, the subject maintained position with an adjustable head stabilizer and bite-board for the 9 min experimental session. During that period he was twice presented with 10 test slides. Each cell appeared randomly as the target four times. Following the offset of the slide, the subject was required to indicate the target cell position by tapping a key the appropriate number of times. This procedure was used because the subject could not respond vocally. The cell data were presented orally by the experimenter.

The slide was presented for 5 sec to allow full inspection of the display. The experimenter's post-stimulus data cue was initiated at slide offset and consisted of five syllables (exceptions being W and 7) voiced in approximately 2.0 sec, for example, "Where was 3, B, J?" The first syllable meaningful for response selection was spoken approximately 1 sec before the end of the last syllable. The instant of the last syllable is denoted as t = 0 for data analysis.

Electrooculographic (EOG) recordings were made with a Coleman-Hitachi 165 Recorder. Drift in the DC signal was effectively countered by introducing a reversible polarity, variable DC power source of very small magnitude into the electrode-recorder circuit. With this device, a signal drift could be balanced with opposing DC current and a reasonably constant zero reference maintained on the chart paper. The EOG was calibrated before each slide. The chart paper speed was 60 mm/min.

Silver/silver chloride surface electrodes, 4 mm in diameter, were placed over the extreme lateral points of both orbital ridges, approximately 1 cm lateral to each external canthus, and on the left ear lobe for recording horizontal eye movements. Prior to electrode placement, the three sites were scrubbed vigorously with a 1:750 aqeous solution of benzalkonium chloride. Electrode paste made of equal parts of bentonite, glycerine, and salt water was used to fill the electrode cups and was also applied to the electrode placement sites on the subject to facilitate signal transmission.

Experimental Design

Forty college student subjects, 24 male and 16 female, were randomly assigned to four groups of 10 with the constraint that each group be equal by sex. The groups were the following:

1. Group N-O (no imaging instructions, eyes-open recall)
2. Group N-C (no imaging instructions, eyes-closed recall)
3. Group I-O (imagining instructions, eyes-open recall)
4. Group I-C (imagining instructions, eyes-closed recall)

Group N-O was instructed to scan the entire stimulus slide during its presentation. Group N-C was instructed in the same way and, in addition, to close its eyes immediately following the termination of each slide. All groups were given identical instructions on answering procedures. All groups were also informed that prior to each slide presentation they would be instructed to look at fixation points marking the centers of specified cells of the stimulus slide. (This procedure was followed in order to facilitate eye movement record scoring by reflecting a running index of stimulus block locations on the chart.)

During the pretest instruction period, Group I-O and I-C subjects were required to develop a visual afterimage by staring for 30 sec at a large black dot on a white sheet of paper. All subjects were able to experience this afterimage. They were informed that they would not be able to form afterimages of the stimulus slides, but that the afterimage they had just formed was a type of visual image — a "seeing" of a stimulus object after the object is removed — and that they were to try to develop and employ memory images for each test trial. The subjects were then given 1–2 sec glimpses of pages containing four meaningless symbols, asked to have images of what they had seen, and queried as to the location of the symbols on the pages. When subjects of both I-O and I-C groups appeared aware of what was involved in forming a visual image, they were considered ready for the experiment. Other instructions to these two groups were identical to those given Groups N-O and N-C.

The experiment was conducted as free visual search. Subjects were given no fixation point and no instructions about where or how to look before, during, or following slide offset. EOGs were recorded continuously from just before the slide onset to 5 sec after the completion of the poststimulus cue. Slide onset and offset, completion of the verbal post-stimulus cue, and the subject's key pressing responses were recorded with event markers. In addition, the onset of the subject's first button-press was timed electronically.

Calibration of the EOG required the subject to fixate the center of positions 3, 1, 5, and 3 prior to each slide presentation. This revealed a distinguishing feature of the eyes-closed eye movement. Eyes-open subjects were able to fixate the arrows on the wall marking the location of stimulus block centers accurately. The eyes-closed subjects, having no reference points to fixate, consistently exaggerated the amount of horizontal eye movement required to move the eyes to blocks 2 and 5. When compared to their eye movements recorded during stimulus slide viewing, the closed-eye movements appeared to exceed the required movement by about 10°. These movements appeared to be quite consistent within subjects and to vary only slightly between subjects. Because the overestimate could be determined on an individual subject basis, and considering the size of the cells of the array, cell positions could be related to eye aiming with no difficulty.

The logic of the experiment required measurement of the timing of the cell position reported as the recall measure in relation to the cell position at which the eye aimed. The latter was analyzed in terms of "eyes at position answered" (EAPA) during recall.

EAPA was determined with regard to the frequency of EAPAs at eight time intervals ranging from t = −2 sec to t = 5 sec. Since t = O was the moment of the last syllable of the experimenter's question, the first cueing syllable which would have permitted a correct response occurred at t = −1 approximately.

An analysis of variance of EAPA frequency in the eight time intervals indicated no main effects of the experimental conditions except that due to the time periods $[F(1, 36) = 11.85, p < .05]$. The interactions of time x eye condition $[F(7, 252) = 3.35, p < .01]$, of instructions x eye conditions $[F(1, 36) = 6.30, p < .05]$, and the triple interaction $[F(7, 252) = 7.60, p < .01]$ were significant. The interaction of instructions x time was not significant.

Figure 2 (upper) presents the percent of the first occurring EAPA as a function of its time of occurrence. Figure 2 (lower) presents the percentage of all of the EAPAs made by time intervals. The figure also presents the mean response latency for the eyes-open and eyes-closed conditions.

Summing EAPA in the upper portion of the figure indicates that with eyes open 62% of the first EAPA occurred before the response, and with eyes closed 78% occurred before the response. After the response occurred, the percentages reversed, that is, there were more EAPAs with eyes open. In fact, the reversal was initiated 1 sec before the response.

The lower figure reveals the same interaction, the percentage of all of the EAPAs that occurred was greater with eyes closed up to the final verbal cue, but greater with eyes open after that. Here 38% of the EAPAs before the responses were made with the eyes open, and 56% with eyes closed. It is apparent that

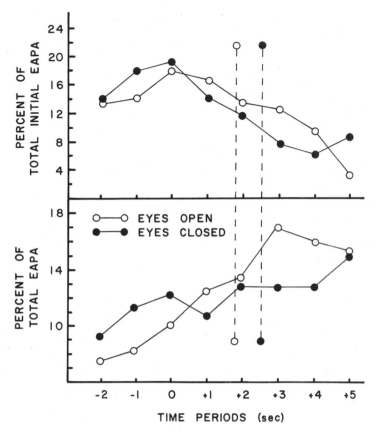

FIG. 2.   Percentage of initial and total occurrences of EAPA following stimulus offset. Dashed vertical lines indicate mean response latencies.

there was a significant movement of the eyes to the position answered before the final cue syllable, but also a substantial effect afterwards.

Major questions of the experiment were whether the eyes move to the answered position without external direction to that position, and whether that eye movement occurs before the response or later. The answer seems to be that most of the EAPAs occur before and that the frequency of first EAPA before the response was somewhat greater with the eyes closed.

Figure 2 also indicates that the response latency of the eyes open group was shorter than that of the eyes closed group. A summary of the latencies by experimental conditions is presented in Table 1. An analysis of variance of the data on which that table is based indicated that each of the main effects was significant: eye condition $F(1, 72) = 19.754$, $p < .01$, instructions $F(1, 72) = 10.32$, $p < .01$ and right vs. wrong responses $F(1, 72) = 9.55$, $p < .01$. None of the interactions were significant. In Table 1, it may be seen that response speed was greater with eyes open and without instructions.

TABLE 1
Mean Response Latency (Seconds)
of Manually-Transmitted Answers

	Instructions		No Instructions	
	Eyes Open	Eyes Closed	Eyes Open	Eyes Closed
Correct Response	1.72	2.50	1.32	2.03
Wrong Response	2.26	3.02	1.85	2.33

	Pooled Latency
Correct Response	1.89
Wrong Response	2.37
No Instructions	1.88
Instructions	2.38
Eyes Open	1.79
Eyes Closed	2.47

Thus, the conditions under which one might expect imagery to be enhanced required a longer information processing time than those in which enhancement was not expected. Table 1 also shows that wrong answers required more processing time than right ones.

An analysis of variance of the correctness of the responses revealed no significant effects. Thus, it appears that the experimental conditions had no significant effect on the accuracy of response, although they did on the latency of response.

Discussion

The results of this experiment appear to indicate that subjects in a partial report paradigm in which there is no cue to position, but in which position recall is required, direct their gaze to the position that represents their response, and do it well before initiation of the response. This was usually, but not always, the case, because after the response 38% of the first EAPAs were with eyes open and 22% with eyes closed. The image-related conditions, instructions to use images and recall with eyes closed, resulted in a greater frequency of the preresponse EAPAs, suggesting a possible relationship between ocular activity and image use.

The results also suggest that instructions to use images during recall, and recall with eyes closed, delayed the selection of a response compared to the absence of such instructions or recall with the eyes open. Accordingly, while we cannot really conclude that images were involved, it does appear that something was going on as the result of those experimental conditions which required more processing time. Whatever it was, it did not affect the accuracy of the report significantly.

We noted earlier that the occurrence of response-indicating eye movements preceding the response could be interpreted as support for the notion that images are constructed and/or scanned. The data of Experiment 1 show a predominance of such occurrences. We also hypothesized, if memory images are both constructed and scanned, that more time might be required to select a response than would be the case if they were not. Assuming that our experimental treatments enhanced the use of images, the data are consistent with the hypothesis. They do not suggest that uninstructed subjects with eyes open do not use images, however, since those subjects also showed a predominance of EPAs before the response. It could be speculated that those subjects receiving the experimental treatments attempted to construct a clearer or more detailed image than the others and, therefore, required more time before the response selection stage.

Although we have not attempted to detail it, it was observed in this experiment that some subjects seemed to characteristically make .a large number of eye movements during inspection, and that others made fewer eye movements with unusually short fixations. These latter subjects tended to sweep the array repeatedly. This observation provokes still another hypothesis, that is, that the pattern of eye movements during inspection affects later recall and/or the construction or use of imagery. The next experiment, therefore, was concerned in part with this new hypothesis.

EXPERIMENT 2

Experiment 2 was an attempt to test the construction and scanning hypotheses more directly by controlling eye movements during inspection and recall. In addition, we wished to explore the possibility that recall phenomena might depend upon the parameters of eye movements during inspection.

The experiment was also intended to improve on certain features of the previous one. Use of the bite-bar had placed a restriction on the duration of testing and required a complex responding method. The nature of the stimuli in conjunction with the nature of the post-stimulus cue, which identified all of the letters in the cell, actually permitted the subject to identify the target cell with just one cell symbol, probably the large centered one. As a result, the array could be thought of as having only five target symbols, each in the presence of smaller irrelevant symbols. This might have made the task too easy although that was not suggested by the results. In any case, Experiment was a methodological improvement in these regards.

Method

The five-celled rectangular array was essentially as before, but their alphanumeric contents were different in that each cell contained two alphanumeric characters separated by one type space. Eight of the 10 characters were upper case consonant letters; one character was a lower case consonant letter, and the remaining one was a digit. The digit, 1, and the lowercase letter, 1, were excluded; the digits used were 2–9. All characters were selected randomly, without replacement, for each slide, except that the digit and the lower case letter never appeared in the same cell together. Each of these two characters appeared equally often in each of the five cells, and the characters were of Gothic type, centered within the cell. Each character subtended a visual angle of approximately 1°6' horizontally and 1°42' vertically. An "empty" slide which contained an outline of the five cells with no characters was projected during recall. Seventy-five "filled" slides were made that differed only in being independent random samples with the restrictions noted.

At the subject's table was mounted a chin and head rest. The bite-bar was not used. Located at the subject's right hand was a response button mounted on a box. When this button was depressed, it terminated a .01 sec timer. There were two pilot lights which were used as fixation points. One was mounted on the wall 4.0° to the right and the other 4.0° to the left of the projected stimulus area. The experimenter operated these lights manually with a toggle switch.

Horizontal eye movements were monitored as before, except that the recorder was a Honeywell Visicorder which permitted the experimenter a visual display of the aiming position of the eye calibrated with respect to the display. Accordingly, the subject's eye movements were easy to monitor on-line.

Exposure times of the slides were controlled by a shutter mounted on the slide projector. The shutter was activated independently of the slide, which was advanced without projecting the material. The opening of the shutter activated a .01 sec timer; that event was also placed on the recorder by a signal marker. There were three separate switches used by the experimenter during the experiment. The first switch opened the shutter to expose the stimulus and simultaneously started the first timer; the second switch closed the shutter, stopped the timer, and advanced the carousel; the third switch opened the shutter to project the "empty" slide and started a second timer. The subject stopped the second timer by pressing the response button, an action which also closed the shutter and advanced the carousel.

Experimental Design

Four major scanning conditions were used in a within-subjects design: Free, Compatible, Incompatible, and Fixated. In the Free condition, the subject was allowed to scan freely as in Experiment 1. In the Compatible conditions, the subject scanned either left to right or right to left during both inspection and recall. For the Incompatible conditions, if the inspection scan were from left to right, then the recall scan proceeded from right to left, and if the inspection scan were from right to left, then the recall span was from left to right. During the Fixated conditions, if the inspection scan were from left to right, the subject

TABLE 2
Experimental Viewing Conditions

Condition	Inspection scan	Recall scan
1. Free	Free	Free
2. Compatible L-R	Left-to-right	Left-to-right
3. Compatible R-L	Right-to-left	Right-to-left
4. Incompatible L-R	Left-to-right	Right-to-left
5. Incompatible R-L	Right-to-left	Left-to-right
6. Fixated L-R	Left-to-right	Fixate right
7. Fixated R-L	Right-to-left	Fixate left

fixated the right light during recall, and if the scan during inspection were from right to left, then during recall the subject fixated the left light. The seven different viewing conditions are shown in Table 2.

Fourteen subjects were randomly assigned, two each, to one of seven independent random orders of the viewing conditions, and to one of seven randomly selected orders of slide presentation. The subjects were male college students paid on an hourly basis for their participation.

Procedure

After the electrodes were applied and the subject's head adjusted in the head-restraining unit, he was asked to relax for a few minutes to permit stabilization of the skin potential. He was then presented with the slide containing only the empty cells. A correspondence was established between the two pilot light fixation points and the two reference channels on the oscillograph, and between the fixation of the middle cell and the central reference marker of the recorder. The central reference point was recalibrated before each trial. At the beginning of the session, the subject was instructed to fixate the borders of each of the five cells, proceeding from left to right as directed by the experimenter. The magnitude of the recorded eye movement was maintained by adjusting the gain on the oscillograph.

The subject's task was to designate the location of an alphanumeric character by vocally indicating its position in one of the five cells and simultaneously pressing the response button. To initiate each trial, the experimenter triggered the shutter and projected the slide; the duration of the stimulus was determined by the subject's visual scan. That is, when the eye movement record indicated that the subject had reached the end of the stimulus array, the slide was removed by closing the shutter. Experimenter reaction time was accounted for by removing the slide as the subject's eyes reached a predesignated position. Upon termination of the slide, the experimenter asked a four-syllable question such as "Where was the F?" This question required approximately 2 sec. As the last syllable of the question was spoken, the experimenter pulsed the shutter that presented the "empty" slide and started the timer. The subject stopped the timer by pressing the response button as he named the cell.

For all of the viewing conditions except Free scanning, the subject was instructed to look at the pilot light when it came on and not to remove his eyes from it until it terminated. He was also instructed to fixate the pilot light before each trial. The experimenter, who was monitoring the eye movement recording, terminated the light only after it was determined that the subject was fixating it. Immediately after the subject's response, a center fixation light was projected onto the blank wall and the subject was instructed to fixate on this light until it went off. As soon as the eye movement recording was recalibrated, the center light was terminated and the next trial was initiated.

During Condition 1, labeled as the Free condition, the subject was given no instructions other than to inspect the presented stimulus. In this condition, no restrictions were imposed on the direction of the eye scan during inspection nor during recall; the subject was allowed to scan freely. For the remaining six conditions, the subject's scan was directed by the two side lights. During Condition 2, the subject was to inspect the stimulus with a left to right scan; therefore, before the slide was presented, the left light was activated. As soon as the subject had fixated the light, it was terminated and simultaneously the stimulus was presented. On termination of the stimulus, the left fixation light was again activated and remained on until the last syllable of the question was spoken by the experimenter. As the side light went off, the empty slide was projected. In the other Compatible condition, Condition 3, the procedure was identical except that the right fixation light was used to direct the eye scan during inspection and recall from right to left.

For the Incompatible conditions, Condition 4 and Condition 5, the recall scan was opposite to the inspection scan. Therefore, in Condition 4, in which the inspection scan was from left to right, the left light was activated and terminated prior to stimulus onset as described for Condition 2. As soon as the stimulus was turned off, the right fixation light was turned on and remained on until the experimenter had asked the question. It was then terminated simultaneously with the projection of the empty slide. Thus, the scan during recall began at the right. For the second Incompatible condition, Condition 5, the subject was to inspect the stimulus with a scan from right to left and to use a left to right scan during recall. The right fixation light was turned on before stimulus onset, and the left light was turned on prior to recall in the manner described above.

The Fixated conditions, Condition 6 and Condition 7, required the subject to fixate one of the side lights during recall. During Condition 6, in which the subject was to use a left to right inspection scan, the left light was turned on before presentation of the stimulus, as described above. However, during recall the right light was activated and remained on until after the subject had responded. For the other fixated condition, Condition 7, the procedure was identical, except that the right light was turned on before the stimulus was presented and the left light was shown during recall. The subject was instructed to keep fixating the light until it was turned off, and not to move his eyes from that position. Compliance with this instruction was determined on line by monitoring the eye movement recording.

The subject was given one 90 min practice session consisting of 50 trials, a block of five trials per condition for 10 conditions. The experimental session, which lasted 60 min, included one rest period and 49 trials — seven blocks of seven trials each. Each block of trials made up one of the seven conditions listed in Table 2. Two additional conditions used during practice were not used during the experiment proper. Those two conditions were: (a) Free—Fixate right and (b) Free—Fixate left. Of the 75 slides available, 20 were used for practice; the remainder constituted the experimental stimuli.

Results

Performance was measured by calculating error scores and response times for each condition. Eye movement data were analyzed in terms of the direction of movements, the number of fixations, the duration per fixation, the number of reversals, and the type of scanning pattern that was used. The eye movement data were analyzed for both inspection and recall. The data from two subjects had to be discarded because those subjects violated the experimental requirement by moving their eyes away from the fixation point during recall in the Fixation condition. Therefore, all analysis was based on the 12 remaining subjects.

The mean number of fixations was calculated for each subject over all the treatments during the inspection period. These 12 obtained values were then inspected for "natural breaks," gaps that might suggest the presence of more than one distribution. One such gap was observed. It was a break of 1.57 fixations which separated a range of 4.6—7.0 fixations from a range of 8.6—14.0 fixations. These two ranges, each of which contained six subjects, were used to define two groups: subjects who used a fast scan (lower range), and subjects who used a slow scan (upper range).

The differences between L—R and R—L scanning were negligible overall. Therefore, the data were averaged over these two categories of treatment. Although the L—R, R—L categories were retained for statistical analysis, they were never significant. They will not appear, therefore, in the results. Figure 3 presents the fixation phenomena for the experimental treatments. The uppermost figure presents the mean number of fixations for each experimental treatment and the data for fast and slow scanners. The figure shows that for both the fast and the slow scanners the mean number of fixations during inspection was nearly constant across all four treatments. The fast scan subjects fixated an average of 5.9 times during inspection at each of the conditions, while the slow scan subjects fixated on average of 10.5 times while inspecting the stimulus during each viewing condition.

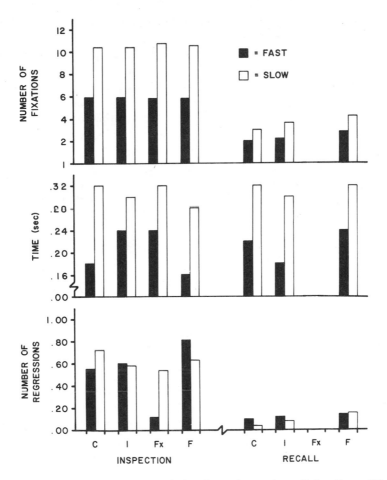

FIG. 3.   Eye movement parameters during inspection and recall for Compatible (C), Incompatible (I), Fixate (Fx), and Free (F) scanning conditions for fast and slow scanning subjects.

In Fig. 3 is also shown the mean number of recall fixations at each condition except for the Fixate group. The figure shows that fewer fixations were made during recall than during inspection for both scanning groups at all of the treatment conditions. The figure also shows that during all of the treatments, the slow scan group made a greater number of fixations than did the fast scan, but the differences between the groups were markedly reduced. For the Free condition, this difference was larger (1.32 fixations) than for the other conditions (0.93, 1.05 fixations). The figure demonstrates that both the fast scan subjects and the slow scan subjects made more recall fixations during the Free condition then during any of the other conditions. In addition, the figure shows that both groups of subjects made the fewest recall fixations during the Compatible condition. The treatment effects are small, but significant, $F(2, 30) = 11.80, p < .01$. Interactions were not significant.

To determine if the fast versus slow scan distinction made for the inspection data was maintained during recall, a Kendall's test for correlation was computed between the mean number of fixations during inspection and the mean number of fixations during recall. The correlation was significant ($p < .05$), suggesting consistency of individuals in their scanning habits during inspection and recall.

The median duration per fixation during inspection for the two subject groups at each treatment condition is also shown in Fig. 3. The figure suggests that fixation duration during both recall and inspection was smallest in the Free and Compatible treatments for fast scanners but was smallest in the Free and Incompatible conditions for the slow scanners. The duration for the slow scan subjects was always longer than that for the fast scan group.

Figure 3 also presents the mean number of eye movements that were regressive during inspection and recall. It can be seen that very few regressions occurred and that they were slightly more frequent under Free scanning in both inspection and recall. The small effect could have been due to the nature of the directed procedures, however, since the subject was instructed to scan systematically. The figure does show that the Incompatible condition was associated with slightly more regressions than the Compatible condition. But, if there are any clear differences, they are that there were fewer regressions during recall than during inspection, and that except during Free scanning in recall, the fast scanners had a slightly, but consistently greater mean number of regressions.

Considering Fig. 3 overall, it is apparent that both during inspection and recall fast scanners made fewer fixations than slow scanners and that their fixations were shorter in duration. In both cases the duration of fixations during recall was the same as during inspection, but the number of fixations was markedly reduced.

Among the experimental treatments, ignoring scanning groups, the Free scan condition was associated with more fixations during recall and those fixations, on the average, were very slightly longer in duration.

Figure 4 presents the total inspection time per condition separately for fast and slow scanners. The figure also presents the mean response time and the percentage of correct responses. The least time was spent in inspection under the Incompatible condition and the most in the Fixate inspection trials. Slow scanners, as would be expected from the previous figure, always required longer inspection times.

An analysis of variance including L–R, R–L comparisons, computed on the reciprocals of response times, but necessarily not including the Free condition, found no significant differences between any of the possible comparisons. A similar analysis which did include the Free condition with the other conditions, averaged over L–R, R–L, found a significant main effect of the treatment conditions, $F(3, 30) = 3.56, p > .05$, and of the Treatment x Subject Groups in-

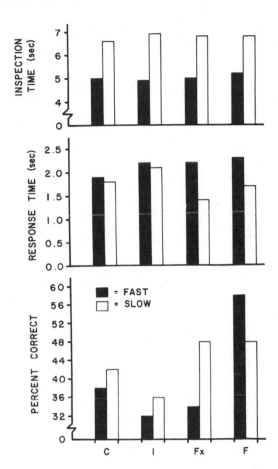

FIG. 4.   Inspection time, response time, and accuracy of response for the four scanning conditions and two subject groups.

teraction $F(3, 30) = 9.38, p > .05$. Thus all effects on response time were due apparently to the Free condition and the scanning groups. Figure 4 shows that fast scanners responded more slowly than slow ones and that the difference between them was markedly increased during the Free condition.

An analysis of variance of a square root transformation of the error data, omitting the Free condition, provided only one significant effect. That was the subject groupings $F(1, 20) = 12.43, p > .01$. Due to the use of a binary (right versus wrong) measure and because the Free condition provided only seven trials per subject, whereas the other conditions provided 14 trials, any statistical comparison between the Free viewing condition and the other three conditions appeared questionable.

Figure 4 suggests that the significant accuracy effects were due to the superiority of the slow scan subjects under the directed viewing conditions. That effect was reversed during the Free condition when the fast scan subjects were more accurate than the slow scan subjects.

TABLE 3

Mean Proportion of Trials in Which There was a Coincidence of
Eye Position and Recall Position, and the Proportion
of Correct Simultaneous Recall and Eye Positioning

Condition	Number of trials	Proportion of coincidence	Proportion of correct recall and eye position	Proportion of correct non-coincidence
Free	7	.66**	.38	.53
Compatible	14	.34**	.27	.43
Incompatible	14	.41**	.22	.37

**$p > .01$.

The data were also analyzed according to the proportion of times the eyes were aimed at the position reported (EAPA) when the subject responded. This was done for the three recall conditions in which eye movements were allowed (Free, Compatible, Incompatible). It was found that the differences in proportions of such fixations between the two subject groups was .04. This difference was considered to be negligible. Therefore, EAPA data were pooled over subject groups. The results are shown in Table 3.

In Table 3 proportions were tested against the probability (.04) that the recalled position and the fixated position would occur simultaneously if they were mutually exclusive, random events. Using the binomial distribution with a one-tailed test, the proportion of times that there was a coincidence between the cell named and where the eyes were looking was significant for each subject for each condition ($p < .01$). It appears, therefore, that as in Experiment 1, there was a tendency for the subject to direct his eyes towards the answered location. The tendency was greatest under the Free condition in which the proportion of coincidence was .66.

The proportion of times in which the subjects looked at the answered cell and were correct is also shown in Table 3. It may be seen that the proportion of those times was small. This result suggests that the coincidence of eye position and recall was independent of the accuracy of recall. Table 3 also shows the proportion of times that the subjects did *not* look at the reported location and were correct. Those proportions are consistently larger than the proportions of correct responses associated with the looked-at location. Thus, the results suggest that the subjects were accurate more often when they did not look at the reported position.

The main results of Experiment 2 can be summarized as follows:

1. There were three kinds of significant effects. One was due to the differences between fast and slow scanning subjects. A second was due to the differences between free scanning and directed ocular activity. The third was an interaction between these two factors.

2. There were no differences in either response time or accuracy of recall among the directed conditions. The slow scan subjects performed about the same over all treatments. They were more accurate than fast scanners and had faster response times in the directed conditions, but in the Free scan condition, fast scanners had about 23% more correct, although they were 150–300 msec slower in their response.

3. There was a significant tendency to aim the eyes at the position being reported. However, that tendency did not result in as great a percentage of correct recall as when the eyes were aimed elsewhere.

GENERAL DISCUSSION

Both experiments showed that there is a strong tendency to move the eyes to the reported position. The timing of these movements suggests that they depend upon some internal process that precedes the occurrence of the response. That phenomenon, then, appears genuine, although it is by no means a certainty that it will happen. The results of Experiment 2 indicate that when it does happen, the recalled position is more likely to be wrong than when the subject does not aim his eyes at the position of his report. Thus, this phenomenon is neither necessary nor useful to recall – in fact, it cannot be trusted as either an indicant of internal scanning or any other retrieval process. Nor is eye aiming a necessary indicant of the individual's response, even under conditions that are assumed to enhance imagery.

Neither experiment provided any suggestion that eye movements were related to the construction of a memory image. Experiment 1 showed that efforts to enhance the use of images result in a delay of the response; from that it may be inferred that a greater use of imagery is possible, but not that it is either necessary or that it aids recall. In fact, the results of Experiment 2 appear clear in showing that eye movements have no effect on recall. Recall is the same whether during recall the eyes are moved in a scan that is compatible or incompatible with the inspection scan. Furthermore, it makes no difference whether the eyes move at all.

Is there any relationship between eye movements and recall? The present results do suggest that there is one, but that it lies entirely in the nature of the scan during inspection. In Experiment 2 there was a close similarity of the inspection scan to the configuration of the display. The number of fixations of those subjects we called slow scanners was approximately the number of characters in the display, whereas those we called fast scanners exhibited approximately the same number of fixations as there were cells in the display. This difference suggests two kinds of encoding strategy. One is a procedure which encodes each character, one at a time in sequential order. Recall from memory might then depend on a sequential retrieval of the encoded items. Position would have to be coded during retrieval, in this case, perhaps, by counting pairs of items. The other strategy is one that encodes first by position and then by pairs of characters, both during inspection. This kind of coding is a form of chunking that requires a two-step decoding process during recall, that is, a retrieval first by position and then within each position. Such decoding should take longer than the character-by-character kind, but for large information loads it should be more effective, since the number of characrers per position will be a smaller memory load than the total of all characters. Miller (1956), of course, has already suggested this for information processing. Our results suggest that eye movements during the inspection of a spatially delineated display or during recall may reflect the nature of the encoding process.

If a two-step encoding is really more effective, why was individual character coding slightly more accurate under the directed conditions of Experiment 2? We can speculate that, at least for memory loads of this size, any condition that forces or restricts eye movements will be interfering, at least in the absence of considerable practice. Under the constraints of what is really a dual task, that is, retrieving from memory and controlling eye movements, the two-step decoding process should be more susceptible to interference. We have already suggested that attempts to use images may also act as a source of interference. In both cases, if interference is what is involved, it will probably be overcome with practice.

The present interpretation may also have implications for the superiority of the Sperling partial report method. The effect may not be the result of a fading memory store, nor of a directed attention, but rather the result of a more efficient encoding strategy that is developed either by instructions or by experience with the partial report procedure.

In summary, it appears that eye movements do have implications for memory, but not as necessary shadows of either a construction or of an image-scanning activity. Instead, their significance to memory lies in their reflection of an encoding process during inspection of the visual scene.

DISCUSSION

KOWLER: I agree that eye movements don't have anything important to do with imagery. I've looked at subjects solving imagery problems like "imagine how many windows there are in your house" and similar kinds of things. The subjects were asked not to make any saccades. I had a device that could detect even the minis and it turns out there weren't any, even when solutions were perfect. What the eye movements may reflect is choice and not necessarily anything important about memory.

V.3

Children and Television: Effects of Stimulus Repetition on Eye Activity[1]

Barbara N. Flagg
Harvard University

One of the most prevalent visual stimuli available to citizens of developed countries is television. Ninety-six percent of American homes have television sets and by the time the average child graduates from high school he has watched television for more hours than he has attended school. Curiously, despite the omnipresence of television in our lives and the many hours spent watching by young children, we have little theory of and even less information about the processing and learning of visual information from television. Most television research is concerned with *after the fact* recall, comprehension, and behavior. We know very little about the moment-to-moment processing of information by the viewer *while* he is watching. We know very little about what controls the viewer's allocation of attention within the television presentation.

The recording of the television viewer's eye movements allows us to examine the way in which he distributes his visual attention over the scene. Eye movement data provide an objective continuous record of the interaction between elements of the dynamic medium and the viewer's perception and cognition. The potential utility of eye movement recording in video communications research has been recognized (Fleming, 1969) but limitations of equipment, time, and money have restricted the use of this methodology.

[1]The work reported here was supported by Dr. Gerald S. Lesser with grants from the Children's Television Workshop and the Spencer Foundation. My grateful thanks go to Leonard Scinto and Ellice Peyton for their aid in data collection and data analysis respectively. Credit should also be given to Children's Television Workshop writers Samuel Gibbon, and David Connell, and to the animator, Susan Rubin, for development of our calibration stimulus.

EYE MOVEMENTS AND DYNAMIC DISPLAYS

The first suggestion for using eye movement recording with dynamic visual displays came from Wendt (1952). He experimented with a primitive eye-camera to record adults' responses to motion pictures. In the 1960s Wendt's idea was applied by Wolf to instructional television displays with junior high and high school students (Guba & Wolf, 1964; Wolf, 1971; Wolf & Knemeyer, 1970; Wolf, Tira, & Knemeyer, 1969). Using a helmet-type Mackworth camera, Wolf attempted to define the types of eye movements of the viewers, the types of visual elements that attracted their attention, and the differences in attention patterns between high IQ and low IQ subjects.

A second wave of eye movement studies of television stimuli was directed by O'Bryan (Mock, 1974; O'Bryan & Silverman, 1972; O'Bryan, 1974, 1975) and sponsored by the Children's Television Workshop, producers of *Sesame Street* and *The Electric Company*. In a number of studies, O'Bryan's group used a Mackworth Stand Camera to examine the eye movements of children, nine to eleven years of age, while they viewed the instructional reading program *The Electric Company*. The children were divided into three groups: good readers, poor readers, and nonreaders. Marked differences in visual scanning were found. In general, the good readers systematically read the printed material undistracted by irrelevant action, and they quickly oriented to new visual material. The poor readers were distracted from the print and showed less skilled reading patterns. The nonreaders displayed random looking patterns in which the printed message was largely ignored. Results of O'Bryan's eye movement studies have led directly to changes in *The Electric Company* program design.

EYE MOVEMENT RECORDING AND TELEVISION

Encouraged by the results of Wolf and O'Bryan, the Children's Television Workshop has supported the development of an eye movement laboratory at Harvard which overcomes the previous limitations of helmets, bite-boards, and manual data analysis. Our facility can examine eye movements of subjects from four years of age to adults, and stimuli ranging from dynamic television presentations to static print and nonprint materials.

The facility is built around a Gulf & Western Eye View Monitor and TV Pupillometer System (Model 1994) which employs a pupil-center/corneal-reflection measurement technique (see Sheena, 1976, for a complete description of this technique). The subject sits in a comfortable adjustable chair, 3 ft away from a 17-inch color television. An invisibly frame-coded audiovisual stimulus is presented via video cassette. The recording camera is approximately 1.5 ft away, at the subject's left side out of his direct field of view. Subjects are aware of the camera but rarely look at it.

Eye position and pupil diameter may be measured as long as the pupil image is within the field of view of the television camera. With the camera position fixed, the subject's eye may move within a 5 cm cube; if the camera position is continually adjusted manually to track the subject's pupil, the cube increases to about 12 cm on a side. Subjects are asked to sit as still as possible during the stimulus presentation. They are aided in this by a padded headrest which fits snugly around the temples and in back of the head. This system restricts gross head movements but allows for verbalizations and small head movements.

Calibration

Calibration was one of our first difficult problems with young children. We wanted to be able to calibrate manually before showing the stimulus material, and we also wanted the ability to calibrate more accurately by computer off-line. Since four-year-olds are not known for their ability to follow instructions, a calibration stimulus was needed that would successfully capture and hold their visual attention at specific points on the screen. To this purpose, we developed a 4 min color Calibration Tape which presents animated "dots" one at a time at five positions on the screen: center, left, right, top, and bottom. The design and activity of the "dots" along with appropriate sound effects attract and hold the child's eyes on the position long enough for the experimenter to calibrate manually. For example, one segment of the Calibration Tape shows a chocolate chip cookie "dot" which gradually disappears by chunks while we listen to Cookie Monster exclaim "Cookie!" and make cookie-gobbling noises. The first half of the tape is used for manual calibration and the second half for off-line computer calibration data.

Data Analysis

The eye movement recording system samples 30 times per sec and produces two data outputs for each subject: (1) a videotape of the stimulus material on which is superimposed a set of cross-hairs whose intersection marks the eyes' fixation point; and (2) a digital tape recording x–y fixation coordinates, pupil diameter, video frame-code information, and experimental and subject codes.

A description of the procedures by which the raw digital data are edited and classified into fixations and saccades is beyond the scope of this particular paper. The general analysis approach is similar to that presented in Lambert, Monty, and Hall (1974), while specific analysis decisions are based on parameters of eye activity as reported in the literature and on examination of data videotapes as well as computer plots of the raw and reduced data. The resulting statistics of fixation duration, interfixation distance, locus of fixation, etc., are used to test various research hypotheses.

CHILDREN AND TELEVISION

The research reported here examines how children of different ages view a television presentation from moment-to-moment and explores what effects the repetition of television segments has on the child's viewing behavior.

Developmental Research

A number of developmental research studies indicate that qualitative and quantitative changes occur over age in the visual scanning of *static* stimuli (Mackworth & Bruner, 1971; Olson, 1970; Whiteside, 1974; Zinchenko, Chzhi-Tsin, & Tarakanov, 1963). In general, these studies conclude that with age children develop the use of systematic organized scanning patterns, view increasingly more area of the stimulus in detail, and focus more on what adults consider the informative areas of the static display. Typically, in scanning the static stimulus the younger subject exhibited fewer eye movements with longer fixations and less focusing on areas providing information appropriate to the task.

These studies do not posit age as a causative factor but imply that age-related variables are involved in visual scanning strategies. One of these variables appears to be simply experience with visual stimuli; familiarity with the stimulus or its class reduces uncertainty so that the material is examined differently. Zinchenko et al. (1963) discovered that after a small amount of increased exposure to the static stimulus, the eye movement patterns of the younger children came to resemble those of the older children.

That familiarity is a factor even in adult scanning is supported by the studies of Antes (1974), Furst (1971), Krugman (1968), and Noton and Stark (1971a,b,c). These studies demonstrate that with long or repeated presentations of static visual stimuli, the adult viewer uses successively fewer fixations on fewer informative areas, and the viewing patterns become more efficient or stereotypic with increasing familiarization.

Stimulus Repetition

The repetition of stimuli is included in the present developmental scanning research in response to the suggestion in the literature that initial age differences in stimulus inspection may simply be a function of familiarity with the stimulus. Repetition effects are particularly appropriate to study with a television stimulus because repetition is a distinctive feature of television. Exact repetition of a whole television show is common, but more often we see repetition of certain formats that may vary in content yet follow characteristic sequences upon each presentation. In commercial television the formats of game shows, situation comedies, and advertisements are repeated. In educational television, the content may change — a different number or letter or reading rule may be presented —

whereas the presentation format remains constant. Commercial television is often criticized for its repetitiveness; conversely, repetition in educational television is endorsed by learning theorists who recommend repetition as an effective teaching method and sometimes as a mechanism for recapturing the child's drifting attention. In support of such shows as *Sesame Street*, Lesser (1974) has advanced the hypothesis that the child's response to each repetition of a segment differs as he explores all aspects of the segment. The initial presentation may offer too many elements or too much information for the child to assimilate at one time. Repeated exposures allow the child to investigate and understand the material.

RESEARCH DESIGN

The eye activity of different age groups was recorded in response to initially unfamiliar television stimuli and to subsequent repeated expsoures of those stimuli.

Subjects

Seventeen four-year-olds (8 male, 9 female) and 22 six-year-olds (11 male, 11 female) participated in the study. The children were white and middle-class drawn from the Cambridge, Massachusetts area.

Procedures

The children were told that a picture was being taken of them while they watched *Sesame Street*, but no specific instructions were given regarding their viewing behavior. Each child viewed two approximately 10-min color videotapes, each comprised of calibration and *Sesame Street* material. A short break was taken between viewings.

Stimulus Materials

The two stimulus videotapes included three short *Sesame Street* segments that had never been aired before or had not been aired for many seasons; these three segments on their initial presentation were new and unfamiliar to all subjects. Each of the experimental segments was repeated in exact form a number of times over the two tapes. Segment A was repeated five times. Segment B was repeated four times and Segment C two times. The *Sesame Street* material interspersed among the repetitions of the three experimental segments was taken from the daily fare of the show and was familiar to most of the children.

Segment A (34 sec) presents the concept of the number three. Scenes of three moving objects (e.g., butterflies) transform into three new objects (e.g., bows)

TABLE 1

Tape 1	Time (Min:Sec)	Tape 2	Time (Min:Sec)
Calibration	4:12	Calibration	4:12
Segment A	:34	Filler Segment	1:53
Segment B	1:05	Segment B	1:05
Filler Segment	1:17	Segment C	:28
Segment A	:34	Segment A	:34
Filler Segment	:30	Filler Segment	2:21
Segment C	:28	Filler Segment	:30
Segment B	1:05	Segment B	1:05
Segment A	:34	Filler Segment	:37
		Segment A	:34
Total	10:19	Total	13:19

to the accompaniment of a spoken poem: "1, 2, 3. 1, 2, 3. Three yellow butter-flies, all in a row. Three birthday presents, each tied with a bow," etc.

Segment B (65 sec) deals with the concept of the word WALK. New York street scenes are edited into a fast paced display of assorted people, children, and dogs walking to the music of the Marine Hymn. Children's voices interrupt the music with the shout of "Walk" each time close-up shots of a crosswalk WALK sign appear briefly on the screen.

Segment C (28 sec) is a short, subdued film of waterfowl. Flamingos strut, swans preen, ducks paddle and feed, all in concert with airy flute music.

Table 1 shows the distribution of the three stimulus segments within the two videotapes.

The stimulus segments were all second-generation copies. Master 2-inch broad-cast tape and film were copied onto videocassettes. The desired segments were then copied and edited onto the experimental cassette in the order shown in Table 1.

Measures

The values of the following eye activity measures were calculated for each subject for each segment repetition:

   Mean Fixation Duration
   Variance of Fixation Duration
   Mean Interfixation Distance
   Variance of Interfixation Distance
   Percent of the Television Screen Area Covered by Fixations

The last measure was derived by dividing the TV screen area into a grid of 400 squares (20 x 20) and determining the percentage of grid squares receiving one or more fixations. Because of the length of the stimulus segments, there are ceiling limits on the percent values. Theoretically, but not practically, the percent ceiling for Segment A is approximately 58%, for Segment B, 100%, and for Segment C, 48%.

Results

The research design was a three-factor experiment with repeated measures on the last factor (Sex x Age x Repetition). Analyses of variance with repeated measures were computed for the five dependent variables for each segment (A, B, and C). No significant main effects or interaction effects were found with respect to sex or age. The main effect for the Repetition factor, however, was statistically significant on three out of the five measures for Segment A ($.017 < p < 0.38$) and on four measures for Segment B ($.003 < p < .038$), but on none of the measures for Segment C. This indicates that there were significant differences among the five means for Segment A and among the four means for Segment B.

Comparisons of successive pairs of means for Segments A and B were performed with t-tests (N = 39;) (Kirk, 1968, p. 292). Figure 1 presents the group

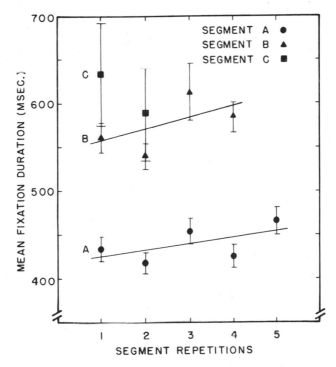

FIG. 1.   Mean fixation duration as a function of repeated presentations of Segments A, B, and C.

mean fixation durations for Segments A, B, and C. The means for Repetition 1 and Repetition 2 do not differ significantly for Segments A, B, and C. Repetition 2 does differ significantly from Repetition 3 for Segment A ($p < .05$) and for Segment B ($p < .01$). Both segments show no differences between Repetitions 3 and 4. Finally, for Segment A, Repetition 4 is significantly different from Repetition 5 ($p < .025$). Linear regression lines were determined by the method of least squares and are shown in Fig. 1. Both segments display an increasing trend in mean fixation duration over repetitions.

In Fig. 2, the mean variances of fixation duration for Repetition 1 do not differ from Repetition 2 for Segments A, B, and C. Repetition 2 differs significantly from Repetition 3 for Segment A ($p < .025$) and for Segment B ($p < .01$). Repetitions 3 and 4 are not significantly different for both segments, and Repetitions 4 and 5 in Segment A also do not differ. Regression lines in Fig. 2 indicate that mean variance of fixation duration tends to increase over repetitions.

For Segments A and C in Fig. 3, the means of interfixation distance show no significant change from Repetition 1 to Repetition 2, but the means for Segment

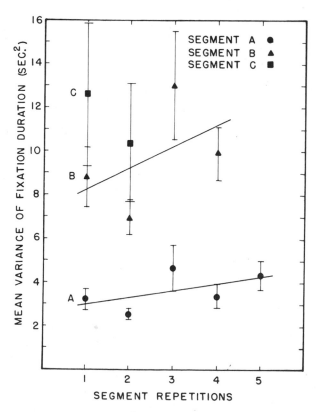

FIG. 2.   Mean variance of fixation duration as a function of repeated presentations of Segments A, B, and C.

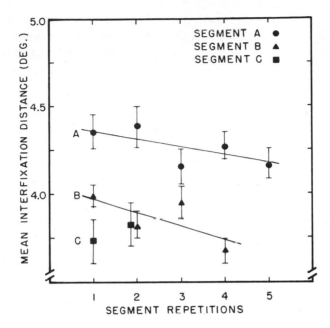

FIG. 3.   Mean interfixation distance as a function of repeated presentations of Segments A, B, and C.

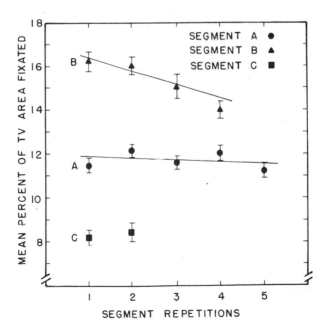

FIG. 4.   Mean percentage of TV area fixated as a function of repeated presentations of Segments A, B, and C.

B do differ significantly ($p < .05$). Repetitions 2 and 3 are significantly different for Segment A ($p < .025$) but not for Segment B, and Repetitions 3 and 4 are significantly different for Segment B ($p < .005$) but not for Segment A. Segment A also shows no change between Repetitions 4 and 5. In Fig. 1 and 2, Segments A, B, and C show the same patterns of change over repetitions. In Fig. 3, Segment B deviates somewhat from the pattern of A and C, yet the overall linear regression lines show a decreasing trend in mean interfixation distance over repetitions for *both* Segments A and B.

In Fig. 4, the mean percentages for Segments A and C do not differ significantly from each other over repetitions. Moreover, the adjacent means in Segment B are not significantly different. The regression lines show a decrease over repetitions in the mean percentage of TV area fixated, although the slope is very small in Segment A.

DISCUSSION OF RESULTS

Age Differences

The static stimulus research suggests that four- and six-year-olds differ significantly in the way they scan a display initially, but after increased exposure to the stimulus the differences disappear. The lack of significant age differences in this study suggests that the television stimulus provides something for the four-year-old that is also provided by increased exposure to the static stimulus. A longer static presentation allows the younger child to determine the informative areas of the display, to assimilate the message presented, and to organize his visual scanning into a more systematic pattern. The six-year-old, it appears, immediately performs these operations and has no need for extra time.

These age differences may not emerge when the stimulus is dynamic because the television stimulus organizes the information *for* the viewer. The message is packaged visually so that it is easily available to the viewer. The four-year-old's visual attention is controlled to a greater extent by the dynamics of the television presentation than by the static display, so that the four-year-old's eye activity is not significantly different from the six-year-old's. This is not to say that the four-year-old is understanding the material in the same way, but only that the younger child looks at the stimulus in a similar fashion.

One could also argue the opposite of the above, that the television stimulus *removes* something for the six-year-old that is provided by the static stimulus. Perhaps the unfamiliar television stimulus pulls the older child down to the younger child's level. This explanation, however, does not hold up when we note that no age differences appear even after *five* repetitions of a stimulus.

The finding of no age differences cannot necessarily be generalized beyond the type of dynamic stimulus used in this study. It is possible that other dynamic stimuli presenting a more complex content or employing a less organized display might yield age group differences in perceptual processing.

Repetition

The discussion of the repetition trends is based on initial data analyses of the group means and any conclusions are considered tentative until substantiated by other analyses currently in progress on individual data.

Examination of the linear regression lines in Fig. 1—4 shows that over four and five repetitions of the same segment, mean fixation duration increases, mean variance of fixation of fixation duration increases, mean interfixation distance decreases, and mean percentage of TV area fixated decreases. These trends are very similar to what has been found in the research on long or repeated presentations of static stimuli.

Furst (1971) presented five trials of six pictures to adults and found over trials an increase in mean fixation duration, a decrease in mean interfixation distance, and a decrease in the mean number of different picture sectors fixated. These results match the patterns we have noted in Fig. 1—4. In addition, Antes (1974) presented ten pictures to adults, each for 20 sec and found that as viewing time increased, mean duration of fixation increased, and mean interfixation distance decreased. He showed that, initially, long saccades were used to fixate high information areas for short durations and subsequently, shorter saccades led to lower information areas for longer durations.

It is possible that scanning patterns similar to those found by Antes (1974) are occurring in our data. During the initial repetitions, the child homes-in on what he conceives of or is lead by the stimulus format to regard as the most informative areas of the segments — those areas which carry the main theme. In the later repetitions, the viewer may be searching for other attention areas, locating less central informative details, or picking up on irrelevant items.

A distinctive change in eye activity patterns on early repetitions from patterns on later repetitions is also supported by the significant differences found between Repetitions 2 and 3 for five out of eight t-tests on Segments A and B. Repetitions 1 and 2 seldom differed significantly and Repetitions 3, and 4, and 5 also showed few differences across the dependent measures. Perhaps similar scanning patterns are being used on Repetitions 1 and 2 and a different sort of scanning pattern on Repetitions 3, and 4, and 5. The children may need two repetitions to assimilate the informative message of the segments, whereas the last two or three repetitions elicit more exploration on secondary information areas or irrelevant details.

SUMMARY

In summary, no significant differences were found between the eye activity patterns of four-year-olds and six-year-olds during the viewing of initially unfamiliar segments of *Sesame Street* and subsequent repeated presentations of the segments. We hypothesized that the *Sesame Street* television display organizes the visual information for the viewer, so that the younger child's attention patterns do not differ from the six-year-old's.

We have also noted in the group data a change in eye activity from the initial repetitions to the later repetitions. The trend over repetitions shows an increase in mean fixation duration and mean variance of fixation duration, and a decrease in mean interfixation distance and mean percentage of television area fixated. We speculated that during the early repetitions the child attends to the "informative" areas of the segments, and during the later repetitions the child scans less relevant details. The changing configuration of the scanning pattern over repetitions needs to be substantiated by an analysis of the fine structure of the individual child's eye activity in relation to the visual stimulus. In addition, the very basic question as to how much the scanning patterns are related to the changing visual structure of the segment, and how much to the content of the segment, remains open for future analysis.

DISCUSSION

STERN: Some time ago I listened to a delightful presentation by Bernard Friedlander on the television watching of 4- and 6 year-old children, and phenomenologically the children appeared to be fascinated by *Sesame Street*. But when Friedlander asked the children what they saw, what they said they saw and what was presented bore little relationship to each other. I wonder whether you're asking the children, in addition to looking at the scan patterns, what it is that they're seeing.

FLAGG: Not yet. That's an obvious next step. This initial study was exploratory and descriptive; we simply recorded the eye activity and tried to deal with what patterns were there. Comprehension is certainly important when one is dealing with educational television materials, and in future studies we plan to investigate the relationship of the viewer's eye movement patterns and his or her comprehension.

RUSSO: I'd like to follow up John Stern's comments and make a suggestion. It's clearly very difficult to interpret the eye fixations for several reasons. Partly, there are long periods to be interpreted. Partly, the task itself isn't very well specified; that is, you haven't instructed the children to do anything, and I think that you don't want to do that by the very nature of your research enterprise. You want the children to do what they would normally do when they watch *Sesame Street*, and you don't know what that is. So, I have a suggestion as to what you might do to help validate your interpretations or discover new ones. I've used a technique that I call "prompt to protocol" in which I record eye fixations and then, immediately after the subject views the task display, I present the same stimulus with the eye fixation superimposed on the stimulus. This prompts a retrospective verbal protocol. You ask the subject to tell you what he or she was thinking during each eye fixation.

FLAGG: Did you do this with adults?

RUSSO: Yes. I have only done it with adults and I do not know how well it will work with younger children, but perhaps a little bit of training might help. But at least it's one suggestion as to what you might do to validate your interpretation and to generate new ones in a task that is very unspecified.

FLAGG: I'll speak to the task question first. The reason the task was unspecified should be obvious. I deal with the mass media — there are millions of children across the country who watch *Sesame Street* twice a day, 365 days a year, and I cannot possibly determine under what task conditions they watch their home television sets. The task was left unstructured in hopes of simulating more closely a home-viewing situation. Certainly the next step in controlled empirical research is to define the task. We could determine a number of tasks that a child brings to home television, set him up for those, and then see what he does.

As for the suggestion of showing the children their eye fixations to elicit verbal protocols, the four-year-olds don't understand what you're talking about when you show them eye fixations superimposed on stimulus tapes. If they are verbal kids, they can give a limited description of what a person thinks about when looking at the picture, but they are too young to reflect on their own thought processes. In the past, to examine comprehension, we have sometimes made cardboard mock-ups of certain scenes from *Sesame Street* — for example, scenes from problem solving segments. And we have asked the children to manipulate these static copies either before and/or after viewing the program. What they do with the models helps us to determine their understanding of the curriculum material.

COOPER: I don't agree with Jay Russo as far as the structuring of the task. I think structuring tasks lead to certain kinds of information, and not structuring the task, looking at what the subject spontaneously does of his own natural accord, leads to different kinds of valuable information. So I personally am in favor of what you're doing.

V.4

Film Cutting and
Visual Momentum[1]

Julian Hochberg
Virginia Brooks
Columbia University

INTRODUCTION

We perceive the world by means of successive sensory samples. In vision, this means by sequences of views. Most view sequences are obtained by the viewer's own perceptuomotor acts. Some view sequences are given to the viewer by a filmmaker, and these often consist of sequences of nonoverlapping views.

There are two general kinds of answers to the question of how we combine our successive glances into a coherent perceptual world: These are (1) the *compensatory,* or subtractive, explanations, whether based on extraretinal signals (cf. Matin, 1976; Sedgwick & Festinger, 1976; Skavenski, 1976) or on the transformations of the visual image (Gibson, 1954, 1957, 1966; Johansson, 1974); and (2) the inferential, expectancy-testing, or schema-testing explanations (Hochberg, 1968; Neisser, 1967; Piaget, 1954).

The compensatory explanations may or may not be fully adequate to explain how we combine view sequences that we obtain by our own perceptuomotor acts, but they simply cannot account for our perception of motion pictures in which scenes are built up by a succession of *nonoverlapping* views.

The inferential or schema-testing theories seem capable in principle of explaining both how we combine our own glances and how we perceive motion picture sequences, but these are still remarkably vague, and we have only rudimentary psychological research on the question of how subjects integrate succes-

[1]The work reported here was supported by a grant from the National Institute of Education, NIE G 74–0099. Paul Roule assisted greatly in the preparation, execution, and analyses of the experiments. Programming and final design and construction of the controlling circuitry were done by Ted Hills.

sive views (Girgus, 1973, 1976; Girgus & Hochberg, 1972; Farley, 1976; Hochberg, 1968; Murphy, 1973). The psychologist is not the first to be concerned with this question, however; the filmmaker has been here before him.

Most cinematic sequences are made up of nonoverlapping views, and that makes the filmmaker's purposes in using such sequences, and his techniques in dealing with them, of interest to us. Conversely, we may be in the position of providing the filmmaker with quantitative information that may be of considerable use to him.

In nonoverlapping sequences of views such as *montages,* or rhythmic series of discontinuous shots, the filmmaker relies on the viewer's knowledge of the world, or on "establishing shots" (e.g., long shots) to provide the "glue" that joins the successive views. This motion picture procedure must draw on the abilities that we normally use in guiding and interpreting our normal purposeful perceptual inquiries. Film editors have, in fact, said that what makes a cut good and rapid to comprehend, is the successful effort of the filmmaker to provide the viewer with the visual answer to a question that he would normally have been about to obtain for himself at that time, were he able to change the scene by his own perceptuomotor acts (as he normally can, of course, but as he cannot do in the movies).

Once the viewer's visual question is answered, there is no further reason for him to explore the scene, and the scene goes "cinematically dead." To the filmmaker, this is a challenge that he can meet by changing to a new camera position, even when there is no need to do so in order to tell the story. To the psychologist, this phenomenon (if he can measure it) is a potential tool for studying how we go about posing and answering visual questions. Such cutting from one view to another merely for the purpose of keeping the screen "alive" is most blatantly evident in television, when a news commentator faces one camera, then another, in order to relieve the viewer's visual boredom or habituation.

This same factor is a central ingredient in the widespread use of *montage* sequences. These sequences are of interest to us here because this motivating factor, which we will call *visual momentum,* should reflect the course of the viewer's perceptual inquiry — the momentary state of his development and testing of schematic maps. This simple form of cutting provides a baseline to study visual momentum; further complexities and varieties will be discussed elsewhere.

When a viewer is first shown a static picture, he looks at the most informative regions (Antes, 1974; Brooks, 1961; Hochberg & Brooks, 1962, 1963; Loftus, 1976; Mackworth & Morandi, 1967; Pollack & Spence, 1968). The glance rate is initially high, and declines rapidly (Curve w, in Fig. 1B, from data of Antes, 1974). In our terms, the viewer takes a few glances to establish the main features or landmarks of the scene, and then his impetus to schema-formation wanes: he knows what he will see, in a general way, wherever he looks, if the scene is a normally redundant one (Biederman, 1972; Loftus, 1976; Reed & Johnsen, 1975). When the eye is exploring a scene at its most rapid rate — say, at 4 to 5 glances per sec — there is clearly no time between glances in which the viewer can sum up what he has seen up to that point, and to decide how many more glances are needed. Something like a rate regulator sounds plausible, perhaps even a mechanism similar to the one recently proposed for reading by Bouma and deVoogd (1974), and Kolers (1976).

If *visual momentum* is the impetus to obtain sensory information, and to formulate and test a schema, it should be reflected by the frequency with which glances are made, and by the viewer's tendency to keep looking within one display *when he is free of external demands to do so*. Visual momentum should, presumably, decline with the length of time that the viewer has been looking at the display, and should increase with the number of different places at which he can look to receive nonredundant information (i.e., to apprehend or comprehend the scene to some level of awareness, which should be task-dependent). These functions ascribed to visual momentum are very similar to those Spottiswoode (1933/1962) attributed to an esthetic arousal variable which he called *affective cutting tone*. Based on the introspective account of his own cinematic experience, he proposed that simple and striking scenes would have their maximum effect early, and then fall off as shown in curve *S* of Fig. 1A, whereas more complex and unexpected scenes would take longer to reach their maximum effect as in curve *C* of Fig. 1A. Sequences of simple scenes would sustain high affective cutting tone when presented at a fast cutting rate, and would be reduced at slower rates, whereas the reverse would be true with the more complex scenes.

We do not know whether these semiquantitative but wholly subjective esthetic functions can be made more objective, but they seem to be sufficiently close to what we have called *visual momentum* that we will return to the question of esthetic judgment (p. 304). We will present and discuss first a set of eye movement experiments designed to provide data on which to base a model of visual momentum; and second, experiments on the ways subjects distribute their glances when they are free to look at one or another (or neither) of two displays.

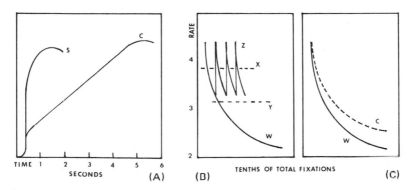

FIG. 1.   (A) Curves *S* and *C* depict Spottiswoode's (1933/1962) introspective account of glance rate or esthetic arousal for simple and complex scenes respectively. (B) and (C) Models of glance rates of subjects looking at static pictures. Curve *W* is from data obtained by Antes (1974).

THE COURSE OF LOOKING AT SEQUENCES OF
SUCCESSIVE VIEWS

If we assume that curve W in Fig. 1B is a rough guide to the course of looking at a single scene, then by repeatedly changing the scene before the glance rate has had a chance to fall very much, we could repeatedly return the glance rate to its peak, and increase the mean rate of looking as represented by line X in Fig. 1B. Again, if *attentional complexity* – the number of places to look at – is increased the curve should not fall sharply, as represented in curve C in Fig. 1C.

Two kinds of experiments using similar apparatus and measurement procedures were performed to test whether these functions in Fig. 1 do indeed obtain. Experiment 1 used sequences of arbitrarily-generated abstract pictures as its stimulus material; Experiment 2 used montages constructed of meaningful, representational photographs assembled in arbitrary orders.

Experiment 1: The Course of Looking at Sequences
of Abstract Views

In this experiment, subjects' eye movements were recorded while they watched sequences of abstract pictures on a rear projection screen. The frequency with which eye movements occurred was a function of the attentional complexity of the views in the sequence, and of the rate at which views were presented. In the first experiment (Hochberg and Brooks, 1974), three degrees of complexity and two cutting rates were used. This was intended as a replication and extension of Brooks and Hochberg (1976), in which sequences of two degrees of view complexity were used at three cutting rates. Results were substantially the same in both experiments, and in accord with the model in Fig. 1B & 1C. The details of the first experiment are as follows.

Stimuli

To pursue research with sequential views, we need a procedure for generating stimulus sequences by some arbitrary process that provides different numbers of places to which the subject's gaze will be drawn. To do this, we drew on an inelegant formula that had been found in earlier research (Hochberg & Brooks, 1962) to account, at least roughly, for where subjects assigned their judgments of "prominence"; it had already been shown (Brooks, 1961; Hochberg & Brooks, 1962) that such prominence judgments were, in turn, correlated with eye movement recordings of where subjects looked (Buswell, 1935). Estimates of prominence may be achieved if a picture is divided into cells, and all of the lines and contours are of approximately equal thickness and contrast; then a simple count of the number of points of inflection and intersection which fall within any cell is an approximate predictor of the mean prominence ratings given that cell. A more cumbersome formula, which provided a better empirical fit to prominence distributions, included a reference point call a *sink*, which is a point having the greatest number of real or *extended* lines passing through it. We drew upon the notion of a sink at the center of the pattern in constructing the present designs.

The unit pattern is shown in Fig. 2. From this, a set of 12 abstract patterns was constructed. Each pattern used four units, located according to a random decision process. The outer dimensions of each unit were also randomly determined, as was the choice among a set of 12 small details, one of which was placed in the center of each unit. When a decision was needed as to which unit would continue and which would end at any intersection that too was randomly determined.

The set of 12 patterns generated in this way was intended to contain four attention centers per view. Again, using a random decision procedure to retain two and one centers per view, two more sets of patterns were generated from the first set. Examples of the 36 patterns are shown in Fig. 3. These three sets of views were each made into motion picture sequences on high contrast 16 mm film, with a 50% random dot matrix inserted before and after each sequence. The sequences were ordered as follows: $1CL_1$, $4CL_1$, $4CS_2$, $2CS_2$, $4CS_1$, $1CS_1$, $2CL_2$, $4CL_2$, $1CL_2$. The notation $1CL_1$ refers to a set of six of the single-center patterns presented for long durations (4 sec/view); $1CL_2$ refers to the remaining set of six of the single-center patterns presented at 4 sec/view, $2CS_1$ refers to a set of the two-center patterns presented at 1 sec/view (i.e., short presentation), and so on.

Subjects and Instructions

Subjects were 10 paid volunteers, graduates and undergraduates, who were naive as to the purpose of the experiments. They were told that we were concerned with their pupilary diameters and other responses in relation to their

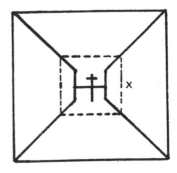

FIG. 2. Typical unit pattern used to construct stimuli for Experiment 1. (The dotted rectangle [X] did not appear in the actual stimuli).

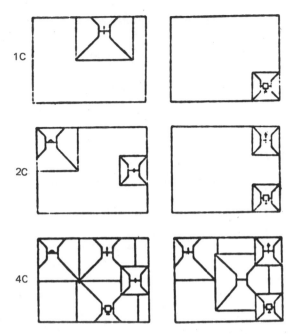

FIG. 3.   Representative stimuli for one, two, and four attention centers per view used in Experiment 1.

esthetic preferences, on which they were to report after the entire series had been viewed. (The pupil diameter data were, in fact, both noisy and uninformative, and the esthetic reports obtained under these conditions were too sketchy to use but, of course, they were not our primary interest.)

Apparatus and Procedure

Stimuli were presented to each subject on a rear-projection screen in a semi-darkened room. Each subject sat with his head in a headrest while his eye movements were recorded by a system built around a Gulf & Western Eye View Monitor (formerly known as the Whittaker, as described by Young & Sheena, 1975) and a computer-coupled 16 mm motion picture camera. Stimulus sequences were projected by a modified L & W 16mm Optical Data Analyzer motion picture projector so arranged that the dimensions of each view were 15.9° horizontal by 12.0° vertical. Subjects viewed the screen from a distance of 65 cm; the direction of the left eye's gaze was monitored by a Gulf & Western Eye-Tracker. A 16mm Bolex camera, driven by a synchronous motor at four frames per sec, recorded the monitor's screen. In addition, in some of the experiments the online computer calculated eye position data 60 times per sec and identified an eye

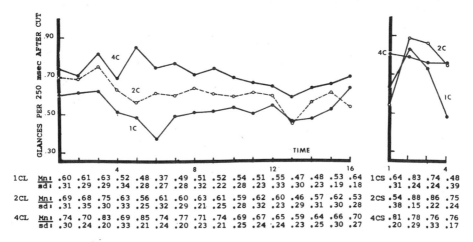

movement as a change taking less than 100 msec (to prevent inclusion of drifts and pursuit movements), and of more than 15° magnitude.

Results and Discussion

The course of looking at each view in each sequence was obtained as follows: The subject's gaze was sampled with a 150 msec photograph 4 times/sec. Starting with the first frame in which a new view was sampled, a change in fixation greater than 1.5° was recorded as an eye movement in the 1/4 second sample in which it first appeared. The 4 sec/view, 2 sec/view, and 1 sec/view sequences were therefore recorded as 16, 8, and 4 samples, respectively. These data are shown in Fig. 4. Note that these graphs are time-locked to the start of each view. Means of the frequencies of eye movements in all samples of each sequence, averaged across views and then across subjects, with the standard deviation of the subjects' means, are given for each cutting rate, and each complexity, in Table 1A. This was done for entire sequences and, for the 4 sec/view sequences, was also done for the first four views and for the remaining views (5−16) separately.

Differences between each subject's mean glance rate for long and short sequences were significant (t = 4.3, df = 9, p < .01), with no interaction effect of complexity (F < 1.0); while effects of complexity on glance rate were significant (F = 8.7, df = 2, 18, p < .01), pooling cutting rates.

The number of fixations falling within 2° x 4° of the center of each unit (cf. the area marked off by the dotted line in Fig. 2) was obtained, and the propor-

		4				8				12				16			1			4
1CL	Mn:	.60	.61	.63	.52	.48	.37	.49	.51	.52	.54	.51	.55	.47	.48	.53	.64	1CS	.64	.83	.74	.48
	sd:	.31	.29	.29	.34	.28	.27	.28	.32	.22	.28	.23	.33	.30	.23	.19	.18		.31	.24	.24	.39
2CL	Mn:	.69	.68	.75	.63	.56	.61	.60	.63	.61	.59	.62	.60	.46	.57	.62	.53	2CS	.54	.88	.86	.75
	sd:	.31	.35	.30	.33	.25	.32	.29	.21	.25	.28	.32	.23	.29	.31	.30	.28		.38	.15	.22	.24
4CL	Mn:	.74	.70	.83	.69	.85	.74	.77	.71	.74	.69	.67	.65	.59	.64	.66	.70	4CS	.81	.78	.76	.76
	sd:	.30	.24	.20	.33	.21	.24	.20	.23	.21	.25	.24	.24	.23	.25	.30	.27		.20	.29	.33	.17

FIG. 4. The means and standard deviation for each time sampled for each view, averaged across subjects for Experiment 1.

TABLE 1
Sequences of Geometrical Patterns

Attentional Complexity:		1 Center			2 Centers			4 Centers		
Samples:		1–16	1–4	5–16	1–16	1–4	5–16	1–16	1–4	5–16
Glance rate, 4 sec/view:	*Mn:*	.53	.59	.51	.60	.69	.59	.66	.73	.70
	sd:	.09	.11	.10	.12	.18	.10	.10	.10	.05
Glance rate, 1 sec/view:	*Mn:*	.	.64			.76			.77	
	sd:		.14			.11			.13	
Accuracy, 4 sec/view:	*Mn:*	.62			.59			.67		
	sd:	.13			.14			.15		

tion of fixations falling within those central areas is also listed under *Accuracy* in Table 1 and did not vary with number of centers per view (F < 1.0). In order to determine how the actual fixations correspond to subjects' prominence judgments, copies of the four-center views were given to two additional groups of subjects, for a total of 27, who marked and ranked what they judged as the most prominent regions in each view. In terms of total area of each view that was included in the designated centers, the proportions were .08, .16, and .32 for the one-, two-, and four-center view sequences, respectively. The proportions of glances that fell in these regions were greater than expected by chance: t = 11.4, 9.7, and 8.5, respectively, all with df = 9. In obtaining the prominence judgments, 15 subjects scored each of the 12 four-center views used, and 12 scored the mirror image of those views. Subjects were asked to indicate at least six and no more than 10 points in each view that were prominent, that is, that attracted and held their attention the most. (Although there might be some doubt as to precisely where within the region indicated by the dotted lines in Fig. 2 subjects may have placed their marks, there was never any doubt as to whether the point lay within the demarcated region; the dotted lines did not appear, of course, on the stimuli that were shown to the subjects.) The sum of the number of subjects who included each designated region in their first four rankings was obtained for each of the 12 views. The mean of the number of such judgments for each view (which with perfect agreement would be 15 × 4 = 60) was 40.50, with a standard deviation of 4.54. This result is significantly greater than the 20 markings one would expect (t = 15.7, df = 11, p < .01). The same analysis performed on the mirror image views (using 12 additional subjects) yielded essentially the same results; in fact, the correlations between the most frequently chosen 10 points in the two groups for each picture ranged from .82 to .98, with a mean r = 0.95 (and a mean rho = 0.86), averaging z transformations. In short, the first four judgments agreed significantly with the points that we had intended to be the attentional centers, and on the average each view had only four points about which subjects agreed.

Discussion and Conclusions

As we expected from the earlier research on single static displays, fixations within the individual views of a sequence are emitted neither randomly nor in a systematic raster, but are directed to points that are also rated as being the most prominent. (Incidentally, this shows that the procedures by which we generated pictures of four attention centers, were at least approximately successful.) The course of looking, within each view of the sequence, is much as Antes (1974) found: *the initial response to each view was an initially high, followed by a declining, glance rate.* The curve derived from Antes' graph in Fig. 1B cannot be directly compared to those obtained here: The abscissa in the former is in tenths of total fixations, whereas the abscissa in the latter is in 250 msec intervals of time so as to allow the course of looking to be time-locked to regular sequences of various frequencies.

As we expected from the simple considerations discussed previously, the rate of active looking is maintained at a higher level when there are more places at which to look, and when the cutting rate is higher. There was no strong interaction between cutting rate (4 sec/view and 1 sec/view) and attentional complexity in these experiments. Because the interaction between complexity and affective cutting tone is an important feature of Spottiswoode's model, and because a decline in glance rate at high cutting rates has been incidentally reported before (e.g., Potter & Levy, 1969), a replication of Experiment 1, including higher cutting rates, was performed (Brooks & Hochberg, 1976) with the same absence of interaction; at 4, 2, 1, and .5 sec/view, respectively, four-center sequences evoked glance rates of .70 (S.D. = .14), .74 (.13), .78 (.18) and .82 (.17), and 1 center sequences evoked glance rates of .48 (.10), .50 (.12), .67 (.18), and .80 (.18).

Within the range in which it applies, the relationship demonstrated here between cutting rate, attentional complexity, and glance rate may make it possible, in principle, to "titrate" cutting rate against attentional complexity, in order to measure the latter. However, we cannot tell from Experiment 1 whether the same kinds of functions will appear when sequences are used that consist of meaningful views instead of abstract arrangements. Experiment 2 was directed to that question.

EXPERIMENT 2: THE COURSE OF ACTIVE LOOKING AT SEQUENCES OF MEANINGFUL PICTURES

Two populations of pictures were obtained by cutting up old magazine illustrations, appliance catalogs, and college yearbooks. From these, sequences of views on 16 mm film were assembled. When projected, they had the format shown in Fig. 5A, B, and C. One population (set *NC*) was chosen to have what appeared to be many centers of attention (one such photograph is represented by the outline drawing in Fig. 5A), whereas the other population (set *SC*) had what we hoped would be a single center (Fig. 5B, C). In set *SC* two sequences consisted of views that occupied the entire format (Fig. 5B), and in which the center of attention might appear to one side or centrally; two other sequences were constructed in which either a series of faces from a yearbook (Fig. 5C) or a sequence of pictures of small household appliances appeared at the same place in each view.

Sequences were all six views in length, and were presented at a rate of either 4 sec/view (*L*ong) or 1 sec/view (*S*hort). These sequences were presented to each of six naive subjects using the same instructions, apparatus, and procedures that had been used in Experiment 1. The order of the sequences for all subjects was as follows: SCL, NCL, SCS, NCS, NCS, SCS, NCL, SCL, SCL, NCL, SCS, NCS, NCS, SCS, NCL, and SCL.

Data were analyzed as they were in the previous experiments. Graphs of the time course of glance rate are shown in Fig. 6; the glance rate data, corresponding to those in Table 1, are summarized in Table 2. As with the abstract pictures, glance rates increased with both cutting rate and attentional complexity. Means and standard deviations of intrasubject differences are as follows: NCL–SCL = .31, s.d. = .08, t = 9.9, df = 5 (p < .01); NCS–SCS = .36, s.d. = .15, t = 5.99,

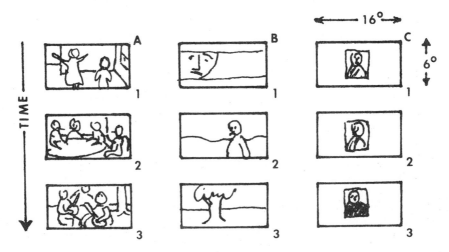

FIG. 5.   Line drawings of typical stimuli, in varying complexity, used in Experiment 2.

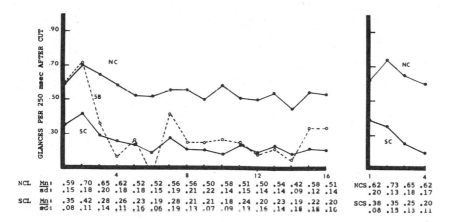

NCL Mn: .59 .70 .65 .62 .52 .52 .56 .56 .50 .58 .51 .50 .54 .42 .58 .51   NCS .62 .73 .65 .62
     sd: .15 .18 .20 .18 .18 .15 .19 .21 .22 .14 .15 .14 .14 .09 .12 .14   .20 .13 .18 .17
SCL Mn: .35 .42 .28 .26 .23 .19 .28 .21 .21 .18 .24 .20 .23 .19 .22 .20   SCS .38 .35 .25 .20
     sd: .08 .11 .14 .11 .16 .06 .19 .13 .07 .09 .13 .16 .14 .16 .16 .16   .08 .15 .13 .11

FIG. 6.   The means and standard deviations for each time sampled for each view, averaged across subjects for Experiment 2.

df = 5 (p < .01); (NCL–SCL) – (NCS–SCS) = –.05, s.d. = .12, t = 1.02. No interaction of complexity and cutting rate were found here, either.

One other aspect of these data should be considered: We can separate two components in the time course of looking, the early peak and the later sustained glance rate. As the graphs suggest, the effects of the difference in cutting rate is significantly greater in the average of the last 3 sec than it is in the first sec, with mean intrasubject differences of $[(SCS–SCL) + (NCS–NCL)]_{1–16} - [(SCS–SCL) + (NCS–NCL)]_{1–4} = .11$, s.d. = .07, t = 3.6, p < .02.

Various explanations can be suggested for this difference. One that follows naturally from the approach we are pursuing is that the initial movements are made to points about which the subject has only the very general information that he can gain by peripheral vision. These movements occur under what we have called elsewhere *peripheral search guidance* (Hochberg, 1970a, b; Hochberg

TABLE 2
Sequences of Meaningful Views

Attentional Complexity:		S Center			N Centers		
Samples:		1–16	1–4	5–16	1–16	1–4	5–16
Glance Rate, 4 sec/view:	Mn:	.24	.33	.21	.55	.64	.53
	sd:	.10	.09	.11	.11	.13	.12
Glance Rate, 1 sec/view:	Mn:		.30			.66	
	sd:		.08			.13	

& Brooks, 1970). After the initial eye movements have established the general nature of the peripherally visible *landmarks* (Hochberg & Gellman, 1977), subsequent saccades are directed to the answers of more cognitively driven questions (*cognitive search guidance,* in the case of meaningful pictures), which sustain inquiry about details near the landmarks. This is similar to suggestions made by Antes (1974), and Loftus (1976). Note, however, that it might be argued, at least as well, that the sustained parts of these curves might arise from an ahistorical recycling, with perturbations, through the points of highest salience (cf. Baker, 1977; Senders, Webb, & Baker, 1955). It is hard to believe that the geometric "scenes" of Experiment 1 can hold much that is of cognitive interest to the viewer after 1 or 2 sec of looking. We will return to this point later, noting here that it makes glance rate, alone, an inadequate index of cognitive search.

It will be remembered that we employed two kinds of simple sequences, that is, views like those in Fig. 5B and in Fig. 5C. In Fig. 5C, successive views all fell in much the same place, so that no large peripheral movements were needed in order to observe succeeding objects or faces. In the sequence of views like Fig. 5B, on the other hand, the viewer would need one or two large initial saccades in order to locate the region at which he might look for the remainder of his viewing time. Compare the graphs of a sequence of views like those in Fig. 5B to those of the whole set of ICL sequences (Fig. 6): The average glance rate is higher (.13) with samples 1–4 than samples 5–16 (.03), t = 3.2, df = 5, p < .05, but this difference is restricted to the first few moments of looking. This raises another difficulty in the use of glance rate to assess perceptual inquiry: the amount of eye movements is strongly dependent on where attentional foci fall in successive views; and a subject might gaze in rapt but immobile attention at successive views that are all most informative at the same place (cf. Potter & Levy, 1969).

We need another measure of visual momentum or tendency to keep looking at a view sequence. We discuss a subjective preference measure in the next section, and turn to a more successful objective measure later.

ESTHETIC PREFERENCE AND VISUAL MOMENTUM

These experiments, described elsewhere in more detail, were quite straightforward attempts to determine whether the sequences of views used in the previous experiments would elicit judgments of preference (other than by chance), and how such preference judgments relate to the variables being investigated. Small groups of two or four subjects, naive as to the hypothesis being tested, were shown the sequences. In each experiment, they were initially shown one sequence to which they were to assign the number 100 as a measure of its *pleasingness.* Tables 3A and 3B show the geometric means of the preferences for the sequences

TABLE 3
Pleasingness Judgments (Geometric Means)

	A. Sequences of Experiment 1		
Attentional Complexity:	1C	2C	4C
Short views	88.0	104.2	131.7
Long views	78.7	97.2	124.2
	B. Sequences of Experiment 2		
Attentional Complexity:	SC		NC
Short views	74.2		88.7
Long views	84.4		125.0

of Experiments 1 and 2, respectively. The effect of complexity is significant, but the effect of cutting rate is not, despite what we expected from Spottiswoode's (1933/1962) model.

It may be that subjects are merely displaying the well-known correlation between esthetic judgments and complexity (cf. Berlyne, 1958; Faw & Nunnally, 1967), without regard to cutting rate: that is, they may simply be reporting the structure they perceive, and the higher cutting rate may merely be an interference — that would certainly be consistent with the *lower* pleasingness of the higher cutting rates. We have not yet run this experiment on subjects steeped in motion picture analysis, and we may yet obtain different results with them. But in any case, we cannot use pleasingness judgments to measure visual momentum. A more objective procedure for measuring the impetus to keep looking was explored in the remaining set of experiments.

PREFERENTIAL FREE LOOKING: SPLIT-FIELD MEASURES OF MOMENTUM

The following experiments are intended to test a measure of the moment-by-moment impetus to look at an extended sequence of views.

Experiments 3—5

The following experiments all have the same basic procedure: Two sequences were displayed simultaneously, one above the other, with the dimensions shown in Fig. 7. We will call these the upper and lower channels. After a relatively small

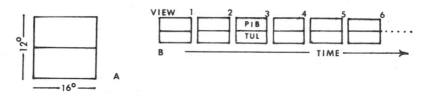

FIG. 7.   (A) Schematic of display with upper and lower channels; (B) Typical view sequence used in Experiments 3–5.

number of pairs of views, a different short typed word appeared briefly in each channel. The sequences of pictorial views in each channel then continued, as shown schematically in Fig. 7B.

Each subject was told that we were concerned with his eye movements under cognitive load, and that he was to attend to the word that would appear in the particular channel specified before each presentation began. He was to note the word, and press a key as quickly as possible as soon as he had read it. After that, he was free to look wherever he wished until the experimenter told him that the next trial was about to begin and in which channel the next target word would appear. When the subject pressed the key, an LED signal was recorded on the motion picture film.

Each pair of sequences was shown twice during the course of each experiment. The channel that had contained the target word on one presentation was the non-attended channel on the other presentation. In all cases, target channels were alternated on initial presentation between subjects. The measure that we were concerned with in each case was the proportion of time spent looking at the nontargeted channel during the "free-looking" period (i.e., after the word). Thus, no task required him to look at that channel, but the distracting or attractive effect of the alternate channel with which it was paired was controlled within subjects, while order was controlled across subjects. Because the looking time for one channel was necessarily affected by the attractiveness of the alternate channel, however, comparisons were made only between sequences that were members of the same pair.

Experiment 3: Preferential Looking at Montages of Geometrical Patterns

The procedure and subjects (N = 10) were as described above. The stimulus sequences were those used in Experiment 1, paired so that the two channels were matched in duration and phase of the view sequences, that is, both were 1 sec/view or 4 sec/view, or paired so that the two channels were equal in complexity but differed in view duration (cutting rate) for a total of 24 possible combinations. A sample of the sequence pairs is as follows: 1CS/4CS, 4CS/4CL, and 1CL/1CS, with the slash (/) separating upper/lower channels.

The means and standard errors of the average proportions of the posttarget time that subjects looked at each category of sequence when it was the nontargeted channel are given in Table 4. When four centers are pitted against one center, it is clear that subjects look longer at the four centers. And when short views (fast sequences) were pitted against long views (slow sequences), the former prevails. Most proportions are less than .50 because there is a tendency to keep looking at the target channel even after the word has been removed. The mean of the differences between each subject's mean of A and B and his mean of C and D, in Table 4, was .23, s.d. = .22, t = 3.21, df = 9, p < .01, indicating a significant effect due to complexity. The mean of the differences between means of E and $F - G$ and H was .24, s.d. = .13, t = 6.03, df = 9, p < .01, indicating a significant effect due to cutting rate. The interaction between complexity of the scene, and cutting rate, is not significant.

Experiments 4A, B, and C: Preferential Looking at Montages and Connected Sequences of Representational Views

The procedure in these experiments was that of Experiment 3, using meaningful pictures (primarily, those of Experiment 2).

Experiment 4A: Effect of Cutting Rate

Two kinds of sequence pairs were presented here, either complex (NC) or simple (SC) views in both upper and lower channel. In each case, the views in one channel were short (.5 sec/view) whereas those in the other were long (3 sec/view). The means and standard deviations for preferential looking (the time spent looking at a channel when the other channel was targeted) are shown in Table 5A. Analyses of intrasubject differences showed that cutting rate clearly affects looking time (pooled t (S/L) = 3.9, df = 7, p < .01), while the effect of cutting rate was not significantly different for the NC and SC view sequences.

TABLE 4
Preferential Looking: Sequences of Geometrical Views[a]

| | Proportion of time spent looking at nontargeted channel | | | | | | | |
| | Short versus Long | | | | 1 Center versus 4 Center | | | |
	A: 4CS	B: 4CL	C: 1CS	D: 1CL	E: 1CL	F: 4CL	G: 1CS	H: 4CS
Mn.	.41	.50	.20	.25	.21	.17	.39	.46
sd	.27	.14	.13	.09	.17	.13	.16	.16

[a]N = 10 in all cases

TABLE 5
Preferential Looking:
Sequences of Meaningful Views

		Proportion of time spent looking at nontargeted channel			
		Experiment 4A. Effect of cutting rate			
4A		1) NCS	2) NCL	3) SCS	4) SCL
	Mn:	.65	.40	.65	.33
	sd:	.22	.20	.16	.24 N = 8
		Experiments 4B and 4C. Effect of attentional complexity			
4B		1) NCS	2) NCL	3) SCS	4) SCL
	Mn:	.28	.53	.22	.34
	sd:	.27	.14	.18	.13 N = 10
4C		1) NCS	2) NCL	3) SCS	4) SCL
	Mn:	.46	.66	.31	.25
	sd:	.27	.18	.25	.15 N = 10

Experiment 4B, C: Effect of Attentional Complexity

In Experiment 4B (N = 10), two kinds of sequence pairs were presented; in both, one channel contained complex views (*NC*) and one contained simple views (*SC*), taken from Experiment 4A. One set of paired sequences was presented at .5 sec/view and the other set was presented at 3 sec/view. In Experiment 4C (N = 10), the same sequences were used as in Eperiment 4B, except that (a) what had been in the upper channel in Experiment 4B was in the lower channel in Experiment 4C, and *vice versa*; and (b) Experiment 4C contained several additional paired sequences as preliminary inquiries for future research, some of which will be referred to later. An ANOVA of subjects' mean scores on NCS, SCS, and SCL for the two groups of Experiments 4B and 4C, showed no difference between the two groups (F = 1.47, df = 1, 54), an interaction between group and sequence which approached significance (F = 2.31, df = 3, 54, p < .10), an effect of complexity which was significant (t = 3.12, df = 18, p < .01), and an effect of the interaction between complexity and cutting rate which was significant (t = 6.40, df = 18, p < .01). It is clear (Table 5B, C) that attentional complexity affects looking time, and that the effect is greater at lower cutting rates.

Discussion.   Experiments 4A–4C give the concept of visual momentum, as a hypothetical construct over and above the measured glance rates obtained in

Experiments 1–3, some plausibility. They do not show, however, that cognitive inquiry, as distinct from stimulus factors such as change and complexity per se, contribute substantially to the sustained component of looking — this is essentially an extension of the question we raised in the course of discussing Experiment 2. That is, movement in the channel that one is not looking at might capture the gaze and account for the greater visual momentum of the channel having the higher cutting rate; and greater complexity might act to hold the gaze simply by increasing the intrachannel transitional probabilities, regardless of any questions of perceptual inquiry.

With respect to the possibility that mere change in pattern accounts completely for visual momentum differences, we have two examples to the contrary, neither of them completely convincing, within the data of the experiments we have already described. If "peripheral capture" were the sole basis of the looking preference measures, a sequence in which the center of attention was in a different place in each view should be looked at more frequently than one in which such displacement did not occur. We have some indication that effects attributable to displacement per se are not a major factor. First, note that the sequence in Fig. 5B, which elicited a higher glance rate during the first second of viewing time, presumably due to the greater displacement from view to view, did not differ from Fig. 5C when the data of Experiment 4C are analyzed specifically with respect to these two sequences, and no differences on the basis of rate were found. We cannot make too much of this point, however, because they had no occasion to be pitted against each other in the same two-channel pair, and we noted that cross-pair comparisons cannot really be made. Second, consider the two sequence pairs in Fig. 8A and 8B. These were designed to induce more eye movement in one channel than in the other, and they were successful in this

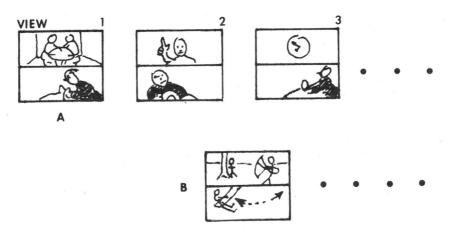

FIG. 8.   Line drawings of typical stimuli used in Experiment 5 to induce more eye movements in one channel than the other.

regard. In sequence A, each channel had a story in the sense that the successive views were designed to represent parts of the same scene, the same "characters" appeared throughout, and the sequence could readily be described in terms of a continuous action narrative. The attention center in the upper channel was designed to fall close to the center on each view; the attention center in the lower channel fell on alternate sides of the view, in successive views. Mean of the momentum differences between upper and lower channels was 0.18, s.d. = .52, $t = 1.09$, df = 9.

In sequence B, the upper channel was a stick-figure animation of the apple-shooting scene in the William Tell story, with occasional cuts and small amounts of continuous movements in the actions of walking, lifting the apple, etc. The movement of the swing in the lower channel was 8°/sec, with a .17 sec pause at each end of the arc. Mean of the differences between momentum for the upper and lower channels was 0.28, s.d. = .35, $t = 2.57$, df = 9, $p < .05$. No differences were found in favor of looking at the lateral-eye movement-inducing channel occurred in either of these two sequence pairs.

If these results are generally reliable, they have some practical importance to filmmakers, who often cut in such a way that the two different foci of attention fall in essentially the same place in two successive views (and maintain the same velocities, if the objects are in motion). This should result in an effectively lowered cutting rate, and in less impetus to keep looking, if peripheral capture were a major component of visual momentum. But if peripheral capture is not the main factor in visual momentum (which is what we are arguing here), then the filmmaker's practice is probably sound for a rather subtle reason: It should delay the viewer's comprehension by several hundred msec (because he lacks the signals that would indicate, rapidly and noncognitively, that changes have occurred), and this delay should sustain visual momentum over a slower cutting rate (cf. Fig. 1A).

This assumes, of course, that cognitive inquiry contributes substantially to visual momentum, an assumption for which we have so far provided only weak support. The next experiment provides better support. The second way in which noncognitive factors might account for visual momentum is by having complexity capture the gaze in the split field experiments regardless of the viewer's experience. This is addressed by Experiment 5.

Experiment 5: The effects of repetition on preferential looking

This experiment is addressed to the same question, within sequences, that Flagg discusses elsewhere in this volume in regard to between-sequence effects. In order to test the possibility that change and complexity per se determine preferential looking, regardless of the viewer's history with the stimuli, new sequences were made from those used in Experiment 4B, with these changes: (1) the sequence length was extended to a total of 18 views past the target word, and (2) the attentionally complex (NC) sequence consisted only of the same two views, alternating repetitively with each other. Eight new subjects were used with these stimuli presented at 1.5 sec/view. Eye movements were recorded and analyzed only during the presentations of the pairs in which the simple sequence (SC) consisted of the extended views (Fig. 5B) as distinguished from the view-sequences of single items (yearbook faces, appliances) centered in each successive view.

Eye movement records were divided into segments corresponding to each cycle (i.e., pair of repeated views) of the NC sequences, and the duration each subject spent in looking at the nontargeted channel within each of the nine cycles was obtained for the presentation in which the NC sequence was the nontargeted channel and that in which the SC sequence was the nontargeted channel. The difference in response between the nine cycles is significant ($F = 3.83$; df = 8, 56; $p < .01$); momentum is significantly greater for SC than for NC in the second half of the sequence: the mean of subjects' differences is .25, s.d. = .17, t = 4.18, df = 7, $p < .01$. The difference in visual momentum (NC–SC), averaged across subjects for each cycle after the target word, is graphed in Fig. 9. The effect of

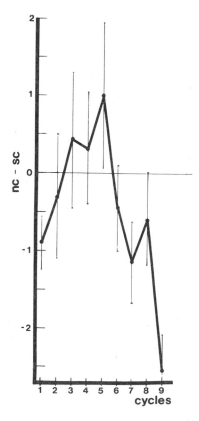

FIG. 9. Time course of differences in visual momentum for a repeating complex view sequence (NC) paired with a nonrepeating simple view sequence (SC). The heavy line is the graph of the differences between durations of looking at the NC and at the SC sequences when each is the nontargeted channel. Thin lines indicate standard errors. The abscissa is the number of the cycle of the repeating NC pair of views after the presentation of the target word; the ordinate is the mean difference in looking times for NC and for SC for that cycle, in terms of number of 250 msec samples.

history is clear and, having seen that the two alternating NC views were the same (to some criterion) from cycle to cycle, subjects reversed the looking preferences they had displayed in the other experiments.

SUMMARY AND CONCLUSIONS

The ways in which people move their eyes while they are watching sequences of changing views, and the proportions of time that they spend in looking at one sequence rather than another, are lawfully related to the characteristics of the views, and to the rates at which they are changed (cutting rates).

We have seen that in general the outcome of experiments on glance rate and experiments on preferential looking at sequences of abstract and representational views (montages) are consistent with the notion of an impetus to gather visual information, which we have called *visual momentum*. The time course of visual momentum as a function of complexity and of cutting rate is quite similar to Spottiswoode's semiquantiative introspective model of what he called affective tone. There are some results that suggest that the course of active looking, and of the visual momentum that presumably impels it, can be partitioned into components: a fast component that brings the eye to those peripherally visible regions that promise to be informative or to act as landmarks, and a more sustained component that directs the eye to obtain more detailed information about the main features that have already been located.

Both of these components of momentum should have theoretical as well as practical interests: practical, because they are important in such applications as film editing; theoretical, because the fast component may be informative about the uses of peripheral vision, and the slow component may reveal the momentary state of schema-formation, using cutting rate (for example) to "titrate" the loss of visual momentum that occurs after the view is comprehended. Such research is now in progress.

DISCUSSION

STARK: Do you think you could put your test words in such a way as to see if the subject was in this peripheral guidance mode or the central schema testing mode and really test out your various hypotheses?

HOCHBERG: We could do that by adding additional probes in the body after the test words have appeared. The initial test words are "covers"; they're used simply to give the subject some task and to mark the start of his free period, after he sees the word he can do what he wants. We can indeed put probes into the free looking period. It is definitely something to do. I have some reservations; that is, I think that will change the mode of the subject's looking. I try to keep the subjects unconstrained, and that's the point of all this elaborate secrecy. For example, the glance rate experiments were presented as experiments in esthetics. We actually did gather some esthetic data, because we're constrained by NIH regulations not to lie to our subjects and some of those data are interesting — unlike the pupillary reflex data, but I can't report them now.

So, the answer is: yes, it can be done, and my guess is that the early component is so robust and probably sufficiently resistant to instructions, that using additional probes would work. We haven't tried it.

NODINE: You've indicated that the early component has to do with peripheral guidance and the later component is more concerned with attention to detail.

HOCHBERG: Maybe, but it would be very possible that there's also a stochastic component as well.

NODINE: Where does expectancy come into this?

HOCHBERG: You set the stage for a paragraph that I had cut out because I didn't have time.

Yes. We've given peripheral search guidance here a new function, namely, because of the nature of unconnected views it has to bring the viewer to some meaningful fixation point to begin with. Now, one of the reasons we use disconnected montage is that it gives us a baseline against which we can refer sequences of views in which the subject does carry over information and expectations from one view to the next.

Part **VI**

PROBLEMS AND APPLICATIONS

VI.1

Studies of Eye Movements and Visual Search in Radiology[1]

Harold L. Kundel
Calvin F. Nodine
Temple University School of Medicine

INTRODUCTION

The major activity of diagnostic radiologists is commonly called film reading. It consists of looking at the x-ray images of people which are generally recorded on films, determining if any abnormal structures or configurations are present in the images, and then making inferences about the conditions or diseases that might cause the abnormal appearances. Like most human endeavors, film reading is subject to error and for the diagnosis of some types of diseases they are surprisingly high. Thirty percent false negatives and 5% false positives are typically found when the diagnosis of tuberculosis (Garland, 1959) or of small lung cancers (Guiss & Kuenstler, 1960) on survey chest films has been studied.

What is the source of these errors? Can they be eliminated? These are the questions that have puzzled us and led us to study visual search and image processing. We will review the role of eye movements in searching chest x-ray films for small lung abnormalities.

DEFINITION OF THE STIMULUS AND THE SEARCH TASK

Film reading is a complicated perceptual and intellectual process that for the sake of analysis can be divided into two distinct, albeit related, components: search—recognition and interpretation. During search and recognition the film

---

[1] This research was supported by U.S. Public Health Service Grant #GM 21474 from the Institute of General Medical Sciences.

reader must decide if any of the normal structures deviate from the accepted limits for size, shape, position, or texture and, in addition, must decide if any new structures that are not normally part of the image are present. Enlargement of the heart is an example of a deviation from normal in size, whereas a lung tumor is an example of a new structure. Once one or more abnormalities have been detected they must be classified into appropriate diagnostic categories. This is interpretation and it usually involves considering clinical information along with the visual data from the x-ray films. Most often it is an assessment of probabilities rather than an absolute diagnosis.

For simplicity, our experimental work has been concentrated on the search—recognition part of film reading and has utilized only one abnormality, a faint, rounded, homogeneous structure called a nodule that is located in the lungs' image on chest film.

This particular abnormality was singled out for study because many nodules are missed on the first reading of the films, and because many of them also turn out to be early lung cancers. Nodules are also convenient to study in the laboratory because they are relatively simple to simulate and we have developed a photographic technique to produce them. The simulated nodules mimic real nodules and have a number of added advantages. Size, shape, texture, edge gradient, contrast, and location on the film can be controlled and the background

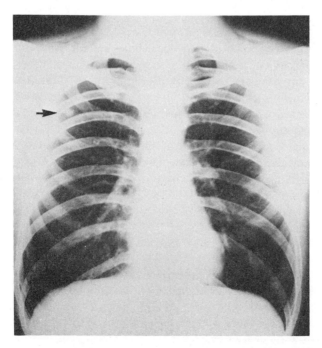

FIG. 1.   An example of a chest film containing a one cm lung nodule.

chest film can be selected as well. Test film series can be made up containing films with and without nodules, and film readers can be asked to search them for nodules. A binary decision, normal or abnormal, can be used and the responses analyzed using statistical decision theory.

A typical lung nodule used in our studies, such as the one shown in Fig. 1, is about one cm in diameter and has a contrast between 2–10%. At a comfortable viewing distance of 70 cm, the nodule subtends a visual angle of about 1° and the entire chest film subtends about 25°.

Recording Eye Movements

We originally used a Mackworth stand camera to record eye movements. The data on 16 mm film are reduced using a X Y plotter interfaced to a LINC-8 computer (Kundel and Nodine, 1973). More recently, we have been using Biometrics glasses on line with a PDP 11/40 computer. The films are reproduced on slides and projected to their natural size with a three-channel tachistoscope that is also interfaced to the computer so that each slide changer and each shutter can be independently controlled.

Visual Scanning as a Sampling Procedure

If one starts with the somewhat naive but nevertheless simple assumption that in order for a nodule to be detected it must be imaged on the fovea, it might be predicted that an effective visual scan would be one that systematically moves the fovea over the entire film. However, scanning patterns are neither very systematic nor very complete. Nodules are typically either detected within the first 10 sec of viewing or missed completely, and in that time a generous fovea of 3° is not scanned over the entire film (Kundel & LaFollette, 1972; Llewellyn-Thomas & Landsdown, 1963).

Scanning patterns that are "typical" for a radiologist viewing a normal chest film and a chest film with a single abnormality are shown in Fig. 2.

The pattern on the normal film begins with a few widely spaced circumferential fixations, as if the entire film was being given a preliminary survey. Frequently this sweep is repeated many times. In a study of five radiologists viewing five different chest films about 40% of the initial patterns were circumferential (Kundel & Wright, 1969). Most of the rest were too complex to analyze. Brandt (1945), who studied hundreds of subjects looking at advertisements from newspapers and magazines, made a similar observation. His subjects appeared to start with a general survey of the pictures and he also noted that no two "ocular patterns" are alike.

Our attempt to classify patterns or to find repeatable sequences of fixation locations has also been unsuccessful. But if sequence is disregarded and only the location of fixations on anatomic regions of the chest film is considered, con-

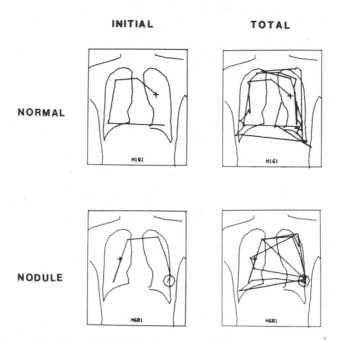

FIG. 2.   Scanpaths of a radiologist viewing a normal film and a film containing a lung nodule for ten seconds. The region of the nodule is indicated as an octagonal zone 4° in diameter. The first few fixations on both of these films are what we call a circumferential pattern.

siderable consistency in fixation distribution emerges. The proportion of the total fixation time spent fixating various anatomic regions of the chest such as the heart, lungs, or rib edges, was consistent between and within film readers. Radiologists tend to fixate the same areas, but not necessarily in the same sequence. Consequently, two patterns with very different overall scanpaths can have very similar fixation distributions.

The distribution of fixation time over the anatomic regions on the chest film could be changed by altering the instructions given to the film readers. Instructions are given in terms of a clinical history. The data in Table 1, taken from Kundel and Wright (1969), show the effect of telling the film readers either that the patient was examined because of the possibility of a lung nodule, or that the film was a routine screening examination.

As would be expected there is a greater concentration on the lungs when the history directs the film reader to the lungs.

The distribution of fixation time was also modified by the presence of an abnormality if it was detected. When a nodule was detected a large and variable proportion of the total fixation time, an average of 14% was spent on the region of the nodule. Because all of the nodules were located in the lungs, the percentage of total time in the lungs was naturally exaggerated. If the time spent in the region of the nodule was subtracted from the total, a new, normalized distribution could be calculated. The percentage of the total time spent in each anatomic region of the normalized distribution was similar to that found when radiologists viewed normal films, given the clinical information that the patient might have a lung nodule (Kundel, 1974).

There is also correlation between subjective estimates of the relative importance of different regions of the chest film and the percentage of the total fixation time spent in those regions when the film readers were shown normal films and given a general search task (Kundel, 1974). These findings are consistent with others who have studied the correlation between fixation time and ratings of informativeness (Antes, 1974; Mackworth & Morandi, 1967). In fact, there is correlation between the fixation time and the subjective ratings of informativeness of laypersons looking at chest films, but they select different areas than do radiologists.

These results suggest that the placement of fixations is organized and highly selective. The search plan does not require either a detached examination of every part of the film or a formalized sequence of data collection. Rather, it is a sampling strategy whose details we are only beginning to understand. Certain regions are selected for sampling to the exclusion of others. The basic sampling distribution is determined in advance and is based on training and experience. The particular sampling distribution that is actually used is a modification of the basic one that takes into consideration clinical information available about the patient before the film is viewed. Further modification is made as abnormalities are recognized and analyzed.

It is common experience that when one looks at a chest film, or indeed anything else, what is perceived is not a number of samples with intervening voids, but a complete image. What we really mean by sampling is selecting some parts of the image for detailed examination and leaving the rest for the less acute peripheral vision and the versatile memory.

TABLE 1

The Effect of Clinical Data on the Viewing Time Spent by Five
Film Readers on Four General Regions of a Normal Chest Film

Region	True Area of Each Region (%)	Clinical Data	
		Routine Chest Film (% time)	Possible Lung Nodule (% time)
Lungs	24	41	60
Heart	26	12	6
Edges	26	29	33
Periphery	24	18	1

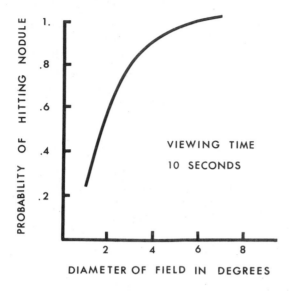

FIG. 3. The relationship between the diameter of the target zone around each fixation called the useful field of view and the probability that the lung nodule will be included in the target zone.

SAMPLING AND THE USEFUL FIELD OF VIEW

A nodule is a small frequently faint target, the area of the lung where a nodule can hide is large, the anatomic fovea is small, and yet the gaze of the radiologist jumps to the region of a nodule very quickly, either interrupting or eliminating the preliminary circumferential scan of the film. Clearly, the portion of the visual field that is capable of detecting a nodule is larger than a 3° fovea. Mackworth (1976) has called this area the useful field of view, and Engel (1971) has called it the conspicuity zone. In both instances it is not a zone of fixed size but is defined operationally or empirically.

How large is the useful field of view when radiologists are searching for nodules? We have made some theoretical calculations that are based on a film reading experiment.

Two experienced film readers were shown a series of ten chest films, six with and four without nodules for 10 sec, and their eye movements were recorded. They were instructed to indicate their decision using a rating scale from 1 to 5 corresponding to 100, 75, 50, 25, and 0% confidence that a nodule was present in a specified location marked by a cross. They were also instructed to discontinue search as soon as a nodule was detected with a confidence of 1. The nodules subtended an angle of 0.7° and had about 8% contrast. The experiment was repeated six times on different days using different starting positions and a randomized film sequence.

The eye movement patterns on the films with nodules that were given a confidence rating of 1 were used to calculate the probability of a fixation hitting a target zone with a specified diameter around each nodule. The diameter was varied from 1–8°, resulting in the curve shown in Fig. 3. The probability of hitting the target zone reaches 1.0 at a target zone diameter of about 6°.

Our recording system is accurate only to about 1°; but, we believe that 5–6° is a good estimate of the limit of the useful field of view.

There is an additional factor that must be considered. Boynton and Bush (1956) and Mackworth (1965) have shown that background complexity decreases the peripheral detectability of visual targets. This is also true for chest films (Kundel, 1975). The ability of film readers to detect lung nodules with peripheral vision decreases sharply with increasing complexity of the normal structures. Therefore, the size of the useful field may vary from fixation to fixation, depending on the complexity of the visual display. The actual limiting factor may be the amount of data that can be processed in the limited time alloted to one fixation.

Five or six degrees may represent an extreme value, and for subsequent calculations we used 4° as the size of the average useful visual field. About 90% of detected nodules are scanned by a field of this size.

Confidence Level and Target Dwell Time

The eye movement data from the experiment described above were also used to calculate the average dwell time of the first cluster of fixations on a 4° target zone. This is analogous to determining how long a 4° diameter useful field of

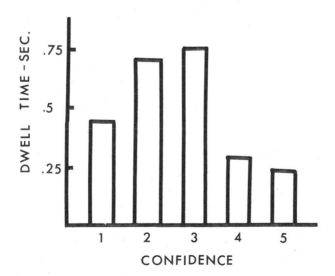

FIG. 4.   The relationship between the average time spent by the first cluster of fixations on the lung nodule and the confidence level of the final decision. The useful visual field was fixed at 4°.

view dwelt on the nodule the first time it was scanned. The data in Fig. 4 show that when no nodule was present and confidence was 4 or 5, dwell time was about 0.25 sec. When the nodule was detected with a confidence of 1, dwell time was about 0.3 sec and it increased for confidence levels 2 or 3. These data will be used later as a basis for separating two classes of error.

SOME SPECULATIONS ABOUT THE FILM READING PROCESS

Searching an x-ray film is a somewhat unusual task because much of the arrangement of the information on the film is fixed; that is, lungs, heart, ribs, and so forth, are almost always found in the same relative position. In this sense film reading is like reading a book where the information is also arranged in a fixed order.

A schematic diagram for the progression of film reading is shown in Fig. 5. The clinical data basically define the search task and, together with the initial visual orientation data gained from the first few fixations, set the sampling priorities.

Very early in film reading, the radiologist must decide if everything is in the right place. This should be a fairly standardized procedure and may account for the early circumferential pattern of fixations. But locating new information such as a nodule is not as standardized, except that clinical experience teaches, first, that nodules are located only in the lungs and, second, that there are certain areas in the lungs where nodules are more likely to be located, or, because of the other anatomic structures, where nodules are more likely to hide. This knowledge exists not only for nodules but also for a large number of other possible abnormalities that are the objects of a radiologist's search. This knowledge is used to develop a priori sampling distributions that provide the format for visual search.

In addition to sampling the appropriate regions of the film, small abnormalities must also be imaged by a critical zone of the visual field within which detection becomes possible. The size of the zone can at present be defined only operationally and depends on properties of the object of search like size, shape, and texture, and on the nature of the background that contains the object of search (Kundel & Revesz, 1976; Revesz, Kundel & Graber, 1974). As the background becomes more complex, a greater processing load is placed on the perceptual system. Within limits, processing time can be increased while maintaining a large useful visual field by increasing fixation duration, but once the limits of time are reached a smaller area must be processed and the useful visual field narrows. The final pattern of fixations or scanpath that is observed results from the dynamic interaction of an a priori sampling distribution and a useful field of view that are both modified from moment to moment in response to the incoming stream of visual data. It is not suprising that no two ocular patterns are alike.

Fixating a nodule with the useful field of view does not insure that it will be detected. A recognition process must disembed the nodule from the surround.

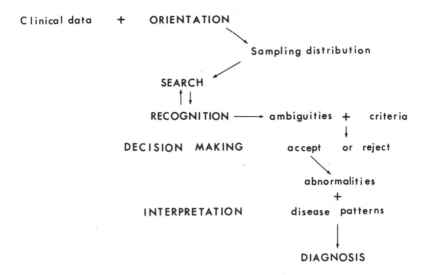

FIG. 5.   A schematic model of the process of film reading.

The flowchart in Fig. 5 indicates that the recognition process may turn up ambiguous areas that are not nodules. Internalized criteria must then be applied to decide if an ambiguous area is or is not a nodule. This is a decision-making step that can result in accepting or rejecting a true nodule or, conversely, accepting or rejecting an ambiguous feature that is not truly a nodule. Once all abnormalities on the film are found, a higher lever of decision making (interpretation) leads to the development of a list of diagnostic possibilities.

Errors in Nodule Detection

Using the model given in flowchart of Fig. 5, three major sources of error can be identified. First, there are search errors where in the useful field of view is not scanned over the nodule. Second, there are recognition errors where in the

TABLE 2
Distribution of Errors

Error Category	Number of Errors	Percentage of Total
Search	2	10
Recognition	6	35
Decision	9	53
Total	20	100

nodule is scanned but not disembedded from the complex surround. Third, there are decision making errors; false negatives when a nodule is rejected as an abnormality, and false positives when an ambiguity is accepted as a nodule.

In a preliminary way, using the error data from only two film readers, we partitioned the errors that were made according to the following criteria. A search error was scored if a 4° diameter useful field of view did not scan the nodule. A recognition error was scored if the nodule was scanned by the useful field of view, but if initial and subsequent dwell times were less than 0.3 sec. A decision making error was scored if the nodule was scanned and if dwell exceeded 0.3 sec. The results are shown in Table 2. For this task, decision-making, not search, appears to be the most important source of error.

CONCLUSION

Our reason for the study of eye movements of radiologists during film reading has been to understand the sources of film reader error. The experiment presented here was the first in a series of studies now in progress, but it represents our model, methodology, and a first approximation of expected final results. We believe that it is important to develop such descriptions and to make them quantitative, because only in this way can the potential value of schemes to reduce error be judged. Eventually, we may be able to do something about these errors, but at present we must be content to describe them in the hope that the detailed description may itself suggest methods for improvement of film reader error.

DISCUSSION

ANON: You refer to a decision-making limitation. What sort of data plots did you come up with?

KUNDEL: There aren't enough data to plot an ROC curve reliably. We've run two subjects for 80 runs. You need hundreds of data points in order to get meaningful curves, and I don't have them. I will in a couple of years.

LLEWELLYN-THOMAS: Have you been able to move on to dynamic presentations at all yet? This is a fascinating use of search and recognition in making a decision, but in fluoroscopy, where the image is changing during search, other factors come into effect.

KUNDEL: No, we have not looked at dynamic displays. Dynamic displays are not commonly used in radiology nowadays. I've tried to stay with a situation that I could understand a little better.

LLEWELLYN-THOMAS: You say they're not common, but how about arteriograms?

KUNDEL: Well, arteriograms are made with serial films and the films are read. Radiologists prefer to read statistic displays.

LLEWELLYN-THOMAS: I know.

KUNDEL: You'll find, in general, that fluoroscopy is done mainly as a means of getting a good film record, and the radiologists make their diagnoses from the static film. We do dynamic studies, particularly in cardiology. Many dynamic studies are done of the heart when one is looking for areas of dyskinesis. But even these are recorded on cine film and for the most part analyzed frame by frame. This is an area where computer processing has become very important.

SNYDER: I'm pleased to see that the kind of numbers you're getting are representative of several studies that were not widely publicized on the inner- and intraobserver reliability of film reading by radiologists. I think we're all aware that much of the work going on in radiology today in the image processing community is with so-called image enhancement and image reconstruction techniques. I'm totally unaware of any research that's been done tying-in good quantitative information extraction studies with various processing algorithms. Could you comment upon your knowledge of that area and anything that has or will be done in that area?

KUNDEL: Processing algorithms for image restoration in CT scanners is a large new field.

SNYDER: This field has mushroomed very greatly without the benefit of any human performance data to justify the techniques which are being used.

KUNDEL: That's right, computerized transaxial tomography (CT) has never been formally studied. You can study the value of diagnostic procedures in three ways. You can look at efficacy in terms of the ability to make a diagnosis. That has been done, and in some areas these machines are better than the other techniques that are available, particularly in the brain. You can look at the next level of efficacy, which asks whether the technique changes the way in which the patient will be treated. It's one thing to make a diagnosis and another thing to do something about it. There are many diagnoses that we can make that we can do absolutely nothing about. The third thing to look at is whether making the diagnosis changes the outcome for the patient at all. None of these data are available.

STARK: Now that you know how the radiologists' scanpaths differ from those of a second year medical student or a layman, are you using that information in your training of residents of radiology?

KUNDEL: No.

SNYDER: Do you think it would be helpful?

KUNDEL: I don't know how to teach people how to scan films. If you'd write down for me how to do it, I'd take it and try it. I think the most important thing is to teach them what they should be looking for, what abnormalities look like, and how abnormalities interact with the surround.

SENDERS: Were the people, who in 1950 missed 50% of the positives, trained radiologists?

KUNDEL: Some of them were and some of them weren't.

SENDERS: I see, but no one knows who did which?

KUNDEL: No, but there are lots of good data with trained radiologists showing that, on the average, false negative rates run around 15—30% and false positive rates about 3—20%.

GOLDBERG: To answer Dr. Stark's question — I've been in Medical School slightly more recently than he, and when I was being taught to look at a chest film, a radiologist said, "Don't look at the heart first, look at the soft tissues, then at the ribs, and then look at the other things in some order," which is pretty much what the scan path of the radiologist was and not what the scanpath of the second year medical student is. So in that sense, the scanpaths are not taught as *scan paths,* but are taught as some kind of anatomical sequence.

VI.2

An Exploratory Investigation of the Stochastic Nature of the Drivers' Eye Movements and Their Relationship to the Roadway Geometry[1]

E.D. McDowell
Oregon State University

T.H. Rockwell
Ohio State University

BACKGROUND

Since it has been estimated (Hartman, 1970), that a driver acquires over 90% of his information visually, an understanding of drivers' visual information acquisition patterns and cues would be not only desirable, but essential to an understanding of the input side of the driving process. If visual driving cues could be identified, they could be explicitly considered both in the formulation of driving models and in the design of the roadway environment. This could have a dual benefit of improving the quality of both.

Two approaches have been used to investigate the visual cues utilized by the driver. One is based on a theoretical analysis of the driver's visual field, and the other involves measurement of the driver's eye movement.

Gordon (1966b), Biggs (1966), and Fry (1968) have used the field theoretic approach to identify cues the driver might utilize. Their approach primarily involves a detailed mathematical analysis that results in a position, a velocity, and an acceleration for every point in the driver's view. From this model they then attempt to identify plausible visual cues.

Although disagreeing on some points, these independent analyses tend to be in general agreement that under steady-state driving conditions, the driver's most likely visual cues are the right or left edge markings, the center line, and

[1]This research was conducted as part of the aims of the Ohio State University Engineering Experimental Station Project EES 428, titled "Improving Driver Performance on Curves in Rural Highways Through Perceptual Changes." This was a cooperative project funded by the Ohio Department of Transportation and the Federal Highway Administration.

the entire roadway. Fry (1968) suggests that the most precise directional information is given by focus of expansion — that point in the moving visual field straight ahead of the driver, where objects appear stationary. This hypothesis would appear to be supported by the results of Mourant and Rockwell (1971), who found that experienced drivers tend to concentrate their fixations close to the focus of expansion.

Similarly, Gordon (1966b) has suggested that a change in perceived position relative to the lane markers may serve as a perceptual cue for corrections in lateral placement. This hypothesis has been supported by Bhise and Rockwell (1971). Their results indicate that lateral vehicle placement can be and is monitored peripherally.

Although helpful in identifying plausible visual cues, this theoretical analysis is somewhat faulty in that it tends to neglect the human being as part of the system, dwelling on the *scene* rather than the *seen.* For example, the visual field is developed in geometric perspective. Although this would, in fact, correspond to the retinal image, it is probably not how the driver actually perceives the world. Perceptual principles like size and shape constancy suggest that the driver's perceptions of the world and retinal image are not homomorphic.

The analysis of the driver's eye fixations is based on the assumption that drivers will fixate their eyes on areas of high information content. This assumption has been supported in the laboratory by Mackworth and Morandi (1967) and Zusne and Michels (1964). Yarbus (1967) has added credibility to this assumption by showing that subjects tend to fixate areas in the visual environment where they expect to find information relevant to their task.

One of the earlier attempts to isolate experimentally the driver's visual inputs by an analysis of his fixation locations was conducted by Gordon (1966a). In this study, subjects were required to drive along a curved road while wearing a specially constructed helmet which allowed only a monocular view of the roadway through either a 9-3/4° or 4° aperture. His results indicated that drivers time-share between scanning the roadway ahead and acquiring lateral position information. The primary source of the lateral position information was the roadway edge markings and the center line (viewed foveally in this case).

In another experimental investigation, Wright (1968), using electrooculographic techniques, investigated subjects' eye movements on both straight and curved rural roadway sections. He found that the fixation frequency varied with roadway type and subject, but that the fixation durations did not. The average eye displacement angle from the roadway center line also varied with the roadway geometry. When compared to straight sections, the eye fixation location moved to the left on left curves, to the right on right curves, and down in both cases. Mourant and Rockwell (1971), in a similar study, found experienced drivers' eye fixation location moved to the right on approaching a right turn but did not show a significant change when approaching a left curve.

The purpose of the following study was to investigate the driver's visual information acquisition activity by exploring the stochastic nature of his eye movement pattern. An ancillary objective was the exploration of the effects of increased speed stress on the driver's visual search activity.

THE RESEARCH SETTING

Because of the complexity of the driving task and the manifold factors affecting the driver's performance, it was necessary to limit the scope of the research. Therefore, the research was restricted to drivers unfamiliar with specific low density rural highways during daylight hours.

Dependent Measures.   Drivers' eye fixation patterns may be characterized in a multitude of ways, each being appropriate for a given situation. The five primary measures selected for analysis were: the duration of the driver's eye fixations, the travel distance in degrees between successive fixation locations, the horizontal coordinate of the fixation, the vertical coordinate of the fixation, and the blink rate.

These measures were recorded using an Eye Marker System installed in a 1970 Chrysler Newport. The Eye Marker System is based on a corneal reflection technique whereby a light spot indicating the point of fixation is superimposed on a scene of the roadway and then recorded. The dependent measures are then encoded for analysis manually, via a superimposed grid system. The interested reader is referred to Rockwell, Bhise, and Mourant (1972) for a more detailed description of the Eye Marker System.

Subject Selection.   The five subjects selected for the research were all paid volunteer college students. Subjects V and P were female. Prior to their selection as subjects, each was submitted to a screening procedure involving a vision test and a questionnaire. The preselection questionnaire was used to examine the volunteer's driving experience and familiarity with the route.

Route Selection.   Several factors that influenced the route selection were the route length, anticipated traffic density, and the roadway geometry. The route selected was comprised of sections of State Routes 315 and 257, and U.S. Route 42, all in Delaware County, Ohio. Eight sections of the roadway were actually used for data collection. Two sections, 1 and 4, were straight or tangent sections with the remaining six sections comprised of curved and straight roadway.

An appropriate characterization was required for the investigation of the relationship between eye movements and the roadway geometry. An economical method for describing the roadway geometry has been suggested by Crossman and Szastak (1968). If we let θ represent the arc length position along the highway from some arbitrary point and $h(\theta)$ the heading of the tangent to the roadway center line at θ, then, since highways are usually constructed of tangent (straight) sections connected by circular arcs, the function $h(\theta)$ is a special kind of stochastic variable whose first derivative, the highway curvature,

$$c(\theta) = dh(\theta)/d\theta \qquad (1)$$

takes on a sequence of randomly chosen constant values for successive sets of ranges of θ. This method of characterizing the roadway was adopted.

Experimental Procedure.   The two independent variables included in the research plan were the vehicle speeds, 40 and 60 mph, and the eight roadway sections. The experimental procedure called for each subject to make two runs over the route, so that the order of presentation of the roadway sections was fixed. The subjects were instructed to maintain 40 mph or 60 mph on each run with the order of the speeds randomly determined. At least two days were allowed to elapse between successive runs for any subject. At the start of each trial, the subject drove the instrumented vehicle to a location about eight-tenths of a mile from the beginning of the first test section. After the Eye Marker System was set up and properly calibrated, the subject was read a set of instructions which included the average speed he was to maintain, and then told to proceed around the route. Precautions were taken to avoid car-following situations.

PRELIMINARY ANALYSIS

An examination of the subjects' average speeds for each section indicated that the instructions were effective. With one exception each of the average speeds for the 60 mph trials were higher than those of the lower speed trials.

The overall average of 38 mph for the low nominal level was quite close to the target value, but the 47.95 mph average was considerably below the higher target value. This would suggest that the high nominal speed level represented a high stress situation because the subjects could not reach or even approach the target speed.

An examination of the individual subjects averages revealed that while subject *S, Z,* and *V* exhibited speed differentials of 14.07, 10.50, and 7.78 mph between the two speed sets respectively, subject *P*'s speed differential was only 4.93 mph. However, with one exception, where there was an exceptionally high 40 mph speed, the subject *P* drove faster at the higher speed than the remaining subjects did at the lower level.

Since six of the possible 16 data points for subject *G* were missing due either to procedural error or to equipment failure, his results were discarded. The addi-

TABLE 1
Results of the Preliminary Analysis
of the Driver's Eye Movements
(Randomized Block Design)

Dependent Measures	Roadway (7)	Speed Set (1)	Roadway x Speed Interaction (7)
Mean Fixation Duration	$p < 0.001$	$p < 0.01$	
Standard Deviation of Fixation Duration	$p < 0.0005$		
Mean Travel Distance	$p < 0.005$	$p < 0.025$	$p < 0.05$
Standard Deviation Travel Distance	$p < 0.005$	$p < 0.05$	
Mean Horizontal Location			
Mean Vertical Location			
Standard Deviation Horizontal Location	$p < 0.005$		
Standard Deviation Vertical Location	$p < 0.005$		
Mean Blink Rate	$p < 0.005$		

tional two missing data points were estimated using Yates procedure, and an analysis of variance was performed on each of the eight dependent measures. The analysis of variance assumed randomized block design and treated the subjects as a random effect and the two treatment factors as fixed effects.

Table 1 shows that the mean and the standard deviation of the fixation duration, the mean and standard deviation of the travel distance, the standard deviation of both the horizontal and vertical eye fixation location, and the mean blink rate were all significantly affected by the roadway geometry. Only the mean horizontal and vertical fixation locations were unaffected.

The plot of standard deviation of horizontal and vertical eye fixation locations versus road geometry, shown in Fig. 1 and 2, indicates that the driver's eye fixation locations were more dispersed on the curved roadway sections. Although the mean travel distance, shown in Fig. 3, was also significantly affected by the roadway type, this relationship is apparently more complex, since the increase was not uniform across all curved sections. There was, as illustrated in Fig. 4, a significant decrease in the driver's eye fixation durations on the curved roadway sections.

The effects of speed stress on the performance measures are not as straightforward as those of the roadway type. An examination of Table 1 suggests that only the mean fixation durations, the mean travel distance, and the standard deviation of the travel distance were significantly affected.

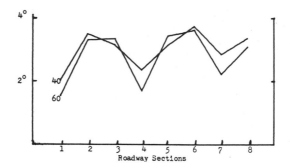

FIG. 1.   Standard deviation of the horizontal eye fixation location.

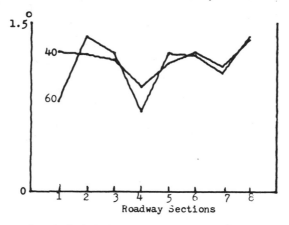

FIG. 2.   Standard deviation of the vertical eye fixation location.

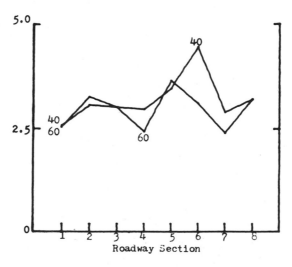

FIG. 3.   Mean eye fixation travel distance.

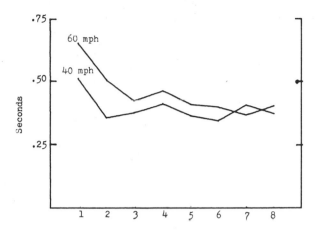

FIG. 4.   Mean fixation duration by roadway and speed.

Since a number of authors, Drew (1951) and Poulton and Gregory (1952), for example, have interpreted blink rates to be a measure of task difficulty or task induced stress, the absence of a significant speed effect on the blink rate was particularly interesting. An examination of the individual blink rates indicated subject S's ($a < 0.01$), subject Z's ($a < .001$), and subject V's ($a < 0.01$) blink rates significantly decreased with increasing speed stress. These three subjects' mean blink rate of 24.62 blinks per min at the 40 mph level dropped to an average of only 4.93 at the higher level. Conversely, the increase in subject P's blink rate from 6.7 blinks per min at the lower level to 14.5 at the higher level was not statistically significant. Thus, it may be concluded that the increased speed stress caused a substantial decrease in the blink rate for three of the four subjects.

Although the analysis of variance failed to show any significant speed effect on the standard deviation of the horizontal eye fixation location, it was felt that the behavior on the two straight sections would be sufficiently different from the other six sections to justify a separate analysis. Here a paired t-test revealed that the increase in speed resulted in a significant ($a \leq 0.0001$) decrease in the standard deviation of the horizontal eye fixation location.

NESTED TIME SERIES ANALYSIS OF THE DRIVER'S EYE MOVEMENTS ON THE STRAIGHT ROADWAY

Because the driver's eye movement records are composed of a sequence of constant eye fixation locations separated by effectively instantaneous movements between locations, certain problems arise in the analysis of these records. The visual technique of sampling the records at equally spaced time intervals will, in this case, have the effect of passing the records through a low-pass filter.

Because of this phenomenon, it was concluded that the eye fixation records should first be analyzed as nested time series; that is, the eye movement records were sampled only when a change in the fixation location occurred. Since substantial differences between the two types of roadway were expected, separate analyses were performed for each.

A similar procedure was utilized for analyzing both the horizontal and vertical eye movement records. For the two straight roadway segments each series was first checked for a trend. If there was a significant ($a < .05$) trend present, then this trend was removed by least squares estimation and the auto-covariance function calculated out of 20 lags. The sample power spectra were then calculated using a rectangular lag window and a lag number of 10. It was interesting to note that 6 of 16 horizontal and 6 of 16 vertical series showed statistically significant ($a < 0.05$) linear trends.

Since the primary hypothesis of interest in this phase of the analysis was the possibility that all the horizontal and all the vertical series of eye fixation locations represented white noise, a simultaneous test of the hypothesis that all the series represented white noise was needed.

To satisfy this need a Chi-squared test for white noise was developed. The test devised is based on Barlett's homogeneity of variance test.

Since the estimated power spectrum, $C(f)$, at frequency f is given by:

$$C(f) = 2\Delta \left[\hat{V}_X(o) + 2 \sum_{k=1}^{L} \hat{V}_X(k)w(k) \cos 2\pi f k \right] \qquad (2)$$

for $0 < f < 1/2$, where Δ represents the sampling interval, $\hat{V}_X(k)$ represents the auto-covariance at lag k and $w(k)$ is the time domain smoothing function; and under the white noise null hypothesis,

$$E[\hat{V}_X(k)] = 0 \text{ for all } k > 0$$

$$= \sigma_X^2 \text{ for } k = 0 \qquad (3)$$

therefore

$$E[C(f)] = 2\Delta \hat{V}_X(0) = 2\Delta \sigma_X^2 \qquad (4)$$

In addition, Jenkins and Watts (1968) have shown that if a rectangular smoothing function is used, then the power spectra estimates $1/(2 L)$ apart, where L is the number of lags, are approximately independent. Since there are $L + 1$ independent estimations in each sample power spectrum, and since Jenkins and Watts (1968) have shown that the quantity

$$\frac{\gamma C_X(f)}{2\Delta \sigma_X^2} ,$$

where γ is the number of degrees of freedom associated with each $C_X(f)$, is approximately distributed as a Chi-Square, with γ degrees of freedom, then the statistic

$$X_L^2 = \ln(10) \, {}^*\gamma^* [(L+1) \log \sigma_X^2 - \sum_{i=0}^{L} \log C_X(f_i) + (L+1) \log(2 \, \Delta)] \quad (5)$$

is distributed approximately as a Chi-square with L degrees of freedom. Moreover independent Chi-Squares may be added to create a new Chi-Squared distribution therey providing the test desired.

When the Chi-Square statistics were calculated and added, the resulting values (each with 150° of freedom) were 309.7 and 237.6 for the horizontal and vertical components respectively. They are both significant at the $a = 0.01$ level. An additional pooled test was also performed on the first lag auto-correlation coefficient with a similar result. The pure white noise hypothesis must be rejected.

The behavior of the drivers, therefore, in selecting next points of regard is constrained. The point chosen is drawn from the domain of possible points with a nonuniform probability distribution. This constraint does not, of course, imply that there is any systematic behavior. In any event, the principle component of the total variability of the performance is random.

A consideration of the processes under study suggests that the linear trends observed in several of the series should be interpreted as a very low frequency component rather than as a trend. This, combined with the high power at low frequencies observed in some of the series, would imply that there is a tendency for the driver's mean fixation location to oscillate slowly.

NESTED ANALYSIS OF THE DRIVER'S EYE MOVEMENT
ON CURVED ROADWAYS

Horizontal Axis.   Since they were not long enough for a detailed analysis, roadway sections 5, and 6, and 7 were omitted from the analysis. This left sections 2, 3, and 8 for analysis.

The analysis for the curved section essentially parallels that for the straight roadway. First, any significant trends were removed via least squares estimation, and the auto-correlation functions were estimated for each subject—roadway combination. The power spectra were estimated using a lag number of 100 and a Tukey smoothing function.

Most of the power spectra exhibited a well-defined peak at a low frequency such as that of subject S at 60 mph on roadway section 2 illustrated in Fig. 5. Several spectra failed to exhibit any well-defined peak.

Since the effects of speed stress and roadway geometry rather than the white noise hypothesis were of interest in this phase of the analysis, summary statistics

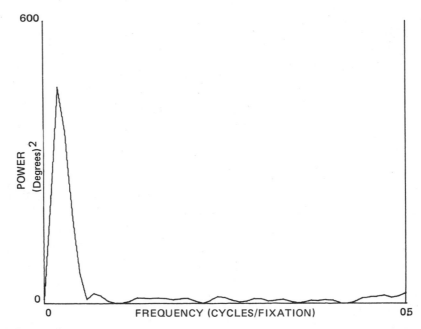

FIG. 5.   The power spectra for the horizontal coordinate for Subject S at 60 miles per hour on roadway section 2.

depicting the series were needed. The four selected were the peak or power density, the frequency at which this peak occurred, the ratio of the peak to the mean power density, and the median frequency (the frequency below which was 50% of the power. These summary statistics are shown in Table 2 for each subject roadway speed combination.

A brief examination of these summary statistics would suggest there were substantial subject differences present. The generally higher peak to mean power ratios 11.93 and 10.09 for S and Z versus 3.80 and 5.94 for V and P would imply the latter subjects' eye movement patterns were more random. Additionally, the average median frequencies of 0.086 and 0.063 for subjects S and Z compared to 0.198 and 0.158 for V and P would imply that the latter subjects' eye fixation locations were changing more rapidly.

In order to assess the statistical significance of the differences, a univariate analysis of variance was performed on each variable. In these analyses, subjects were assumed to be a random effect and the treatments to be fixed effects. In each case the subject and subject-by-speed interaction terms dominated the partitioned sum of squares with only the subject-by-speed interaction approaching statistical significance. This interaction was significant for the peak power $[F(3, 6) = 8.4, p < 0.025)$, frequency of the peak power $[F(3, 6) = 5.55, p < 0.05]$, and the peak to mean power ratio $[F(3, 6) = 3.42, p < 0.05]$; the median frequency was not statistically significant. These significant interactions suggest

TABLE 2
Summary Statistics for the Time Series Analysis for
the Horizontal Component of the Eye Movement Record

Roadway	Section 2		3		8	
Speed	40	60	40	60	40	60
Subject	Peak to Mean Power Ratio					
S	11.88	13.68	10.21	17.92	3.19*	14.86
Z	6.97	13.15	11.83	12.44	6.67	9.52
V	5.05*	6.78	1.77*	3.90	2.83*	2.48
P	7.19	3.20*	5.11	6.13	11.23*	2.78
	Median Frequency					
S	.03	.03	0.6	.04	.28*	.08
Z	.06	.04	.08	.04	.15	.10
V	.17*	.17	.25*	.18	.17	.25
P	.12	.28*	.13	.16	.03*	.23
	Frequency of Peak Power					
S	.015	.022	.010	.014	.009	.014
Z	.016	.027	.010	.014	.014	.016
V	.031*	.021	.037*	.014	.023*	.020
P	.020	.020*	.016	.020	.025	.023
	Peak Power					
S	285	465	204	430	83*	386
Z	121	341	201	298	213	266
V	161*	203	60*	187	130*	104
P	359	96*	153	135	561*	116

*Estimated from short records

that the effects of speed stress on driver's eye movement patterns are substantially mediated by individual differences.

While subjects V and P failed to show any consistent effects of increased speed stress, S and Z did. Each showed an increase in the peak power frequency with increased speed while simultaneously exhibiting a decrease in the median frequency. This, along with the systematic increase in the peak power and the peak-to-mean power ratio, implies that the main effects of speed stress on these two subjects was an elimination of the noise from their visual information acquisition patterns.

This suggests they were utilizing a larger proportion of their total visual information acquisition capacity to acquire information relevant to the driving task at the higher speeds, and eliminating the nondriving related activity. This conclusion is consistent with the earlier conclusion about the effects of speed stress on visual information acquisition behavior on straight roadways.

Vertical Axis.   A similar analysis was performed for the vertical coordinate of the eye fixation location. The subject-by-speed interaction was statistically significant for the peak power [$F(3,6) = 3.9, p < 0.1$] and the median frequency [$F (3, 6) = 7.76, p < 0.01$] and the subject-by-roadway interaction was significant for the peak-to-mean power ratio [$F (6, 6) = 5.05, p < 0.05$]. None of the main effects or interactions was statistically significant for the frequency of the peak power.

It has been hypothesized that the frequency of the peak power in the vertical axis would be approximately double that of the horizontal axis, since it was believed that the driver would reduce his preview distance, that is, lower his point of regard, on both right and left hand curves as suggested by Wright (1968). An examination of the peak power frequencies for both axes did not support this position. No consistent effects of speed stress were evidenced in the vertical eye fixation data.

RELATIONSHIP BETWEEN THE DRIVER'S EYE MOVEMENTS AND THE ROADWAY GEOMETRY

The objective of the final phase of the analysis was a better understanding of the nature of the relationship between the driver's eye movements and the roadway geometry. Since eye movement records with a high signal to noise ratio were desired for this analysis, only the eye movement records for subjects S and Z for the 60 mph trial on roadway sections 2 and 3 were analyzed.

As previously noted, the roadway was characterized in terms of the rate of change of the center line tangent with distance, similar to the method suggested by Crossman and Szastak (1968). The actual units used were degrees per one hundredth mile. Each roadway record was then translated into a description by estimating the time at which the driver entered and exited each curve.

This description along with the horizontal and vertical eye movement records were digitized at 0.2 sec time intervals. The auto- and cross-correlations (between highway and fixation locations) and the cross spectra were then estimated from the sampled data.

Although spurious cross-correlations may be developed between low frequency stochastic processes, an examination of the cross-correlations in Table 3 would suggest a close relationship did exist. It may be observed from this table that the maximum cross-correlation coefficients all occurred at positive lags of from 1.0 to 2.8 sec.

TABLE 3
The Cross-Correlation Between the Roadway
and the Eye Fixation Location

Subject Roadway Section	S		Z	
	2	3	2	3
Horizontal				
Zero lag Cross-Correlation	.6694	.3193	.4719	.3624
Maximum Cross-Correlation	.8157	.6116	.7460	.6741
Lead Time of Max. Cross-Correlation (Sec.)	1.0	2.4	2.8	1.8
Vertical				
Zero lag Cross-Correlation	−.5606	−.1304	−.0550	−.0683
Maximum Cross-Correlation	−.6238	−.4094	−.4344	−.2123
Lead Time of Max. Cross-Correlation (Sec)	1.0	2.0	2.6	1.4

From the estimated cross spectra, the frequency response function for the roadway geometry and horizontal eye movement system was estimated. In this process the roadway was considered the input and the eye fixation location as the output.

The estimated squared coherencies illustrated in Fig. 6 in the frequency range 0.025 to 0.150 Hz, with the exception of several values at or above 0.125, were all statistically significant at the $a = 0.05$ level. It should be observed that the squared coherencies were high whenever the input (roadway) power was high.

Further insight into the relationship may be gained by examining the gain functions as shown in Fig. 7. Again the two subjects appeared similar, although there are substantial differences between the two roadway sections.

Both subjects' gain functions for roadway section 3 are entirely above the corresponding estimates for section 2. The most likely source of this gain change is the substantial difference in curve amplitudes of the sections. The curves of roadway section 2 were appreciably greater than those for 3. Thus a nonlinear gain function would result in the behavior observed.

The phase angles shown in Fig. 8 between the horizontal eye movements and the roadway suggest that the driver's scan patterns actually led the roadway

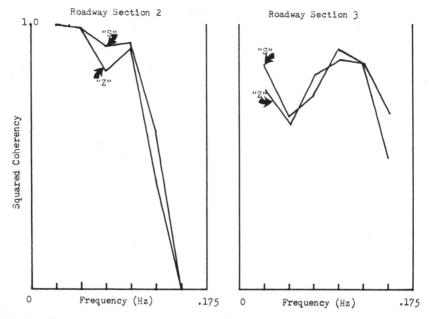

FIG. 6.   The squared coherency between the horizontal component of the driver's eye fixation location and the roadway.

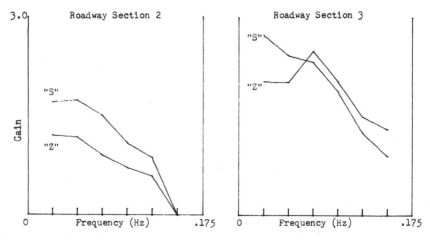

FIG. 7.   The gain between the roadway geometry and the horizontal component of the fixation location.

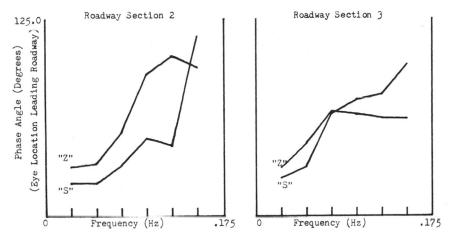

FIG. 8. The phase angle between the horizontal component of the driver's eye location and the roadway.

by 1.5 to 2 sec. In this case no differences between the two roadway sections were observed.

A similar analysis of the relationship between the vertical component of the eye fixation locations and roadway geometry was performed. As expected, this relationship was not as strong as that for the horizontal fixations. Only one subject's squared coherence was significant at the 0.05 level. For this reason the results of this analysis are not discussed further.

CONCLUSIONS

The results of the analysis suggest that whereas neither the horizontal nor the vertical component of the driver's eye fixation location may be considered a white noise process when driving on straight roadway sections, the nonwhite noise component, or constraint, accounted for only a small portion of the total behavior.

The major effect of introducing variable roadway geometry on the eye movement pattern is an increased dispersion of the eye fixation locations with a concomitant decrease in the mean fixation duration. The increased dispersion is, however, due primarily to a low frequency high amplitude component reflecting the roadway geometry.

The results engender several observations about the effects of speed stress on the driver's visual information acquisition behavior. Prior to the study it was hypothesized that drivers' mean eye fixation durations would decrease with increased speed due to their need to increase information processing rates. Quite the opposite results were observed; the drivers' mean fixation durations actually increased with increased speed.

The most plausible explanation of this phenomenon is that the drivers are making finer discriminations at the higher speeds, and that these demand longer fixation durations. This interpretation would be consistent with the model of visual information acquisition behavior developed and later validated by Senders (1955, 1964). Gould (1973) and others have also suggested that the need to make finer discriminations will usually result in longer fixation durations.

To understand better how the driver adapts to increased speed stress, one can consider the driver's information processing capacity as divided among processing driving-related visual information, nondriving-related visual information, and nonvisual information. In this additive model, an increase in the rate of processing of driving-related information would be accompanied by a decrease in other categories.

Thus the increased driver concentration, as reflected in the decrease in the standard deviation of the eye fixation location on straight roadways, and an increase in the peak to mean power ratios on curved roadway sections, may be interpreted as being indicative of an increase in the driver's rate of processing driving-related information.

The analysis of the relationship between the driver's horizontal eye movements and the roadway geometry indicated that the driver's eye movement pattern was leading the geometry by 1 to over 2½ sec. This amount of lead is surprising in light of the findings of Weir and McRuer (1968), McLean and Hoffman (1973), and Hoffman and Joubert (1966) that there is a critical preview time is reduced below this critical value, significant changes in driver behavior begin to occur. The lead times observed would suggest these drivers were operating close to or possibly below this critical value, leaving only a small margin for error. However, if there are two parallel visual processing systems, it could still be the case that we have been dealing primarily with the peripheral processor and its driving of horizontal movements in the curves.

DISCUSSION

ZWAHLEN: First, when you look at horizontal and vertical eye movements (H & Z) separately, you're ripping apart the process. Are H and V independent in driving?

McDOWELL: I never claimed that they were independent.

ZWAHLEN: Why didn't you run a cross-correlation between them.

McDOWELL: We did other things. I didn't attempt to run a cross-correlation on H and V, though it had occurred to me. One reason is that the earlier literature suggested that V does not vary linearly with H. We expect, for example,

V to show a decrease on both left and right curves, or perhaps no change at all on left curves and a decrease on right curves. Naturally, H goes to the right on right curves and to the left on left curves. So, I didn't expect any significant correlation between the two.

GIBBON: You indicated that the eye movements were less frequent and smaller at 60 mph than at 40 mph. I wondered if the subjects were spending more of their time looking at the expansion point of the field and having less time to look foveally at other points.

McDOWELL: That's a very good point. The effects of speed stress of behavior were interesting; we found that when speed went up concentration went up. This happened both on the curves and on the straight roadways. On the curves, the significant increase in the squared coherency indicated stronger concentration. The increased fixation duration at the higher speeds is more difficult to interpret. I would simply suggest that two things are happening. One is that the driver is inputting more information with each fixation, processing cues or signals with greater accuracy requiring longer fixation durations. The other thing that may be happening is the eliminating of noise from the visual process. I believe Senders, Christofferson, Levinson, Dietrich, and Ward (1966) showed that around 50% of drivers' fixations are probably not necessary. Their visual capacity isn't needed to watch the roadway all the time but as the demands went up a higher percentage of capacity was devoted to driving.

Part **VII**

REFERENCES

References

Abrams, S. G., & Zuber, B. L. Some temporal characteristics of information processing during reading. *Reading Research Quarterly,* 1972, *8,* 42–51.

Allington, R. L. *Developmental trends in the discrimination of high frequency words.* Paper presented at the annual meeting of the National Reading Conference, Atlanta, Ga., December 1976.

Alpern, M. Metacontrast. *Journal of the Optical Society of America,* 1953, *43,* 648–657.

Alpern, M. Movements of the eyes. In H. Davson (Ed.), *The Eye* (Vol. 3): *Muscular Mechanism.* New York: Academic Press, 1962.

Anderson, I. H. Studies of the eye-movements of good and poor readers. *Psychological Monographs,* 1937, *48,* 1–35.

Antes, J. R. The time course of picture viewing. *Journal of Experimental Psychology,* 1974, *103,* 62–70.

Astruc, J. Cortifugal connections of area 8 (frontal eye field) in *Macaca mulatta. Brain Research,* 1971, *33,* 241–256.

Bahill, A. T., & Stark, L. Overlapping saccades and glissades are produced by fatigue in the saccadic eye movement system. *Experimental Neurology,* 1975, *48,* 95–106.

Bahill, A. T., Clark, M. R., & Stark, L. Dynamic overshoot in saccadic eye movements caused by neurological control signal reversal. *Experimental Neurology,* 1975, *48,* 107–122.

Baker, M. A. *A model for predicting duration, location, and sequence of eye-fixation for metric polygons.* Paper presented at US Army Human Engineering Laboratory Conference, Eye Movements and Psychological Processes II: The higher functions, Monterey, Ca., February, 1977.

Bayle, E. The nature and causes of regressive movements in reading. *Journal of Experimental Education,* 1942, *11,* 16–36.

Becker, W., & Fuchs, A. F. Further properties of the human saccadic system: Eye movements and correction saccades with and without visual fixation points. *Vision Research,* 1969, *9,* 1247–1258.

Becker, W., & Jurgens, R. Saccadic reactions to double-step stimuli: Evidence for model feedback and continuous information uptake. In G. Lennerstrand & P. Bach-y-Rita (Eds.), *Basic Mechanisms of Ocular Motility and Their Clinical Implications*. New York: Pergamon, 1975.

Bender, L. Specific reading disability as a maturational lag. *Bulletin of the Orton Society*, 1957, *7*, 9–18.

Berlyne, D. E. The influence of complexity and novelty in visual figures on orienting responses. *Journal of Experimental Psychology*, 1958, *55*, 289–296.

Bertelson, P. The time course of preparation. *Quarterly Journal of Experimental Psychology*, 1967, *19*, 272–279.

Bhise, V. C., & Rockwell, T. H. The role of peripheral vision and time sharing in driving. *Proceedings of the Annual Meeting of the American Association for Automotive Medicine*, New York, 1971.

Biederman, I. Perceiving real-world scenes. *Science*, 1972, *177*, 77–80.

Biggs, N. L. Directional guidance of motor vehicles — A preliminary survey and analysis. *Ergonomics*, 1966, *9*, 193–202.

Bischof, N., & Kramer, E. Untersuchungen und überlegungen zur richtungswahrnehmung bei willkürlichen skkadischen augenbewegungen. *Psychologische Forschung*, 1968, *32*, 185–218.

Bizzi, E. Discharge of frontal eye field neurons during saccadic and following eye movements of unanesthetized monkey. *Experimental Brain Research*, 1968, *6*, 69–80.

Bizzi, E. The coordination of eye-head movements. *Scientific American*, 1974, *231*, 100–106.

Bizzi, E., & Schiller, P. H. Single unit activity in the frontal eye fields of unanesthetized monkeys during eye and head movement. *Experimental Brain Research*, 1970, *10*, 151–158.

Blair, W. C. Measurement of observing responses in human monitoring. *Science*, 1958, *128*, 255–256.

Blakemore, C., & Tobin, E. A. Lateral inhibition between orientation detectors in the cat's visual cortex. *Experimental Brain Research*, 1972, *15*, 439–440.

Bossom, J. Movement without proprioception. *Brain Research*, 1974, *71*, 285–296.

Bouma, H., & deVoogd, A. H. On the control of eye saccades in reading. *Vision Research*, 1974, *14*, 273–284.

Bouma, H., & Legein, Ch. P. Foveal and parafoveal recognition of letters and words by dyslexics and by average readers. *Neurophyschologia*, 1977, *15*, 69–79.

Bower, G. Mental imagery and associative learning. In L. Gregg (Ed.), *Cognition in learning and memory*. New York: Wiley, 1972.

Bower, G. H. Cognitive psychology: An Introduction. In W. K. Estes (Ed.), *Handbook of Learning and Cognitive Processes* (Vol. 1). Hillsdale, N.J.: Lawrence Erlbaum Associates, 1975.

Boynton, R. M., & Bush, W. R. Recognition of forms against a complex background. *Journal of the Optical Society of America*, 1956, *46*, 758–764.

Brandt, H. F. *The psychology of seeing*. New York: Philosophical Library. 1945.

Breitmeyer, B. G. A relationship between the detection of size, rate, orientation and direction in the human visual system. *Vision Research*, 1973, *13*, 41–58.

Breitmeyer, B. G. Simple reaction time as a measure of the temporal response properties of transient and sustained channels. *Vision Research*, 1975, *15*, 1411–1412.

Breitmeyer, B. G., & Ganz, L. Implications of sustained and transient channels for theories of visual pattern masking, saccadic suppression, and information processing. *Psychological Review*, 1976, *83*, 1–37.

Breitmeyer, B. G., & Ganz, L. Temporal integration as a function of spatial frequency. *Vision Research*, 1977, *17*, 861–865.

Breitmeyer, B., & Julesz, B. The role of on and off transients in determining the psychophysical spatial frequency response. *Vision Research*, 1975, *15*, 411–415.

Bridgeman, B., Hendry, D., & Stark, L. Failure to detect displacement of the visual world during saccadic eye movements. *Vision Research*, 1975, *15*, 719–722.

Brindley, G. S., & Merton, P. A. The absence of position sense in the human eye. *Journal of Physiology*, (London), 1960, *153*, 127–130.

Broadbent, D. E. *Perception and Communication*. Oxford: Pergamon, 1958.

Brooks, B. A. Vision and the visual evoked response during saccadic eye movement. In preparation.

Brooks, B. A., & Fuchs, A. F. Influence of stimulus parameters on visual sensitivity during saccadic eye movement. *Vision Research*, 1975, *15*, 1389–1398.

Brooks, B. A., & Jung, R. Neuronal physiology of the visual cortex. In R. Jung (Ed.), *Handbook of sensory physiology* (Vol. 7, Part 3). Berlin: Springer-Verlag, 1973.

Brooks, B. *An exploratory comparison of some measures of attention*. Unpublished master's thesis, Cornell University, 1961.

Brooks, V., & Hochberg, J. Control of active looking by motion picture cutting rate. *Proceedings of the Eastern Psychological Association*, 1976, *49*. (Abstract).

Bryden, M. P. The role of post-exposural eye movements in tachistoscopic perception. *Canadian Journal of Psychology*, 1961, *15*, 220–225.

Bugelski, B. R. Words and things and images. *American Psychologist*, 1970, *25*, 1001–1012.

Buswell, G. T. *How people look at pictures*. Chicago: University of Chicago Press, 1935.

Buswell, G. T. How adults read. *Supplementary Educational Monographs*, No. *45*, Chicago, Ill.: University of Chicago Press, 1937.

Byrne, B. Item concreteness vs. spatial organization as predictors of visual imagery. *Memory & Cognition*, 1974, *2*, 53–59.

Campbell, F. W. Correlation of accommodation between the two eyes. *Journal of the Optical Society of America*, 1960, *50*, 738.

Campbell, F. W., & Wurtz, R. H. Saccadic omission: Why we don't see a grey-out during a saccade eye movement. *Vision Research* (in press).

Carpenter, P. A., & Just, M. A. Linguistic influences on picture scanning. In R. A. Monty & J. W. Senders (Eds.), *Eye movements and psychological processes*. Hillsdale, N.J.: Lawrence Erlbaum Associates, 1976.

Carpenter, P. A., & Just, M. A. Reading comprehension as eyes see it. In M. A. Just & P. A. Carpenter (Eds.), *Cognitive processes in comprehension*. Hillsdale, N.J.: Lawrence Erlbaum Associates, 1977. (a)

Carpenter, P. A., & Just, M. A. Integrative processes in comprehension. In D. LaBerge & J. Samuels (Eds.), *Basic processes in reading: Perception and comprehension*. Hillsdale, N.J.: Lawrence Erlbaum Associates, 1977. (b)

Clark, H. H. Bridging. In R. Schank & B. Nash-Webber (Eds.), Theoretical issues in natural language processing. *Proceedings of a conference at the Massachusetts Institute of Technology*, June, 1975.

Cleland, B. G., Dubin, M., & Levick, W. R. Sustained and transient neurones in the cat's retina and lateral geniculate nucleus. *Journal of Physiology*, 1971, *217*, 473–496.

Cleland, B. G., Levick, W. R., & Sanderson, K. J. Properties of sustained and transient cells in the cat retina. *Journal of Physiology*, 1973, *228*, 649–680.

Coleman, J. C. Perceptual retardation in reading disability. *Perceptual and Motor Skills*, 1959, *9*, 117.

Collewijn, H., van der Mark, F., & Jansen, T. C. Precise recording of human eye movements. *Vision Research*, 1975, *15*, 447–450.

Cooper, L. A. Mental rotation of random two-dimensional shapes. *Cognitive Psychology*, 1975, *7*, 20–43.

Cooper, L. A., & Podgorny, P. Mental transformations and visual comparison processes: Effects of complexity and similarity. *Journal of Experimental Psychology: Human Perception and Performance,* 1976, *2,* 503–514.

Cooper, L. A., & Shepard, R. N. Chronometric studies of the rotation of mental images. In W. G. Chase (Ed.), *Visual information processing.* New York: Academic Press, 1973.

Cooper, L. A., & Shepard, R. N. Mental transformations in the identification of left and right hands. *Journal of Experimental Psychology,* 1975, *104,* 48–56.

Cornsweet, T. N. Determination of the stimuli for involuntary drifts and saccadic eye movements. *Journal of the Optical Society of America,* 1956, *46,* 987–993.

Cornsweet, T. N., & Crane, H. D. Servo-controlled infrared optometer. *Journal of the Optical Society of America,* 1970, *60,* 548–554.

Cornsweet, T. N., & Crane, H. D. Accurate two-dimensional eye tracker using first and fourth Purkinje images. *Journal of the Optical Society of America,* 1973, *63,* 921–928.

Craik, F. I. M., & Lockhart, R. S. Level of processing: A framework for memory research. *Journal of Verbal Learning and Verbal Behavior,* 1972, *11,* 671–684.

Crane, H. D., & Clark, M. R. A three-dimensional visual stimulus deflector. *Applied Optics,* 1978, *17,* 706–714.

Crane, H. D., & Steele, C. M. An accurate three-dimensional eyetracker. *Applied Optics,* 1978, *17,* 691–705.

Crossman, E., & Szastak, H. *Man-machine models for car steering.* Paper presented at the Fourth NASA/University Conference on Manual Control, University of Michigan, 1968.

Crovitz, H. F., & Daves, W. Tendency to eye movement and perceptual accuracy. *Journal of Experimental Psychology,* 1962, *63,* 495–498.

Cumming, G. D. Eye movements and visual perception. In E. C. Carterette & M. Friedman (Eds.), *Handbook of Perception* (Vol. VIII). New York: Academic Press, 1976.

Cynader, M., & Berman, N. Receptive-field organization of monkey superior colliculus. *Journal of Neurophysiology,* 1972, *35,* 187–201.

Dallos, P. J., & Jones, R. W. Learning behavior of the eye fixation control system. *IEEE Transactions on Automatic Control,* 1963, *AC-8,* 218–227.

Daneš, F. *Papers on functional sentence perspective.* The Hague: Mouton, 1974.

Davidson, M. L., Fox, M. J., & Dick, A. O. Effect of eye movements on backward masking and perceived location. *Perception and Psychophysics,* 1973, *14,* 110–116.

Dickinson, J. *Proprioceptive Control of Human Movement,* Princeton, N.J.: Princeton Book Co., 1974.

Ditchburn, R. W. Eye-movements in relation to retinal action. *Optica Acta,* 1955, *1,* 171–176.

Ditchburn, R. W. *Eye-Movements and Visual Perception,* Oxford: Claredon Press, 1973.

Ditchburn, R. W., & Ginsborg, B. L. Vision with a stabilized retinal image. *Nature* (London), 1952, *170,* 36–37.

Dodge, R. Visual perception during eye movement. *Psychological Review,* 1900, *7,* 454–465.

Dodge, R. The illusion of clear vision during eye movement. *Psychological Bulletin,* 1905, *2,* 193–199.

Dodge, R. An experimental study of visual fixation. *Psychological Monographs,* 1907, *8,* (No. 35), 1–92.

Dow, B. M. Functional classes of cells and their laminar distribution in monkey visual cortex. *Journal of Neurophysiology,* 1974, *37,* 927–946.

Drew, G. C. Variations in reflex blink rate during visual motor tasks. *Quarterly Journal of Experimental Psychology,* 1951, *3,* 73–88.

Duffy, F. H., & Burchfiel, J. L. Eye movement-related inhibition of primate visual neurons. *Brain Research,* 1975, *80,* 121–132.

Engel, F. L. Visual conspicuity, directed attention, and retinal locus. *Vision Research,* 1971, *11,* 563–576.

Enroth-Cugell, C., & Robson, J. G. The contrast sensitivity of retinal ganglion cells of the cat. *Journal of Physiology*, 1966, *187*, 517–552.

Erdmann, B., & Dodge, R. *Psychologische untersuchungen über das lesen*. Halle: Niemeyer, 1898.

Farley, A. M. A computer implementation of constructive visual imagery and perception. In R. A. Monty & J. W. Senders (Eds.) *Eye movements and psychological processes*. Hillsdale, N.J.: Lawrence Erlbaum Associates, 1976.

Faw, T. T., & Nunnally, J. C. The effects on eye movements of complexity, novelty and affective tone. *Perception and Psychophysics*, 1967, *2*, 263–267.

Fehrer, E., & Biederman, I. A comparison of reaction and verbal report in the detection of masked stimuli. *Journal of Experimental Psychology*, 1962, *64*, 126–130.

Fehrer, E., & Raab, D. Reaction time to stimuli masked by metacontrast. *Journal of Experimental Psychology*, 1962, *63*, 143–147.

Ferrier, D. The localization of function in the brain. *Proceedings of the Royal Society, B*, 1874, *22*, 229–232.

Festinger, L. Eye movements and perception. In P. Bach-y-Rita, C. C. Collins, & J. E. Hyde (Eds.), *The control of eye movements*. New York: Academic Press, 1971.

Festinger, L., & Canon, L. K. Information about spatial location based on knowledge about efference. *Psychological Review*, 1965, *72*, 373–384.

Festinger, L., & Easton, A. M. Inferences about the efferent system based on a perceptual illusion produced by eye movements. *Psychological Review*, 1974, *81*, 44–58.

Festinger, L., Sedgwick, H. A., & Holtzman, J. D. Visual perception during smooth pursuit eye movements, *Vision Research*, 1976, *16*, 1377–1386.

Fillmore, C. J. The case for case. In E. Bach & R. T. Harms (Eds.), *Universals in linguistic theory*. New York: Holt, Rinehart and Winston, 1968.

Finlay, B. L., Schiller, P. H., & Volkman, S. L. Quantitative studies of single-cell properties in monkey striate cortex, IV Corticotectal cells. *Journal of Neurophysiology*, 1976, *39*, 1352–1361.

Fisher, D. F. Dysfunctions in reading disability: There's more than meets the eye. In L. Resnick, & Weaver, P. (Eds.), *Theory and Practice in Beginning Reading Instruction* (Vol. 1). Hillsdale, N.J.: Lawrence Erlbaum Associates (in press).

Fisher, D. F. Spatial factors in reading and search: The case for space. In R. A. Monty & J. W. Senders (Eds.), *Eye movements and psychological processes*. Hillsdale, N.J.: Lawrence Erlbaum Associates, 1976.

Flagg, B. N., Allen, B. D., Geer, A. H., & Scinto, L. F. *Children's visual response to Sesame Street: A formative research report*. Unpublished report to Children's Television Workshop, Boston, 1976.

Fleming, D. G., Vossius, G. W., Bouman, G., & Johnson, E. L. Adaptive properties of the eye-tracking system as revealed by moving-head and open loop studies. *Annals of the New York Academy of Science*, 1969, *156*, 825–850.

Fleming, M. Eye movement indices of cognitive behavior. *Audio-visual Communications Review*, 1969, *17*, 383–398.

Ford, A., White, C. T., & Lichtenstein, M. Analysis of eye movements during free search. *Journal of the Optical Society of America*, 1959, *49*, 287–292.

Fribas, J. On defining the theme in functional sentence analysis. In J. Vachek (Ed.), *Travaux Linguistiques de Prague*. Alabama: University of Alabama Press, 1966.

Fribas, J. On the thematic and the non-thematic section of the sentence. In H. Ringborn (Ed.), *Style and Text*. Stockholm: Skriptor, 1975.

Fry, F. A. The use of the eyes in steering a car on straight and curved roads. *Journal of Optometry*, 1968, *45*, 374–391.

Fuchs, A. F. Saccadic and smooth pursuit eye movements in the monkey. *Journal of Physiology*, (London), 1967, *191*, 609–631.

Fuchs, A. F. The saccadic system. In P. Bach-y-Rita, C. C. Collins, & J. E. Hyde (Eds.), *The control of eye movements*. New York: Academic Press, 1971.

Fuchs, A. F. The neurophysiology of saccades. In R. A. Monty & J. W. Senders (Eds.), *Eye Movements and Psychological Processes.* Hillsdale, N.J.: Lawrence Erlbaum Associates, 1976.

Fukada, Y. Receptive field organization of cat optic nerve fibers with special reference to conduction velocity. *Vision Research,* 1971, *11,* 209–226.

Furst, C. J. Automatizing of visual attention. *Perception and Psychophysics,* 1971, *10,* 65–70.

Gaarder, K. Interpretive study of evoked responses elicited by gross saccadic eye movements. *Perceptual and Motor Skills,* 1967, *27,* 683–703.

Gaarder, K. *Eye movements, vision and behavior.* New York: Wiley, 1975.

Gagné, E. D., & Rothkopf, E. Z. Text organization and learning goals. *Journal of Educational Psychology,* 1975, *67,* 445–450.

Gardner, G. T. Evidence for independent parallel channels in tachistoscopic perception. *Cognitive Psychology,* 1973, *4,* 130–155.

Garland, L. H. Studies on the accuracy of diagnostic procedures. *American Journal of Roentgenology,* 1959, *82,* 25–38.

Gatev, V. Studies on the temporal characteristics of the saccadic eye movements in normal children. *Experimental Eye Research,* 1968, *7,* 63–72.

Gentles, W., & Llewellyn-Thomas, E. Commentary: effect of benzodiazepides upon saccadic eye movements in man. *Clinical Pharmacology Therapy,* 1971, *12,* 563–574.

Gerathewohl, S. J., & Strughold, H. Time consumption of eye movements and high-speed flying. *Aviation Medicine,* 1954, *3,* 38–45.

Gerrits, H. J. M., & Vendrik, A. J. H. Eye movements necessary for continuous perception during stabilization of retinal images. *Bibliotheca Ophthalmologica,* 1972, *82,* 339–347.

Gerrits, H. J. M., & Vendrik, A. J. H. The influence of stimulus movements on perception in parafoveal stabilized vision. *Vision Research,* 1974, *14,* 175–180.

Gibbon, S. Y. *Report on the Conference of Visual Information Processing Research and Technology to the National Institute of Education.* Washington, D.C.: National Institute of Education, 1975.

Gibson, E. J. *Principles of perceptual learning and development.* New York: Appleton-Century-Crofts, 1969.

Gibson, J. J. The visual perception of objective motion and subjective movement. *Psychological Review,* 1954, *61,* 304–314.

Gibson, J. J. Optical motions and transformations as stimuli for visual perception. *Psychological Review,* 1957, *64,* 288–295.

Gibson, J. J. *The Senses Considered as Perceptual Systems.* Boston: Houghton Mifflin, 1966.

Girgus, J. A developmental approach to the study of shape processing. *Journal of Experimental Child Psychology,* 1973, *16,* 363–374.

Girgus, J. A developmental study of the effect of eye movement on shape perception in a sequential viewing situation. *Journal of Experimental Child Psychology,* 1976, *22,* 386–399.

Girgus, J. & Hochberg, J. Age differences in shape recognition through an aperture in a free-viewing situation. *Psychonomic Science,* 1972, *28,* 237–238.

Gippenreiter, Yu. B., Romanov, V. Ia., & Smirnov, S. D. Eye and hand movements in the process of counting the elements of a test object. *Psikhologicheski Issledovaniya,* 1969, *1,* 51–56.

Goldberg, M. E., & Robinson, D. L. Visual responses of neurons in monkey inferior parietal lobule: The physiologic substrate of attention and neglect. *Neurology,* 1977, *27,* 350.

Goldberg, M. E. & Wurtz, R. H. Activity of superior colliculus in behaving monkey, I: Receptive fields of single neurons. *Journal of Neurophysiology,* 1972, *35,* 542–559. (a)

Goldberg, M. E. & Wurtz, R. H. Activity of superior colliculus in behaving monkey, II: Effect of attention on neuronal responses. *Journal of Neurophysiology,* 1972, *35,* 560–574. (b)

Goltz, T. H. Comparison of the eye movements of skilled and less-skilled readers. Unpublished doctoral dissertation, Washington University, St. Louis, Missouri, 1975.

Goodman, K. S. The psycholinguistic nature of the reading process. In K. S. Goodman (Ed.), *The psycholinguistic nature of the reading process,* Detroit: Wayne State University Press, 1968.

Goodwin, W. W., & Fender, D. H. The interaction between horizontal and vertical eye rotations in tracking tasks. *Vision Research,* 1973, *13,* 1701–1712.

Gordon, D. A. Experimental isolation of the driver's visual input. *Highway Research Record,* 1966, *122,* 129–137. (a)

Gordon, D. A. Perceptual basis of Vehicular Guidance. *Public Roads,* 1966, *34,* 53–68. (b)

Gordon, I. E. Eye movements during search through printed lists. *Perceptual and Motor Skills,* 1969, *29,* 683–686.

Gould, J. D. *Eye movements during visual search.* IBM Research Report. Yorktown Heights, New York, 1973.

Gould, J. D. Eye movements during visual search and memory search. *Journal of Experimental Psychology,* 1973, *98,* 184–195.

Gould, J. D. Looking at pictures. In R. A. Monty & J. W. Senders (Eds.), *Eye movements and psychological processes.* Hillsdale, N.J.: Lawrence Erlbaum Associates, 1976.

Gould, J. D., & Dill, A. B. Eye-movement parameters and pattern discrimination. *Perception and Psychophysics,* 1969, *6,* 311–320.

Gracfe, T. M., & Vaughan, J. Saccadic and manual reaction times to stimuli initiated by eye or finger movements. *Bulletin of the Psychonomic Society,* 1978, *11,* 97–99.

Gray, C. T. The anticipation of meaning as a factor in reading ability. *The Elementary School Journal,* 1923, 614–626.

Gregory, M., & Poulton, E. C. Even versus uneven right-hand margins and the rate of comprehension in reading. *Ergonomics,* 1970, *13,* 427–434.

Gregory, R. L. Eye movements and the stability of the visual world. *Nature,* 1958, *182,* 1214.

Gregory, R. L. *Eye and brain.* London: World University Press, 1966.

Gregory, R. L. The confounded eye. In R. L. Gregory & E. H. Gombrich (Eds.), *Illusion in nature and art.* London: Duckworth & Co., Ltd., 1973.

Growney, R. L. The function of contour in metacontrast. *Vision Research,* 1976, *16,* 253–262.

Guba, E., & Wolf, W. *Perception and television: Physiological factors of television viewing.* (ERIC Document Reproduction Service No. ED 003 610) Columbus, Ohio: Ohio State University Research Foundation, 1961-64.

Guiss, L. W., & Kuenstler, P. A retrospective view of survey photofluorograms of persons with lung cancer. *Cancer,* 1960, *13,* 91–95.

Guitton, D., & Mandl, G. The effect of frontal eye field stimulation on unit activity in the superior colliculus of the cat. *Brain Research,* 1974, *68,* 330–334.

Haber, R. N. Control of eye movements during reading. In R. A. Monty & J. W. Senders (Eds.), *Eye movements and psychological processes.* Hillsdale, N.J.: Lawrence Erlbaum Associates, 1976.

Haber, R. N. & Hershenson, M. *The psychology of visual perception.* New York: Holt, Rinehart and Winston, 1973.

Haddad, G. M., & Steinman, R. M. The smallest voluntary saccade: Implications for fixation. *Vision Research,* 1973, *13,* 1075–1086.

Hall, D. C. Eye movements in scanning iconic imagery. *Journal of Experimental Psychology,* 1974, *103,* 825–830.

Hallett, P. E., & Lightstone, A. D. Saccadic eye movements towards stimuli triggered by prior saccades. *Vision Research,* 1976, *16,* 99–106. (a)

Hallett, P. E. & Lightstone, A. D. Saccadic eye movements to flashed targets. *Vision Research,* 1976, *16,* 107–114. (b)

Hammill, D. Training visual perceptual processes. *Journal of Learning Disabilities,* 1972, *5,* 39–46.

Hansen, R. M., & Skavenski, A. A. Accuracy of eye position information for motor control, *Vision Research,* 1977, *17,* 919–926.

Hartmen, E. *Driver vision requirements.* 1970 International Automobile Safety Conference, New York: SAE, Inc. 1970.

Hawley, T. F., Stern, J. A., & Chen, S. C. Computer analysis of eye movements during reading. *Reading World,* 1974, *XIII,* 307–317.

Hebb, D. O. Concerning imagery. *Psychological Review,* 1968, *75,* 466–477.

Heilman, K. M., & Valenstein, E. Frontal lobe neglect in man. *Neurology,* 1972, *22,* 660–664.

Helmholtz, H., von. Handbuch der physiologischen optik (3rd ed.). In J. P. C. Southall (Ed. and trans.), *A treatise on physiological optics* (Vol. III). New York, Dover, 1962. (Originally published, 1909.)

Helmholtz, H., von. *Handbuch der physiologischen optik* (2nd ed.). Hamburg: G. Voss, 1896.

Hendry, D. P. Saccadic velocities determined by a new perceptual method. *Vision Research,* 1975, *15,* 149–151.

Hirschfeld, A. *The world of Hirschfeld.* New York: H. N. Abrams, Inc., 1970.

Hochberg, J. In the mind's eye. In R. N. Haber (Ed.), *Contemporary theory and research in visual perception.* New York: Holt, Rinehart, and Winston, 1968.

Hochberg, J. Attention, organization and consciousness. In D. I. Mostofsky (Ed.), *Attention: Contemporary theory and analysis.* New York: Appleton-Century-Crofts, 1970. (a)

Hochberg, J. Components of literacy: Speculation and exploratory research. In H. Levin & J. P. Williams (Eds.), *Basic studies on reading.* New York: Basic Books, 1970. (b)

Hochberg, J. Toward a speech-plan eye movement model of reading. In R. A. Monty & J. W. Senders (Eds.), *Eye movements and psychological processes.* Hillsdale, N.J.: Lawrence Erlbaum Associates, 1976.

Hochberg, J. & Brooks, V. The psychophysics of form: reversible-perspective drawings of spatial objects. *American Journal of Psychology,* 1960, *73,* 332–334.

Hochberg, J. & Brooks, V. The prediction of visual attention to designs and paintings. *American Psychologist,* 1962, *17,* 7. (Abstract)

Hochberg, J. & Brooks, V. Geometrical vs. directional factors in the prediction of attention distributions. *American Psychologist,* 1963, *18,* 437. (Abstract)

Hochberg, J. & Brooks, V. Reading as intentional behavior. In H. Singer (Ed.), *Theoretical Models and Processes of Reading.* Newark, Delaware: International Reading Association, 1970.

Hochberg, J., & Brooks, V. *The maintenance of perceptual inquiry: Quantitative tests of some simple models.* Paper read at the Spring 1974 meetings of the Society of Experimental Psychologists.

Hochberg, J. and Gellman, L. Feature saliency, "mental rotation" times, and the integration of successive views. *Memory and Cognition,* 1977, *5,* 23–26.

Hoffman, E. R., & Joubert, P. N. The effect of changes in some vehicle handling variables on driver steering performance. *Human Factors,* 1966, *8,* 245–263.

Holt, E. B. Eye-movement and central anaesthesia, I: The problem of anaesthesia during eye-movement. *Psychological Monographs,* 1903, *4,* 3–46.

Howarth, C. I., Beggs, W. D. A., & Bowden, J. M. The relationship between speed and accuracy of movement aimed at a target. *Acta Psychologica,* 1971, *35,* 207–218.

Hubel, D. H., & Wiesel, T. N. Receptive fields, binocular interaction and functional architecture in the cat's visual cortex. *Journal of Physiology,* 1962, *160,* 106–154.

Hubel, D. H. & Wiesel, T. N. Receptive fields and functional architecture of monkey striate cortex. *Journal of Physiology,* 1968, *195,* 215–243.

Huey, E. B. *The psychology and pedagogy of reading.* New York: MacMillan, 1908.

Humphrey, N. K. Responses to visual stimuli of units in the superior colliculus of rats and monkeys. *Experimental Neurology* 1968, *20,* 312–340.

Hyvärinen, J., & Poranen, A. Function of the parietal associative area 7 as revealed from cellular discharges in alert monkeys. *Brain,* 1974, *97,* 673–692.

Irvine, S. R., & Ludvigh, F. Is ocular proprioceptive sense concerned in vision? *Archives of Opthamology,* 1936, *15,* 1037–1049.

Jacoby, J., Chestnut, R. W., Fisher, W. A., & Weigl, K. C. Simulating nondurable purchase: individual differences and information acquisition behavior. *Purdue Papers in Consumer Psychology,* 1976, No. 153.

Jacoby, J., & Chestnut, R. W. Amount, type, and order of package information acquisition in purchasing decisions. Monograph in preparation [Final report to the National Science Foundation (GI-43687), 1977].

Jeannerod, M., & Chouvet, G. Saccadic displacement of the retinal image: Effects on the visual system in the cat. *Vision Research,* 1973, *13,* 161–169.

Jenkins, G. M., & Watts, D. G. *Spectral analysis and its application.* San Francisco: Holden-Day, 1968.

Johansson, G. *Spatio-temporal differentiation and integration in visual motion perception.* (Report #160). Uppsala, Sweden, Department of Psychology, 1974.

Jones, L., & Higgins, G. Photographic granularity and graininess, III: Some characteristics of the visual system of importance in the evaluation of graininess and granularity. *Journal of the Optical Society of America,* 1947, *37,* 217–263.

Jones, L., & Higgins, G. Photographic granularity and graininess, IV: Visual acuity thresholds, dynamic versus static assumptions. *Journal of the Optical Society of America,* 1948, *38,* 398–405.

Just, M. A., & Carpenter, P. A. Eye fixations and cognitive processes. *Cognitive Psychology,* 1976, *8,* 441–480. (a)

Just, M. A., & Carpenter, P. A. The role of eye-fixation research in cognitive psychology. *Behavior Research Methods and Instrumentations,* 1976, *8,* 139–143. (b)

Just, M. A., & Carpenter, P. A. The role of eye-fixation research in cognitive psychology. *Behavior Research Methods and Instrumentation,* 1976, *8,* 139–143. (c)

Kahneman, D. Temporal summation in an acuity task at different energy levels – A study of the determinants of summation. *Vision Research,* 1964, *4,* 557–166.

Kahneman, D. Method, findings, and theory in studies of visual masking. *Psychological Bulletin,* 1968, *70,* 404–425.

Kahneman, D. *Attention and effort.* Englewood Cliffs, N.J.: Prentice-Hall, Inc., 1973.

Kahneman, D., & Lass, N. Eye position in tasks of association and memory. Unpublished manuscript, Hebrew University, Jerusalem, 1971.

Kahneman, D., & Norman, J. The time-intensity relation in visual perception as a function of observer's task. *Journal of Experimental Psychology,* 1964, *68,* 215–220.

Kantowitz, B. H. Double stimulation. In B. H. Kantowitz (Ed.), *Human Information processing: Tutorials in performance and cognition.* Hillsdale, N.J.: Lawrence Erlbaum Associates, 1974.

Kaplan, R. M. Transient processing load in relative clauses. Unpublished doctoral dissertation, Harvard University, 1974.

Kaplan, R., & Rothkopf, E. Z. Instructional objectives as directions to learners: Effect of passage length and amount of objective-relevant content. *Journal of Educational Psychology*, 1974, *66*, 448–456.

Katz, J. *The language of thought.* Cambridge: MIT Press, 1975.

Kaufman, E. L., Lord, M. W., Reese, T. W. & Volkmann, J. The discrimination of visual number. *American Journal of Psychology*, 1949, *62*, 498–525.

Keesey, U. T. Effects of involuntary eye movements on visual acuity. *Journal of the Optical Society of America*, 1960, *50*, 769–774.

Keesey, U. T. Flicker and pattern detection: A comparison of thresholds. *Journal of the Optical Society of America*, 1972, *62*, 446–448.

Keesey, U. T., & Jones, R. M. The effect of micromovements of the eye and exposure duration on contrast sensitivity. *Vision Research*, 1976, *16*, 481–488.

Kirk, R. E. *Experimental design: Procedures for the behavioral sciences.* Belmont, Ca.: Brooks/Cole Publishing Co., 1968.

Kolers, P. *Aspects of motion perception.* Oxford: Pergamon Press, 1972.

Kolers, P. A. Buswell's discoveries. In R. A. Monty & J. W. Senders (Eds.), *Eye movements and psychological processes.* Hillsdale, N.J.: Lawrence Erlbaum Associates, 1976.

Kolers, P. Experiments in reading. *Scientific American*, 1972, *227*, 84–91.

Kolers, P. A., & Katzman, M. T. Naming sequentially presented letters and words. *Language and Speech*, 1966, *9*, 84–95.

Kolers, P. A., & Lewis, C. L. Bounding of letter sequences and the integration of visually presented words. *Acta Psychologica*, 1972, *36*, 112–114.

Kornmuller, A. E. Eine experimentelle anesthesie der auberen augenmuskein am menschen und ihre auswirKugen. *Journal für Psychologie und Neurologie*, 1930, *41*, 354–366.

Kowler, E. *Scanning in the microcosm, or, the role of small saccades in counting.* Paper presented at the U.S. Army Human Engineering Laboratories symposium, Eye movements and psychological processes II: The higher functions. Monterey, Ca., 1977.

Kowler, E., & Steinman, R. M. The role of small saccades in counting. *Vision Research*, 1977, *17*, 141–146.

Krauskopf, J., Graf, V., & Gaarder, K. Lack of inhibition during involuntary saccades. *American Journal of Psychology*, 1966, *79*. 73–78.

Krugman, H. E. Processes underlying exposure to advertising. *American Psychologist*, 1968, *23*, 245–53.

Kuffler, S. W. Discharge patterns and functional organization of mammalian retina. *Journal of Neurophysiology*, 1953, *16*, 37–68.

Kulikowski, J. J., & Leisman, G. The effect of nitrous oxide on the relation between the evoked potential and contrast threshold. *Vision Research*, 1973, *11*, 2079–2086.

Kulikowski, J. J., & Tolhurst, D. J. Psychophysical evidence for sustained and transient detectors in human vision. *Journal of Physiology*, 1973, *232*, 149–162.

Kundel, H. L. Visual sampling and estimates of the location of information on chest films. *Investigative Radiology*, 1974, *9*, 87–93.

Kundel, H. L. Peripheral vision, structural noise, and film reader error. *Radiology*, 1975, *144*, 269–273.

Kundel, H. L., & LaFollette, P. S. Visual search patterns and experience with radiological images. *Radiology*, 1972, *103*, 523–528.

Kundel, H. L., & Nodine, C. F. A computer system for processing eye movement records. *Behavior Research Methods and Instrumentation*, 1973, *5*, 147–152.

Kundel, H. L., & Revesz, G. Lesion conspicuity, structured noise, and film reader error. *American Journal of Roentgenology*, 1976, *126*, 1233–1238.

Kundel, H. L., & Wright, D. J. The influence of prior knowledge on visual search strategies during the viewing of chest films. *Radiology*, 1969, *93*, 315–320.

Künzle, H., Akert, K., & Wurtz, R. H. Projection of area 8 (frontal eye field) to superior colliculus in the monkey: An autoradiographic study. *Brain Research*, 1976, *117*, 487–492.

Laberge, D., & Samuels, S. J. Toward a theory of automatic information processing in reading. *Cognitive Psychology*, 1974, *6*, 293–323.

Lahey, B. B., & Lefton, L. A. Discrimination of letter combinations in good and poor readers. *The Journal of Special Education*, 1976, *10*, 205–210.

Lahey, B. B., & McNees, M. P. Letter discrimination errors in kindergarten through third grade: Assessment and operant training. *Journal of Special Education*, 1975, *9*, 191–199.

Lahey, B. B., McNees, M. P., & Brown, C. C. Modification of deficits in reading comprehension. *Journal of Applied Behavior Analysis*, 1973, *6*, 475–480.

Lahey, B. B., Sperduto, G. R., Beggs, V. E., & Lefton, L. A. *Comparison of letter discrimination of learning disabled and normal children under untimed classroom-like conditions.* Manuscript submitted for publication, 1978.

Lambert, R. H., Monty, R. A., & Hall, R. J. High speed data processing and unobtrusive monitoring of eye movements. *Behavior Research Methods and Instrumentation*, 1974, *6*, 525–530.

Landolt, E. Nouvelles recherches sur la physiologie des mouvements des yeaux. *Archives d'Ophtalmologie*, 1891, *11*, 385–395.

Larsen, S. C., & Hammill, D. The relationship of selected visual-perceptual abilities in school learning. *Journal of Special Education*, 1975, *9*, 282–291.

Latour, P. L. Visual threshold during eye movements. *Vision Research*, 1962, *2*, 261–262.

Latour, P. L. *Cortical control of eye movements.* Unpublished doctoral thesis, Institute for Perception RVO–TNO, Soesterberg, The Netherlands, 1966.

Lefton, L. A. Metacontrast: A review. *Perception and Psychophysics*, 1973, *13*, 161–171.

Leisman, G. Conditioning variables in attentional handicaps. *Neuropsychologia*, 1973, *11*, 199–205.

Leisman, G. The relationship between saccadic eye movements and the alpha rhythm in attentionally handicapped patients. *Neuropsychologia*, 1974, *12*, 209–218.

Leisman, G. Characteristics of saccadic eye movements in attentionally handicapped patients. *Perceptual and Motor Skills*, 1975, *40*, 803–809.

Leisman, G. The neurophysiology of visual processing: Implications for learning disability. In G. Leisman (Ed.), *Basic visual processes and learning disability.* Springfield, Ill.: Charles C Thomas, 1976. (a)

Leisman, G. The role of visual processes in attention and its disorders. In G. Leisman (Ed), *Basic visual processes in learning disability.* Springfield, Ill.: Charles C Thomas, 1976. (b)

Leisman, G. Functional cortical analtomy in relation to visual processing and learning disability. In G. Leisman (Ed.), *Basic visual processes in learning disability.* Springfield, Ill.: Charles C Thomas, 1976. (c)

Leisman, G. A note on the effect of stabilized retinal image on active visual memory in brain damaged patients. *Neuropsychologia*, 1977, *16*, 449–450. (a)

Leisman, G. Return sweep latency in reading with a paralyzed eye. *Perceptual Motor Skills*, 1977, *44*, 1169–1170. (b)

Leisman, G. Ocular-motor factors in visual perceptual response efficiency. *Human Factors*, 1978 (in press).

Leisman, G., & Schwartz, J. Ocular-motor variables in reading discorders. In R. M. Knights & D. K. Bakker (Eds.), *The neuropsychology of learning disorders: Theoretical approaches.* Baltimore, Md.: University Park Press, 1976.

Leisman, G., & Schwartz, J. Ocular-motor function and visual information processing: Implications for the reading process. *International Journal of Neuroscience,* 1977, *8,* 7—15.

Leisman, G., Sprung, L., Ashkenazi, M., & Schwartz, J. Aetiologic factors in dyslexia; II. Ocular-motor programming, *Perceptual Motor Skills* (in press).

Lesser, G. S. *Children and television: Lessons from Sesame Street.* New York: Random House, 1974.

Leushina, L. I. On estimation of position of photostimulus and eye movements. *Biofizika,* 1965, *10,* 130—136.

Levin, H., & Kaplan, E. L. Grammatical structure and reading. In H. Levin & J. P. Williams (Eds.), *Basic studies on reading,* New York: Basic Books, Inc., 1970.

Llewellyn-Thomas, E., & Landsdown, E. L. Visual search patterns of radiologists in training. *Radiology,* 1963, *81,* 288—292.

Loftus, G. R. A framework for a theory of picture recognition. In R. A. Monty & J. W. Senders (Eds.), *Eye Movements and Psychological Processes.* Hillsdale, N.J.: Lawrence Erlbaum Associates, 1976.

Lotze, R. H. *Medicinische Psychologie.* (Reprinted) Amsterdam: Bonet, 1966. (Originally published, 1852.)

Ludvigh, E. Possible role of proprioception in the extra ocular muscles. *A.M.A. Archives Ophthalmology,* 1952, *48,* 436—441. (a)

Ludvigh, E. Control of ocular movements and visual interpretation of environment. *A.M.A. Archives Ophthalmology,* 1952, *48,* 442—448. (b)

Luria, S. M., & Strauss, M. S. Eye movements during search for coded and uncoded targets. *Perception and Psychophysics,* 1975, *17,* 303—308.

Lyle, J. G. Reading retardation and reversal tendency: A factorial study. *Child Development,* 1969, *40,* 833—843.

Mach, E. *The analysis of sensations.* (C. M. Williams, trans.) New York: Dover, 1959.

Mack, A. An investigation of the relationship between eye and retinal image movement in the perception of motion. *Perception and Psychophysics,* 1970, *8,* 291—298.

Mack, A., & Herman, E. Position constancy during pursuit eye movement: An investigation of the Filehne illusion, *Quarterly Journal of Experimental Psychology,* 1973, *25,* 71—84.

MacKay, D. M. Elevation of visual threshold by displacement of retinal image. *Nature* (London), 1970, *225,* 90—92.

MacKay, D. M. Visual stability. *Investigative Ophthalmology,* 1972, *11,* 518—524.

MacKay, D. M. Visual stability and voluntary eye movements. In R. Jung (Ed.), *Handbook of Sensory Physiology* (Vol. 7, part 3: *Central Processing of Visual Information*). Berlin: Springer-Verlag, 1973.

Mackworth, N. H. Visual noise causes tunnel vision. *Psychonomic Science,* 1965, *3,* 67—68.

Mackworth, N. H. Personal communication, 1973.

Mackworth, N. H. Stimulus density limits the useful field of view. In R. A. Monty, & J. W. Senders, (Eds.), *Eye movements and psychological processes.* Hillsdale, N.J.: Lawrence Erlbaum Associates, 1976.

Mackworth, N. H., & Bruner, J. S. How adults and children search to recognize pictures. *Human Development,* 1971, *13,* 149—177.

Mackworth, N., & Morandi, A. J. The gaze selects informative details within pictures. *Perception and Psychophysics,* 1967, *2,* 547—552.

Marshall, W., & Talbot, S. Recent evidence for neural mechanisms in vision leading to a general theory of sensory acuity. In J. Cattell (Ed.), *Biological Symposia* (Vol. 8). Lancaster, Pa.: Cattell Press, 1942.

Mateeff, St., Yakimoff, N., & Mitrani, L. Some characteristics of the visual masking by moving contours. *Vision Research,* 1976, *16,* 489—492.

Matin, E. Saccadic suppression: A review and an analysis. *Psychological Bulletin,* 1974, *81,* 899–917.

Matin, E. The two-transient (masking) paradigm. *Psychological Review,* 1975, *82,* 451–461.

Matin, E. Saccadic suppression and the stable world. In R. A. Monty, & J. W. Senders, (Eds.), *Eye movements and psychological processes.* Hillsdale, N.J.: Lawrence Erlbaum Associates, 1976.

Matin, E., Clymer, A., & Matin, L. Metacontrast and saccadic suppression. *Science,* 1972, *178,* 179–182.

Matin, L. Eye movements and perceived visual direction. In D. Jameson & L. Hurvich (Eds.), *Handbook of sensory physiology* (Vol. 7, Pt. 4): *Visual psychophysics.* New York: Academic Press, 1972.

Matin, L. Saccades and extraretinal signal for visual direction. In R. A. Monty & J. W. Senders (Eds.), *Eye movements and psychological processes.* Hillsdale, N.J.: Lawrence Erlbaum Associates, 1976.

Matin, L., Matin E., & Pearce, D. G. Visual perception of direction when voluntary saccades occur: I. Relation of visual direction of a fixation target extinguished before a saccade to flash presented during the saccade. *Perception and Psychophysics,* 1969, *5,* 65–80.

Matin, L., Matin E., & Pola, J. Visual perception of direction when voluntary saccades occur. II. Relation of visual direction of a fixation target extinguished before a saccade to a subsequent test flash presented before the saccade, *Perception and Psychophysics,* 1970, *8,* 9–14.

McLean, J. R., & Hoffman, E. R. The effects of restricted preview on driver steering control and performance. *Human Factors.* Vol. *15,* 1973, 421–430.

McConkie, G. W. The use of eye movement data in determining the perceptual span in reading. In R. A. Monty & J. W. Senders (Eds.). *Eye movements and psychological processes.* Hillsdale, N.J.: Lawrence Erlbaum Associates, 1976.

McConkie, G. W., & Rayner, K. *The span of the effective stimulus during fixations in reading.* Paper presented at the American Educational Research Association meetings, New Orleans, 1973.

McIlwain, J. T. Visual receptive fields and their images in superior colliculus of the cat. *Journal of Neurophysiology,* 1975, *38,* 219–230.

Mehler, J., Bever, T. G., & Cary, P. What we look at when we read. *Perception and Psychophysics,* 1967, *2,* 213–218.

Merton, P. A. The accuracy of directing the eye and the hand in the dark. *Journal of Physiology* (London), 1961, *156,* 555–577.

Metzler, J., & Shepard, R. Transformational studies of the internal representation of three-dimensional objects. In R. Solso (Ed.), *Theories in cognitive psychology: The loyola symposium.* Potomac, Md.: Lawrence Erlbaum Associates, 1974.

Miller, G. A. The magical number seven, plus or minus two. *Psychological Review,* 1956, *63,* 81–97.

Miller, G. A., & Johnson-Laird, P. N. *Perception and Language.* Cambridge: Harvard University Press, 1976.

Millodot, M. Foveal and extra-foveal acuity with and without stabilized retinal images. *British Journal of Physiological Optics,* 1966, *23,* 75–106.

Milldot, M. Variation of visual acuity in the central region of the retina. *British Journal of Physiological Optics,* 1972, *27,* 24–28.

Mitrani, L., Mateeff, St., & Yakimoff, N. Smearing of the retinal image during voluntary saccadic eye movements. *Vision Research,* 1970, *10,* 405–409. (a)

Mitrani, L., Mateeff, St., & Yakimoff, N. Temporal and spatial characteristics of visual suppression during voluntary saccadic eye movement. *Vision Research,* 1970, *10,* 417–422. (b)

Mitrani, L., Mateeff, St., & Yakimoff, N. Is saccadic suppression really saccadic? *Vision Research,* 1971, *11,* 1157–1161.

Mitrani, L., Radil-Weiss, T., Yakimoff, N., Mateeff, St., and Bŏzkov, V. Deterioration of vision due to contour shift over the retina during eye movements. *Vision Research,* 1975, *15,* 877–878.

Mitrani, L., Yakimoff, N., & Mateeff, St. Saccadic suppression in the presence of a structured background. *Vision Research,* 1973, *13,* 517–521.

Mock, K. *The relationship of audio-visual attention factos and reading ability to children's television viewing strategies.* Unpublished manuscript, Ontario Institute for Studies in Education, 1974.

Mohler, C. W., Goldberg, M. E., & Wurtz, R. H. Visual receptive fields of frontal eye field neurons. *Brain Research,* 1973, *61,* 385–389.

Mohler, C. W., & Wurtz, R. H. Effects of striate cortical and tectal lesions on saccadic eye movements. *Journal of Neurophysiology,* 1977, *40,* 74–94.

Monty, R. A., & Senders, J. W. (Eds.) *Eye Movements and Psychological Processes.* Hillsdale, N.J.: Lawrence Erlbaum Associates, 1976.

Morton, J. The effects of context upon speed of reading, eye movements and eye-voice span. *Quarterly Journal of Experimental Psychology,* 1964, *16,* 340–354.

Mountcastle, V. B. The world around us: Neural command functions for selective attention. *Neurosciences Research Program Bulletin,* 1976, *14,* 1–47.

Mountcastle, V. B., Lynch, J. C., Georgopoulos, A., Sakata, H., & Acuna, D. Posterior parietal association cortex of the monkey: Command functions for operations within extrapersonal space. *Journal of Neurophysiology,* 1975, *38,* 871–908.

Mourant, R. R., & Grimson, C. G. Predictive head-movements during automobile mirror-sampling. *Perceptual and Motor Skills,* 1977, *44,* 283–286.

Mourant, R. R., & Rockwell, T. H. *Visual scan patterns of novice and experienced drivers.* International Symposium on Psychological Aspects of Driver Behavior, Noordwjkerhout, The Netherlands, 1971.

Murphy, R. Recognition memory for sequentially presented pictorial and verbal spatial information. *Journal of Experimental Psychology,* 1973, *100,* 327–334.

Neisser, U. *Cognitive Psychology,* New York: Appleton, 1967.

Neisser, U. Visual imagery as a process and experience. In J. Antrobus (Ed.), *Cognition and affect.* Boston: Little, Brown, 1970.

Neisser, U. *Cognition and Reality.* San Francisco: W. H. Freeman & Co., 1976.

Newell, A., & Simon, H. A. *Human Problem Solving.* Englewood Cliffs, N.J.: Prentice-Hall, 1972.

Nodine, C. F., & Simmons, F. G. Processing distinctive features in the differentiation of letterlike symbols. *Journal of Experimental Psychology,* 1974, *103,* 21–28.

Norman, D. A. *Memory and attention* (2nd ed.). New York: Wiley, 1976.

Norman, D. A., & Bobrow, D. G. On data-limited and resource-limited processes. *Cognitive Psychology,* 1975, *7,* 44–64.

Norman, D. A., & Rumelhart, D. E. *Explorations in cognition.* San Francisco: W. H. Freeman and Co., 1975.

Noton, D., & Stark, L. Eye movements and visual perception. *Scientific American,* 1971, *224,* 34–43. (a)

Noton, D., & Stark, L. Scanpaths in eye movements during pattern perception. *Science,* 1971, *171,* 308–311. (b)

Noton, D., & Stark, L. Scanpaths in saccadic eye movements while viewing and recognizing patterns. *Vision Research,* 1971, *11,* 929–942. (c)

O'Bryan, K. G. *Summary of research findings from eye movement studies of children's reading strategies.* Unpublished manuscript, Ontario Educational Communications Authority, 1974.

O'Bryan, K. G. *Eye movement research and the development of educational technology in programmes for the slow reader.* Unpublished manuscript, Ontario Institute for Studies In Education, 1975.

O'Bryan, K. G. & Silverman, H. *Report on children's television viewing strategies.* Children's Television Workshop, 1972.

Olson, D. R. *Cognitive development: The child's acquisition of diagonality.* New York: Academic Press, 1970.

O'Regan, J. K. *Structural and contextual constraints on eye movements in reading.* Unpublished doctor dissertation, University of Cambridge, 1975.

Pachella, R. G. The interpretation of reaction time in information processing research. In B. H. Kantowitz (Ed.), *Human information processing: Tutorials in performance and cognition.* Hillsdale, N.J.: Lawrence Erlbaum Associates, 1974.

Paivio, A. Psychophysiological correlates of imagery. In F. J. McGuigan & R. A. Schoonover (Eds.), *The psychophysiology of thinking: Studies of covert processes.* New York and London: Academic Press, 1973.

Pantle, A. J. Adaptation to pattern spatial frequency effects on visual movement sensitivity in humans. *Journal of the Optical Society of America,* 1970, *60,* 1120–1124.

Parker, R. E. *Picture processing during recognition.* Unpublished manuscript, University of California, San Diego, 1977.

Pearce, D., & Porter, E. Changes in visual sensitivity associated with voluntary saccades. *Psychonomic Science,* 1970, *19,* 225–227.

Piaget, J. *The construction of reality in the child.* (Margaret Cook, trans.) New York: Basic Books, 1954.

Piaget, J., & Inhelder, B. *The child's conception of space.* New York: Norton, 1967.

Pola, J. *Visual direction of a flash presented during or following saccades of variable length to an 8° peripheral target.* Paper presented at the Eastern Psychological Meeting, New York City, 1971.

Pollack, I., & Spence, D. Subjective pictorial information and visual search. *Perception and Psychophysics,* 1968, *3* (1-B), 41–44.

Polyak, S. L. *The retina.* Chicago: University of Chicago Press, 1941.

Potter, M. C. Short-term conceptual memory for pictures. *Journal of Experimental Psychology: Human Learning and Memory,* 1976, *2,* 509–522.

Potter, M. C., & Levy, E. I. Recognition memory for a rapid sequence of pictures. *Journal of Experimental Psychology,* 1969, *81,* 10–15.

Poulton, E. C. Peripheral vision, refractoriness and eye movements in fast oral reading. *British Journal of Psychology.* 1962, *53,* 409–419.

Poulton, E. C. Engineering psychology. *Annual Review of Psychology,* 1966, *17,* 177–200.

Poulton, E. C., & Gregory, R. L. Blinking during visual tracking. *Quarterly Jounal of Experimental Psychology,* 1952, *4,* 57–65.

Rashbass, C., & Westheimer, G. H. Disjunctive eye movements. *Journal of Physiology,* 1961, *159,* 149–170.

Ratliff, F., & Riggs, L. A. Involuntary motions of the eye during monocular fixation. *Journal of Experimental Psychology,* 1950, *40,* 687–701.

Rayner, K. *The perceptual span and peripheral cues in reading.* Reading and Learning Series Research Report, Department of Education, Cornell University, 1974.

Rayner, K. The perceptual span and peripheral cues in reading. *Cognitive Psychology,* 1975, *7,* 65–81.

Rayner, K., & McConkie, G. W. What guides a reader's eye movements? *Vision Research.* 1976, *16,* 829–837.

Reed, S. K., & Johnsen, J. A. Detection of parts in patterns and images. *Memory and Cognition,* 1975, *3,* 569–575.

Revesz, G., Kundel, H. L., & Graber, M. A. The influence of structured noise on the detection of radiologic abnormalities. *Investigative Radiology,* 1974, *9,* 479–486.

Richards, W. Saccadic suppression. *Journal of the Optical Society of America,* 1969, *59,* 617–623.

Richmond, B. J., & Wurtz, R. H. Visual responses during saccadic eye movement: A corollary discharge to superior colliculus. *Neuroscience Abstracts,* 1977, *3,* 574.

Riggs, L. A., Merton, P. A., & Morton, H. B. Suppression of visual phosphenes during saccadic eye movements. *Vision Research,* 1974, *14,* 997–1010.

Riggs, L. A., Ratliff, F., Cornsweet, J. C., & Cornsweet, T. N. The disappearance of steadily fixated visual test objects. *Journal of the Optical Society of America,* 1953, *43,* 495–501.

Robinson, D. A. A method of measuring eye movements using a scleral search coil in a magnetic field. *IEEE Transactions on Biomedical Electronics,* 1963, *10,* 137–145.

Robinson, D. A. The mechanics of human saccadic eye movement. *Journal of Physiology* (London), 1964, *174,* 245–264.

Robinson, D. A. Eye movements evoked by collicular stimulation in the alert monkey. *Vision Research,* 1972, *12,* 1975–1808.

Robinson, D. A. Oculomotor control signals. In P. Bach-y-Rita and G. Lennerstrand (Eds.), *Basic mechanism of ocular motility and their clinical implications.* New York: Pergamon Press, 1975.

Robinson, D. A., & Fuchs, A. F. Eye movements evoked by stimulation of frontal eye fields. *Journal of Neurophysiology* 1969, *32,* 637–649.

Robinson, D. L., & Goldberg, M. E. Visual properties of neurons in the parietal cortex of the awake monkey. *Invest. Ophthal. Vis. Sci.,* 1977, *16* ([Suppl.] 156).

Robinson, D. L., & Wurtz, R. H. Use of an extraretinal signal by monkey superior colliculus neurons to distinguish real from self-induced stimulus movement. *Journal of Neurophysiology,* 1976, *39,* 852–870.

Robinson, G. H., Erikson, D. J., Thurston, G. L. & Clark, R. L. Visual search by automobile drivers. *Human Factors,* 1972, *14,* 315–323.

Robinson, G. H., Koth, B. W., & Ringenback, J. P. Dynamics of the eye and head during an element of visual search. *Ergonomics,* 1976, *19,* 691–709.

Rockwell, T. H., Bhise, D., & Mourant, R. R. *A television system to record eye movements of automobile drivers.* Paper presented at the annual meeting of the Society of Photo-optical Instrument Engineers, Detroit, 1972.

Rosen, L. D. *Memory influence during reprocessing.* Unpublished doctoral dissertation, University of California, San Diego, 1975.

Rosen, L. D. *Memory-controlled task repetition: The eyes see but the mind knows.* Paper presented at U.S. Army Human Engineering Laboratory Conference Eye Movements and Psychological Processes II: The higher functions. Monterey, Ca., February, 1977.

Ross, A. O. *Psychological aspects of learning disabilities and reading disorders.* New York: McGraw-Hill Book Company, 1976.

Rothkopf, E. Z. Experiments on mathemagenic behavior and the technology of written instruction. In E. Z. Rothkopf & P. E. Johnson (Eds.), *Verbal learning research and the technology of written instruction.* New York: Columbia University Teachers College Press, 1971.

Rothkopf, E. Z. Structural text features and the control of processes in learning from written material. In R. O. Freedle & J. B. Carroll (Eds.), *Language Comprehension and The Acquisition of Knowledge.* Washington, D. C.: V. H. Winston & Sons, 1972.

Rothkopf, E. Z. Writing to teach and reading to learn: A perspective on the psychology of written instruction. In N. L. Gage (Ed.), *The psychology of teaching methods, The Seventy-fifth Yearbook of the National Society for the Study of Education, Part I.* Chicago: National Society for the Study of Education, 1976.

Rothkopf, E. Z., & Billington, M. J. A two-factor model of the effect of goal-descriptive directions on learning from text. *Journal of Education Psychology*, 1975, *67*, 692–704. (a)

Rothkopf, E. Z., & Billington, M. J. Relevance and similarity of text elements to descriptions of learning goals. *Journal of Educational Psychology*, 1975, *67*, 745–750. (b)

Rothkopf, E. Z., & Billington, M. J. *Goal-guided learning from written discourse: A descriptive processing model inferred from inspection time measures.* Manuscript submitted for publication, 1978. (a)

Rothkopf, E. Z., & Billington, M. J. *Effects of task demands on eye movements during goal-guided reading.* Manuscript submitted for publication, 1978. (b)

Rothkopf, E. Z. & Billington, M. J. Individual reading style in two learning tasks. Unpublished manuscript, 1977.

Rothkopf, E. Z., & Kaplan R. An exploration of the effect of density and specificity of instructional objectives on learning from text. *Journal of Educational Psychology*, 1972, *63*, 295–302.

Rothkopf, E. Z., & Krudys, J. Copying span as a measure of the information burden in written language. Unpublished manuscript, 1978.

Russo, J. E., & Dosher, B. A. *Dimensional evaluation: A heuristic for binary choice.* Unpublished manuscript, Carnegie-Mellon University, 1976.

Russo, J. E. & Rosen, L. D. An eye fixation analysis of multi-alternative choice. *Memory and Cognition*, 1975, *3*, 267–276.

St. Cyr, G. J., & Fender, D. H. The interplay of drifts and flick in binocular fixation. *Vision Research*, 1969, *9*, 245–265. (a)

St. Cyr, G. J., & Fender, D. H. Nonlinearities of the human oculomotor system: Gain. *Vision Research*, 1969, *9*, 1235–1246. (b)

St. Cyr, G. J., & Fender, D. H. Nonlinearities of the human oculomotor system: Time delay. *Vision Research*, 1969, *9*, 1491–1503. (c)

Sakitt, B. Iconic memory. *Psychological Review*, 1976, *83*, 257–276.

Salapatek, P., & Kessen, W. Visual scanning of triangles by the human newborn. *Journal of Experimental Child Psychology*, 1966, *3*, 155–167.

Sanders, G. A. On the natural domain of grammar. University of Indiana Linguistics Club, 1969.

Schank, R. C. Identification of conceptualizations underlying natural language. In R. C. Schank & K. M. Colby (Eds.), *Computer models of thought and language.* San Francisco: W. H. Freeman and Co., 1973.

Schiller, P. H., & Koerner, F. Discharge characteristics of single units in superior colliculus of the alert rhesus monkey. *Journal of Neurophysiology*, 1971, *34*, 920–936.

Schiller, P. H., & Stryker, M. Single-unit reading and stimulation in superior colliculus of the alert rhesus monkey. *Journal of Neurophysiology*, 1972, *35*, 915–924.

Schneider, G. Two visual systems. *Science*, 1969, *163*, 895–902.

Schober, H. A. W., & Hilz, R. Contrast sensitivity of the human eye for square-wave gratings. *Journal of the Optical Society of America*, 1965, *55*, 1086–1091.

Schoonard, J. W., Gould, J. D. & Miller, L. A. Experimental studies of visual inspection (Tech. Rep. RC 3085 [#14168]). IBM Research Center, Yorktown Heights, N.Y., October, 1970.

Scinto, L. F. Textual competence: A preliminary analysis of orally generated texts, *Linguistics*, 1977.

Sedgwick, H. A., & Festinger, L. Eye movements, efference and visual perception. In R. A. Monty, & J. W. Senders (Eds.), *Eye movements and psychological processes.* Hillsdale, N.J.: Lawrence Erlbaum Associates, 1976.

Senders, J. W. Man's capacity to use information from complex displays. In H. Quastler (Ed.), *Information theory in Psychology,* Glencoe, Ill.: Free Press, 1955.

Senders, J. W. The human operator as a monitor and controller of multi degree systems. *IEEE Transactions of Human Factors in Electronics*, HFE-5. 1964, 2–5.

Senders, J. W., Christofferson, A. B., Levinson, W. H., Dietrich, C. W., & Ward, J. L. An investigation of automobile driver information processing (Report #1335). Cambridge, Mass.: Bolt, Beranek & Newman. April, 1966.

Senders, J. W., Webb, I. B., & Baker, C. A. The peripheral viewing of dials. *Journal of Applied Psychology*, 1955, *39*, 433–436.

Sheena, D. Pattern-recognition techniques for extraction of features of the eye from a conventional television scan. In R. A. Monty & J. W. Senders (Eds.), *Eye movements and psychological processes*. Hillsdale, N.J.: Lawrence Erlbaum Associates, 1976.

Shepard, R., & Metzler, J. Mental rotation of three-dimensional objects. *Science*, 1971, *171*, 701–703.

Sherrington, C. S. On the anatomical constitution of nerves of skeletal muscles: with remarks on recurrent fibers in the ventral spinal nerve-root. *Journal of Physiology* (London), 1894, *17*, 211–258.

Sherrington, C. S. Further note on the sensory nerves of the eye muscles, *Proceedings of the Royal Society*, 1898, *64*, 120–121.

Sherrington, C. S. *The integrative action of the nervous system*. London: Constable, 1906.

Singer, W., & Creutzfeldt, O. D. Reciprocal lateral inhibition of on-and off-center neurons in the lateral geniculate body of the cat. *Experimental Brain Research*, 1970, *10*, 311–330.

Skavenski, A. A. Inflow as a source of extraretinal eye position information. *Vision Research*, 1972, *12*, 221–229.

Skavenski, A. A. The nature and role of extraretinal eye position information in visual localization. In R. A. Monty, & J. W. Senders (Eds.), *Eye Movements and Psychological Processes*. Hillsdale, N.J.: Lawrence Erlbaum Associates, 1976.

Skavenski, A. A., Haddad, G., and Steinman, R. M. The extraretinal signal for the visual perception of direction. *Perception and Psychophysics*, 1972, *11*, 287–290.

Skavenski, A. A., & Steinman, R. M. Control of eye position in the dark. *Vision Research*, 1970, *10*, 193–203.

Sperling, G. The information available in brief visual presentations. *Psychological Monographs*, 1960, *74*(Whole No. 498), 1–29.

Sperling, G., Budiansky, J., Spivak, J. G., & Johnson, M. C. Extremely rapid visual search: The maximum rate of scanning letters for the presence of a numeral. *Science*, 1971, *174*, 307–311.

Sperry, R. W. Neural basis of the spontaneous optokinetic response produced by visual inversion. *Journal of Comparative and Physiological Psychology*, 1950, *43*, 482–489.

Spottiswoode, R. *A grammar of the film*. Berkeley, Calif.: University of California Press, 1962. (Originally published, 1933.)

Stark, L. The control system for versional eye movements. In P. Bach-y-Rita & C. C. Collins (Eds.), *The Control of Eye Movements*. New York: Academic Press, 1971.

Stark, L., Kong, R., Schwartz, S., Hendry, D., & Bridgeman, B. Saccadic suppression of image displacement. *Vision Research*, 1976, *16*, 1185–1187.

Stark, L., Michael, J. A., & Zuber, B. L. Saccadic suppression: a product of the saccadic anticipatory signal. In C. R. Evans & T. B. Mulholland (Eds.), *Attention in Neurophysiology*. London: Butterworths, 1969.

Steinman, R. M., Haddad, G. M., Skavenski, A. A., & Wyman, D. Miniature eye movement. *Science*, 1973, *181*, 810–819.

Stern, J. A., & Bynum, J. A. Analysis of visual search activity in skilled and novice helicopter pilots. *Aerospace Medicine*, 1970, *41*, 300–308.

Sternberg, S. The discovery of processing stages: Extension of Donder's method. In W. G. Koster (Ed.), *Attention and Performance II*, Amsterdam: North Holland, 1969. (Reprinted from *Acta Psychologica*, 1969, *30*.)

Stevens, J. K., Emerson, R. C., Gerstein, G. L., Kallos, T., Neufeld, G. R., Nichols, C. W., & Rosenquist, A. C. Paralysis of the awake human: Visual perceptions. *Vision Research*, 1976, *16*, 93–98.

Stoper, A. Apparent motion of stimuli presented stroboscopically during pursuit movement of the eye. *Perception and Psychophysics*, 1973, *13*, 201–211.

Sutton, S., Tueting, P., Zubin, J., & John, E. R. Information delivery and the sensory evoked potential. *Science*, 1967, *155*, 1436–1439.

Taylor, E. A. The spans: Perception, apprehension and recognition as related to reading and speed reading. *American Journal of Ophthamology*, 1957, *44*, 105–505.

Taylor, E. A. Ocular-motor processes and the act of reading. In G. Leisman (Ed.), *Basic visual processes and learning disability*. Springfield, Ill.: Charles C Thomas, 1976.

Taylor, S. E., Frackenpohl, H., & Pettee, J. L. *Grade level norms for the components of the fundamental reading skill* [EDL Research and Information Bulletin No. 3]. Huntington, N.Y.: Educational Developmental Laboratories, 1960.

Taylor, W. L. 'Cloze" readability scores as indices of individual differences in comprehension and aptitude. *Journal of Applied Psychology*, 1957, *41*, 19–26.

Thomas, E. L. The eye movements of a pilot during aircraft landing. *Aerospace Medicine*, 1963, *34*, 424–426.

Thomas, E. L. Search behavior. *Radiologic Clinics of North America*, 1969, *7*, 403–417.

Tinker, M. A. Reliability and validity of eye-movement measures of reading. *Journal of Experimental Psychology*, 1939, *19*, 732–746.

Tinker, M. A. Fixation pause duration in reading. *Journal of Educational Research*, 1951, *44*, 471–479.

Tinker, M. A. Recent studies of eye movements in reading. *Psychological Bulletin*, 1958, *55*, 215–231.

Tolhurst, D. J. Separate channels for the analysis of the shape and the movement of a moving visual stimulus. *Journal of Physiology*, 1973, *231*, 385–402.

Townsend, J. T. Issues and models concerning the processing of a finite number of inputs. In B. Kantowitz (Ed.), *Human information Processing. Tutorials in performance and cognition*. Hillsdale, N.J.: Lawrence Erlbaum Associates, 1974.

Travers, J. R. The effects of forced serial processing on identification of words and random letter strings. *Cognitive Psychology*, 1973, *5*, 109–137.

Travers, J. R. Forced serial processing of words and letter strings: A re-examination. *Perception and Psychophysics*, 1975, *18*, 447–452.

Trevarthen, C. B. Two mechanisms of vision in primates. *Psychologische Forschung*, 1968, *31*, 299–337.

Triesman, A. Verbal cues, language and meaning in attention. *American Journal of Psychology*, 1964, *77*, 206–214.

Uttal, W. R., & Smith, P. Recognition of alphabetic characters during voluntary eye movements. *Perception and Psychophysics*, 1968, *3*, 257–264.

Vachek, J. *Travaux linguistiques de Prague*. Alabama: University of Alabama Press, 1966.

Van Dijk, T. *Some aspects of text grammars*. The Hague: Mouton, 1972.

Vaughan, H. G., Jr., The role of stimulus pattern in suppression of vision during eye movements. In V. Zikmund (Ed.), *The oculomotor system and brain functions*. London: Butterworths, 1973.

Vaughan, J., & Graefe, T. M. Delay of stimulus presentation after the saccade in visual search. *Perception and Psychophysics*, 1977, *22*, 201–205.

Vernon, M. D. *Backwardness in reading. A study of its nature and origin*. Cambridge, Mass.: Cambridge University Press, 1957.

Volkmann, F. C. Vision during voluntary saccadic eye movements. *Journal of the Optical Society of America*, 1962, *52*, 571–578.

Volkmann, F. C. Saccadic suppression: A brief review. In R. A. Monty & J. W. Senders (Eds.), *Eye movements and psychological processes.* Hillsdale, N.J.: Lawrence Erlbaum Associates, 1976.

Volkmann, F. C., & Riggs, L. A. *Contrast sensitivity during saccadic eye movements.* Paper presented at the Association for Research in Vision and Ophthalmology. Sarasota, Florida, May, 1975.

Volkmann, F. C., Schick, A. M. L., & Riggs, L. A. Time course of visual inhibition during voluntary saccades. *Journal of the Optical Society of America,* 1968, *58,* 562–569.

von Holst, E. Relations between the central nervous system and the peripheral organs. *British Journal of Animal Behaviour,* 1954, *2,* 89–94.

von Holst, E. & Mittelstaedt, H. Das reafferenzprinzip: Wechselwirkungen zwischen zentral nervensystem und peripherie. *Naturwissen,* 1950, *37,* 464–476.

Walker, R. Y. The eye movements of good readers. *Psychological Monographs,* 1933, *44,* 95–117.

Walls, G. L. The evolutionary history of eye movements. *Vision Research,* 1962, *2,* 69–80.

Walter, K. *The Measurement of verbal information in psychology and education.* Berlin, Heidelberg: Springer-Verlag, 1971.

Walter, W. G. Slow potential waves in the human brain associated with expectancy, attention and decision. *Archives Psychiatrie Und Nervenkranken.* 1964, *208,* 309–322.

Wanat, S. *Linguistic structure and visual attention in reading.* Newark, Del.: International Reading Association, 1971.

Weber, R. B., & Daroff, R. B. The metrics of horizontal saccadic eye movements in normal humans. *Vision Research,* 1971, *11,* 921–928. (a)

Weber, R. B., & Daroff, R. B. Corrective movements following refixation saccades: Type and control system analysis. *Vision Research,* 1971, *12,* 467–475. (b)

Weir, D. H., & McRuer, D. T. A theory for driver steering control of motor vehicles. *Highway Research Record,* 1968, No. *247,* 7–39.

Weisstein, N. Metacontrast. In D. Jameson & L. M. Hurvich (Eds.), *Handbook of sensory physiology* (Vol. 7, part 4): Visual psychophysics. New York: Springer-Verlag, 1972.

Weitzenhoffer, A. A case of pursuit like eye movements directly reflecting dream content during hypnotic dreaming. *Perceptual and Motor Skills,* 1971, *32,* 701–702.

Wendt, P. Development of an eye camera for use with motion pictures. *Psychological Monographs: General and Applied,* 1952, *66,* No. 339.

Westheimer, G. H. Eye movement responses to horizontally moving visual stimulus. *Archives of Ophthalmology,* 1954, *52,* 932–943.

Westheimer, G. Oculomotor control: The vergence system. In R. A. Monty & J. W. Senders (Eds.), *Eye movements and psychological processes.* Hillsdale, N.J.: Lawrence Erlbaum Associates, 1976.

Weymouth, F., Andersen, E., & Averill, H. Retinal mean local sign: A new view of the relation of the retinal mosaic to visual perception. *American Journal of Physiology,* 1923, *63,* 410–411.

Weymouth, F. W., Hines, D. C., Acres, L. H., Raaf, J. E., & Wheeler, M. C. Visual acuity within the area centralis and its relation to eye movements and fixation. *American Journal of Ophthalmology,* 1928, *11,* 947–960.

White, A. T. *Aesop's fables retold by Ann Terry White.* New York: Random House, 1964.

White, C. W. Visual masking during pursuit eye movements. *Journal of Experimental Psychology: Human Perception and Performance,* 1976, *2,* 469–478.

White, C. W., & Lorber, C. M. Spatial frequency specificity in visual masking. *Perception and Psychophysics,* 1976, *19,* 281–284.

Whiteside, J. A. Eye movements of children, adults, and elderly persons during inspection of dot patterns. *Journal of Experimental Child Psychology,* 1974, *18,* 313–332.

Williams, L. G. The effect of target specification on objects fixated during visual search. *Perception and Psychophysics*, 1966, *1*, 315–318.

Winnick, W. A., & Dornbush, R. L. Pre- and post-exposure processes in tachistoscopic identification. *Perceptual and Motor Skills*, 1965, *20*, 107–113.

Winterson, B. J., & Collewijn, H. Microsaccades during finely guided visuomotor tasks. *Vision Research*, 1976, *16*, 1387–1390.

Wisher, R. A. *The role of expectations in reading.* Unpublished doctoral dissertation, University of California, San Diego, 1976. (a)

Wisher, R. A. The effects of syntactic expectations during reading. *Journal of Educational Psychology*, 1976, *68*, 597–602. (b)

Wolf, W. Perception of visual displays. *Viewpoints: Bulletin of the School of Education, Indiana University*, 1971, *47*, 112–140.

Wolf, W. & Knemeyer, M. *A study of eye movements in television viewing* (ERIC Document Reproduction Service No. ED 046 254). Columbus, Ohio: Ohio State University Research Foundation, 1970.

Wolf, W., Tira, D. E., & Knemeyer, M. *Children's eye movement responses to dynamic fields: A study of IQ and stimulus characteristics.* Paper presented at the meeting of the American Educational Research Association, 1969.

Woodworth, R. S. Vision and localization during eye movements. *Psychological Bulletin*, 1906, *3*, 68–70.

Wright, K. Driver eye fixation patterns while steering a curved test course. Human Factors Working Paper, Department of Industrial Engineering and Operations Research, University of California, Berkeley, 1968.

Wurtz, R. H. Visual receptive fields of striate cortex neurons in awake monkeys. *Journal of Neurophysiology*, 1969, *32*, 727–742. (a)

Wurtz, R. H. Comparison of effects of eye movements and stimulus movements on striate cortex neurons of the monkey. *Journal of Neurophysiology*, 1969, *32*, 987–994. (b)

Wurtz, R. H., & Goldberg, M. E. Activity of superior colliculus in behaving monkey, IV: Effects of lesions on eye movements. *Journal of Neurophysiology*, 1972, *35*, 587–596.

Wurtz, R. H., & Mohler, C. W. Organization of monkey superior colliculus: Enhanced visual response of superficial layer cells. *Journal of Neurophysiology*, 1976, *39*, 745–765. (a)

Wurtz, R. H., & Mohler, C. W. Enhancement of visual response in monkey striate cortex and frontal eye fields. *Journal of Neurophysiology*, 1969, *39*, 766–772. (b)

Yarbus, A. L. *Eye movements and vision.* New York: Plenum Press, 1967.

Yasui, S., & Young, L. R. Eye movements during after-image tracking under sinusoidal and random vestibular stimulation. In R. A. Monty & J. W. Senders (Eds.), *Eye Movements and Psychological Processes.* Hillsdale, N.J.: Lawrence Erlbaum Associates, 1976.

Young, L. R., & Sheena, D. *Survey of eye movement recording methods.* Conference on Eye Movement Research and Technology, Task Force on Essential Skills, National Institute of Education, July, 1974.

Young, L. R., & Sheena, D. Survey of eye movement recording methods. *Behavior Research Methods and Instrumentation*, 1975, *1*, 397–429.

Young, L. R., & Stark, L. Variable feedback experiments testing a sampled data model for eye tracking movements. *IEEE Transactions*, 1963, *HFE-4*, 38–51.

Zach, L., & Kaufman, J. How adequate is the concept of perceptual deficit for education? *Journal of Learning Disabilities*, 1972, *5*, 351–356.

Zavalishin, N. V. Hypothesis concerning the distribution of eye fixation points during the examination of pictures. *Automatic Remote Control*, 1964, *29*, 1944–1951.

Zee, D. S., Optican, L. M., Cook, J. D., Robinson, D. A., & Engel, W. K. Slow saccades in spinocerebellar degeneration. *Archives of Neurology*, 1976, *33*, 243–251.

Zinchenko, V. P., Chzhi-Tsin, B., & Tarakanov, V. V. The formation and development of perceptual activity. *Soviet Psychology and Psychiatry*, 1963, *2*, 3–12.

Zuber, B. L., Crider, A., & Stark, L. *Saccadic suppression associated with microsaccades.* Quarterly Progress Reports, Research Laboratory of Electronics, Cambridge, Mass.: MIT, 1964.

Zuber, B. L., & Stark, L. Saccadic suppression: Elevation of visual threshold associated with saccadic eye movements. *Experimental Neurology,* 1966, *16,* 65–79.

Zusne, L., & Michels, K. M. Nonrepresentational shapes and eye movements. *Perceptual and Motor Skills,* 1964, *18,* 11–20.

Author Index

Numbers in *italics* refer to pages on which the complete references are listed.

A

Abrams, S. G., 106, 110, 196, 197, 206, *349*
Acuna, D., 11, *362*
Akert, K., 8, *359*
Allen, B. D., 71, *353*
Allington, R. L., 233, *349*
Alpern, M., 48, 55, 195, *349*
Anderson, I. H., 159, *349*
Antes, J. R., 243, 246, 250, 252, 256, 282, 289, 295, 304, 321, *349*
Ashkenazi, M., 197, *360*
Astruc, J., 8, *349*

B

Bahill, A. T., 82, 93, *349*
Baker, C. A., 304, *366*
Baker, M. A., 304, *349*
Bayle, E., 102, *349*
Becker, W., 26, 92, *349, 350*
Beggs, V. E., 226, *359*
Beggs, W. D. A., 30, *357*
Bender, L., 226, *350*
Berlyne, D. E., 305, *350*
Berman, N., 3, *352*

Bertelson, P., 139, *350*
Bever, T. G., 176, *361*
Bhise, D., 331, *364*
Bhise, V. C., 330, *350*
Biederman, I., 56, 295, *350, 353*
Biggs, N. L., 329, *350*
Billington, M. J., 210, 213, 214, 215, 218, 219, 220, *364, 365*
Bischof, N., 22, *350*
Bizzi, E., 8, 10, 106, *350*
Blair, W. C., 106, *350*
Blakemore, C., 59, *350*
Bobrow, D. G., 107, *362*
Bossom, J., 202, *350*
Bouma, H., 140, 141, 142, 234, 295, *350*
Bouman, G., 198, 201, 206, *353*
Bowden, J. M., 30, *357*
Bower, G. H., 90, 261, *350*
Boynton, R. M., 323, *350*
Božkov, V., 48, *362*
Brandt, H. F., 243, 319, *350*
Breitmeyer, B. G., 35, 37, 48, 50, 53, 55, 57, 58, 59, 60, *350, 351*
Bridgeman, B., 36, 37, 53, *351, 366*
Brindley, G. S., 16, 202, *351*
Broadbent, D. E., 192, *351*
Brooks, B. A., 37, 48, 49, 51, 52, 205, 295, 297, *351*

371

Subject Index